Wilderness and Environmental Medicine

Editors

ERIC A. WEISS
DOUGLAS G. SWARD

EMERGENCY MEDICINE CLINICS OF NORTH AMERICA

www.emed.theclinics.com

Consulting Editor
AMAL MATTU

May 2017 • Volume 35 • Number 2

ELSEVIER

1600 John F. Kennedy Boulevard • Suite 1800 • Philadelphia, Pennsylvania, 19103-2899

http://www.theclinics.com

EMERGENCY MEDICINE CLINICS OF NORTH AMERICA Volume 35, Number 2
May 2017 ISSN 0733-8627, ISBN-13: 978-0-323-52836-8

Editor: Katie Pfaff

Developmental Editor: Casey Potter

Emergency Medicine Clinics of North America (ISSN 0733-8627) is published quarterly by Elsevier Inc., 360 Park Avenue South, New York, NY, 10010-1710. Months of issue are February, May, August, and November. Business and Editorial Offices: 1600 John F. Kennedy Boulevard, Suite 1800, Philadelphia, PA 19103-2899. Customer Service Office: 6277 Sea Harbor Drive, Orlando, FL 32887-4800. Periodicals postage paid at New York, NY, and additional mailing offices. Subscription prices are $100.00 per year (US students), $323.00 per year (US individuals), $608.00 per year (US institutions), $220.00 per year (international students), $455.00 per year (international individuals), $747.00 per year (international institutions), $220.00 per year (Canadian students), $389.00 per year (Canadian individuals), and $747.00 per year (Canadian institutions). International air speed delivery is included in all *Clinics'* subscription prices. All prices are subject to change without notice. **POSTMASTER:** Send address changes to *Emergency Medicine Clinics of North America*, Elsevier Periodicals Customer Service, 11830 Westline Industrial Drive, St. Louis, MO 63146. Customer Service (orders, claims, online, change of address): Elsevier Periodicals **Customer Service, 11830 Westline Industrial Drive, St. Louis, MO 63146. Tel: 1-800-654-2452 (U.S. and Canada); 314-453-7041 (outside U.S. and Canada). Fax: 314-453-5170. E-mail: journalscustomerservice-usa@elsevier.com (for print support);** **journalsonlinesupport-usa@elsevier.com (for online support).**

Reprints. For copies of 100 or more of articles in this publication, please contact the Commercial Reprints Department, Elsevier Inc., 360 Park Avenue South, New York, NY 10010-1710. Tel.: 212-633-3874; Fax: 212-633-3820; E-mail: reprints@elsevier.com.

Emergency Medicine Clinics of North America is covered in *MEDLINE/PubMed (Index Medicus), Current Contents/Clinical Medicine, EMBASE/Excerpta Medica, BIOSIS, SciSearch, CINAHL, ISI/BIOMED,* and *Research Alert.*

Contributors

CONSULTING EDITOR

AMAL MATTU, MD
Professor and Vice Chair, Department of Emergency Medicine, University of Maryland School of Medicine, Baltimore, Maryland

EDITORS

ERIC A. WEISS, MD, FACEP
Professor of Emergency Medicine, Founder and Director Emeritus, Stanford Wilderness Medicine Fellowship, Department of Emergency Medicine, Stanford University School of Medicine, Director, Wilderness & Travel Medicine, Stanford, California

DOUGLAS G. SWARD, MD, FACEP
Clinical Assistant Professor, Emergency Medicine, Division of Hyperbaric Medicine, Program in Trauma, Attending Physician, Department of Emergency Medicine, University of Maryland School of Medicine, Baltimore, Maryland

AUTHORS

KENTON L. ANDERSON, MD
Director, Emergency Ultrasound Research and Scholarly Activity; Clinical Assistant Professor, Department of Emergency Medicine, Stanford University School of Medicine, Stanford, California

PAUL S. AUERBACH, MD, MS
Redlich Family Professor, Department of Emergency Medicine, Stanford University School of Medicine, Stanford, California

BRAD BENNETT, PhD
Uniformed Services University of the Health Sciences, Bethesda, Maryland

DOMINIQUE BUTEAU, MD
Medical Director, CISSS Chaudière-Appalaches (CHAU-Hôtel-Dieu de Lévis), Hyperbaric Medicine Unit, Emergency Department, Lévis, Quebec, Canada; Associate Clinical Professor, Family Medicine and Emergency Medicine Department, School of Medicine, Université Laval, Quebec City, Quebec, Canada

FRANK K. BUTLER, MD
Committee on Tactical Combat Casualty Care, Joint Trauma System, US Army Institute of Surgical Research, JBSA Fort Sam Houston, Texas

NAVNEET CHEEMA, MD
Assistant Professor & Assistant Program Director, Section of Emergency Medicine, University of Chicago, Chicago, Illinois

RICHARD F. CLARK, MD
Professor of Clinical Emergency Medicine, Division of Medical Toxicology, Department of Emergency Medicine, UC San Diego Health, San Diego, California

BRYAN CORBETT, MD
Toxicology Fellow, Division of Medical Toxicology, Department of Emergency Medicine, UC San Diego Health, San Diego, California

CHRISTOPHER DAVIS, MD, DiMM, DTMH
Department of Emergency Medicine, Assistant Professor, University of Colorado School of Medicine, Aurora, Colorado

VALERIE A. DOBIESZ, MD, MPH
Director of External Programs, STATRUS Center for Medical Simulation, Department of Emergency Medicine, Brigham & Women's Hospital, Harvard Humanitarian Initiative, Harvard Medical School, Boston, Massachusetts

HOWARD J. DONNER, MD, CFI (Certified Flight Instructor)
National Wilderness Medicine Conferences, Palo Alto, California; Medical Operations, NASA Johnson Space Center, Houston, Texas

TIMOTHY B. ERICKSON, MD, FACEP, FACMT, FAACT
Chief, Division of Medical Toxicology, Department of Emergency Medicine, Brigham and Women's Hospital, Harvard Humanitarian Initiative & Harvard Medical School, Boston, Massachusetts

LALEH GHARAHBAGHIAN, MD
Director, Emergency Ultrasound Program; Clinical Associate Professor, Department of Emergency Medicine, Stanford University School of Medicine, Stanford, California

PETER HACKETT, MD
Institute for Altitude Medicine, Telluride, Colorado

CHARLES HANDFORD, MBChB (Hons), MRCS, DMCC
General Duties Medical Officer, 2 Medical Regiment, St George's Barracks, North Luffenham, Oakham, Rutland, United Kingdom

SETH C. HAWKINS, MD
Assistant Professor, Department of Emergency Medicine, Wake Forest University School of Medicine, Medical Director, Burke County EMS Special Operations Team, Morgantown, North Carolina

KIRSTEN B. HORNBEAK, MD
Resident, Department of Emergency Medicine, Stanford Kaiser Emergency Medicine Residency, Stanford, California

RWO-WEN HUANG, MD
Fellow, Emergency Ultrasound Program; Clinical Instructor, Department of Emergency Medicine, Stanford University School of Medicine, Stanford, California

CHRISTOPHER H.E. IMRAY, MB BS, DiMM, MSc, PhD, FRCS, FRCP, FRGS
Professor, Department of Vascular Surgery, University Hospital Coventry and Warwickshire NHS Trust, Warwick Medical School and Coventry University, Coventry, United Kingdom

VIVETA LOBO, MD
Associate Director, Emergency Ultrasound Program; Clinical Assistant Professor, Department of Emergency Medicine, Stanford University School of Medicine, Stanford, California

SWAMINATHA V. MAHADEVAN, MD
Chair, Department of Emergency Medicine, Stanford University School of Medicine, Stanford, California

MICHAEL G. MILLIN, MD, MPH
Associate Professor, Department of Emergency Medicine, Johns Hopkins University School of Medicine, Medical Director, Maryland Search and Rescue, Baltimore, Maryland

PHI D. NGUYEN, MD
Emergency Medicine Resident, Stanford/Kaiser Emergency Medicine Residency Program, Stanford, California

CORI McCLURE POFFENBERGER, MD
Faculty, Emergency Ultrasound Program, Clinical Assistant Professor, Department of Emergency Medicine, Stanford University School of Medicine, Stanford, California

NEAL W. POLLOCK, PhD
Associate Professor, Department of Kinesiology, Université Laval, Quebec City, Quebec, Canada

MATTHEW C. STREHLOW, MD
Director, Stanford Emergency Medicine International, Department of Emergency Medicine, Stanford University School of Medicine, Stanford, California

WILLIAM SULLIVAN, DO, JD
Department of Emergency Medicine, University of Illinois, Chicago; St. Margaret's Hospital, Spring Valley; Law Office of William Sullivan, Frankfort, Illinois

OWEN THOMAS, MBChB (Hons), BMedSc (Phys), DTM&H
Anaesthetic trainee, Department of Anaesthetics, Musgrove Park Hospital, Taunton, Somerset, United Kingdom

COLONEL IAN WEDMORE, MD
Madigan Army Medical Center, Tacoma, Washington

KEN ZAFREN, MD
Emergency Programs Medical Director, State of Alaska, Juneau, Alaska; Vice President, International Commission for Mountain Emergency Medicine (ICAR MEDCOM); Clinical Professor, Department of Emergency Medicine, Stanford University Medical Center, Stanford, California; Staff Emergency Physician, Alaska Native Medical Center, Anchorage, Alaska

Contents

> High altitude illness encompasses a spectrum of clinical entities to include: acute mountain sickness, high altitude cerebral edema, and high altitude pulmonary edema. These illnesses occur as a result of a hypobaric hypoxic environment. Although a mild case of acute mountain sickness may be self-limited, high altitude cerebral edema and high altitude pulmonary edema represent critical emergencies that require timely intervention. This article reviews recent advances in the prevention and treatment of high altitude illness, including new pharmacologic strategies for prophylaxis and revised treatment guidelines.

> Accidental hypothermia is an unintentional drop in core temperature to 35°C or below. Core temperature is best measured by esophageal probe. If core temperature cannot be measured, the degree should be estimated using clinical signs. Treatment is to protect from further heat loss, minimize afterdrop, and prevent cardiovascular collapse during rescue and resuscitation. The patient should be handled gently, kept horizontal, insulated, and actively rewarmed. Active rewarming is also beneficial in mild hypothermia but passive rewarming usually suffices. Cardiopulmonary resuscitation should be performed if there are no contraindications to resuscitation. CPR may be delayed or intermittent.

> Deep frostbite is a thermal injury associated with significant morbidity. Historically, this has been associated with military personnel; however, increasingly it is becoming an injury that afflicts the civilian population. The use of intravenous iloprost or intra-arterial thrombolytics has led to promising tissue salvage. This article provides an up-to-date understanding of frostbite pathophysiology, classification, prevention, and management. It also highlights the role of telemedicine in optimizing patient outcomes. To further the understanding of optimal frostbite management,

and lakes. Although arthropods are most intrusive during warmer months, many are active throughout the winter, particularly indoors. Arthropods are also nocturnal and often bite unsuspecting victims while they are sleeping. Encounters with humans are generally defensive, accidental, or reactive. An individual stung by an insect or bitten by an arachnid may experience pain and local swelling, an anaphylactic reaction, or life-threatening toxicity. This review discusses the clinical presentation and latest treatment recommendations for bites and stings from spiders, scorpions, bees, ants, ticks and centipedes of North America.

Wilderness emergency medical services (WEMS) are designed to provide high quality health care in wilderness environments. A WEMS program should have oversight by a qualified physician responsible for protocol development, education, and quality improvement. The director is also ideally fully trained as a member of that wilderness rescue program, supporting the team with real-time patient care. WEMS providers function with scopes of practice approved by the local medical director and regulatory authority. With a focus on providing quality patient care, it is time for the evolution of WEMS as an integrated element of a local emergency response system.

Tactical Combat Casualty Care (TCCC) is a set of evidence-based, best-practice prehospital trauma care guidelines customized for use on the battlefield. Military units that have trained all of their unit members in TCCC have now documented the lowest incidence of preventable deaths in the history of modern warfare and TCCC is now the standard for battlefield trauma care in the US Military. TCCC and wilderness medicine share the goal of optimizing care for patients with trauma in austere environments that impose significant challenges in both equipment and evacuation capability. This article reviews the current battlefield trauma care recommendations in TCCC and discusses their applicability to the wilderness setting.

 Video content accompanies this article at http://www.emed. theclinics.com.

With the advent of portable ultrasound machines, point-of-care ultrasound (POCUS) has proven to be adaptable to a myriad of environments, including remote and austere settings, where other imaging modalities cannot be carried. Austere environments continue to pose special challenges to ultrasound equipment, but advances in equipment design and environment-specific care allow for its successful use. This article describes the technique and illustrates pathology of common POCUS

EMERGENCY MEDICINE
CLINICS OF NORTH AMERICA

FORTHCOMING ISSUES

August 2017
Observation Medicine
R. Gentry Wilkerson and Christopher
Baugh, *Editors*

November 2017
Vascular Disasters
Alex Koyfman and Brit Long, *Editors*

February 2018
Trauma
Christopher Hicks and
Andrew Petrosoniak, *Editors*

RECENT ISSUES

February 2017
**Severe Sepsis Care in the Emergency
Department**
Jack Perkins and Michael E. Winters,
Editors

November 2016
Neurological Emergencies
Jonathan Edlow and Michael Abraham,
Editors

August 2016
Geriatric Emergencies
Brendan G. Magauran Jr,
Kalpana N. Shankar, and Joseph H. Kahn,
Editors

RELATED INTEREST

Medical Clinics of North America, March 2016 (Vol. 100, Issue 2)
Travel and Adventure Medicine
Paul S. Pottinger and Christopher A. Sanford, *Editors*

THE CLINICS ARE NOW AVAILABLE ONLINE!
Access your subscription at:
www.theclinics.com

PROGRAM OBJECTIVE

The goal of *Emergency Medicine Clinics of North America* is to keep practicing emergency medicine physicians and emergency medicine residents up to date with current clinical practice in emergency medicine by providing timely articles reviewing the state of the art in patient care.

LEARNING OBJECTIVES

Upon completion of this activity, participants will be able to:

1. Review updates in care of evenomation, illnesses due to extreme weather and altitudes, and other topics in wilderness medicine.
2. Recognize advances in wilderness medicine and trauma care in austere environments.
3. Discuss medical-legal issues in wilderness medicine.

ACCREDITATION

The Elsevier Office of Continuing Medical Education (EOCME) is accredited by the Accreditation Council for Continuing Medical Education (ACCME) to provide continuing medical education for physicians.

The EOCME designates this enduring material for a maximum of 15 *AMA PRA Category 1 Credit*(s)™. Physicians should claim only the credit commensurate with the extent of their participation in the activity.

All other health care professionals requesting continuing education credit for this enduring material will be issued a certificate of participation.

DISCLOSURE OF CONFLICTS OF INTEREST

The EOCME assesses conflict of interest with its instructors, faculty, planners, and other individuals who are in a position to control the content of CME activities. All relevant conflicts of interest that are identified are thoroughly vetted by EOCME for fair balance, scientific objectivity, and patient care recommendations. EOCME is committed to providing its learners with CME activities that promote improvements or quality in healthcare and not a specific proprietary business or a commercial interest.

The planning committee, staff, authors and editors listed below have identified no financial relationships or relationships to products or devices they or their spouse/life partner have with commercial interest related to the content of this CME activity:

Kenton L. Anderson, MD; Paul S. Auerbach, MD, MS; Brad Bennett, PhD; Dominique Buteau, MD; Frank K. Butler, MD; Navneet Cheema, MD; Richard F. Clark, MD; Bryan Corbett, MD; Christopher Davis, MD, DiMM, DTMH; Valerie A. Dobiesz, MD, MPH; Howard J. Donner, MD, CFI (Certified Flight Instructor); Timothy B. Erickson, MD, FACEP, FACMT, FAACT; Anjali Fortna; Laleh Gharahbaghian, MD; Peter Hackett, MD; Charles Handford, MBChB (Hons), MRCS, DMCC; Seth C. Hawkins, MD; Kirsten B. Hornbeak, MD; Rwo-Wen Huang, MD; Christopher H.E. Imray, MB BS, DiMM, MSc, PhD, FRCS, FRCP, FRGS; Indu Kumari; Viveta Lobo, MD; Swaminatha V. Mahadevan, MD; Amal Mattu, MD; Phi D. Nguyen, MD; Katie Pfaff; Cori McClure Poffenberger, MD; Neal W. Pollock, PhD; Matthew C. Strehlow, MD; William Sullivan, DO, JD; Douglas G. Sward, MD, FACEP; Owen D. Thomas, MBChB (Hons), BMedSc (Phys), DTM&H; Colonel Ian Wedmore, MD; Eric A. Weiss, MD, FACEP; Katie Widmeier; Ken Zafren, MD.

The planning committee, staff, authors and editors listed below have identified financial relationships or relationships to products or devices they or their spouse/life partner have with commercial interest related to the content of this CME activity:

Michael G. Millin, MD, MPH is the co-director of the National Wildnerness Medical Directors Course through Elsevier.

UNAPPROVED/OFF-LABEL USE DISCLOSURE

The EOCME requires CME faculty to disclose to the participants:

1. When products or procedures being discussed are off-label, unlabelled, experimental, and/or investigational (not US Food and Drug Administration [FDA] approved); and
2. Any limitations on the information presented, such as data that are preliminary or that represent ongoing research, interim analyses, and/or unsupported opinions. Faculty may discuss information about pharmaceutical agents that is outside of FDA-approved labelling. This information is intended solely for CME and is not intended to promote off-label use of these medications. If you have any questions, contact the medical affairs department of the manufacturer for the most recent prescribing information.

TO ENROLL

To enroll in the *Emergency Medicine Clinics* Continuing Medical Education program, call customer service at 1-800-654-2452 or sign up online at http://www.theclinics.com/home/cme. The CME program is available to subscribers for an additional annual fee of $235 USD.

METHOD OF PARTICIPATION

In order to claim credit, participants must complete the following:

1. Complete enrolment as indicated above.
2. Read the activity.
3. Complete the CME Test and Evaluation. Participants must achieve a score of 70% on the test. All CME Tests and Evaluations must be completed online.

CME INQUIRIES/SPECIAL NEEDS

For all CME inquiries or special needs, please contact elsevierCME@elsevier.com.

Foreword

Wilderness and Environmental Medicine

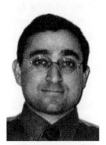

Amal Mattu, MD
Consulting Editor

"We need a doctor!"

I went into emergency medicine because I wanted to be the person who could respond to this plea. Whether the setting was a restaurant, an airplane, a hiking path, or a roadside accident, I wanted to be the kind of doctor who was trained to step forward and provide effective care. Unfortunately, emergency medicine residency didn't quite teach me how to accomplish that goal. Instead, residency training taught me how to provide care in the cocoon of a well-stocked and well-staffed emergency department. Outside of that cocoon, however, I wasn't much better than any other bystander. Sure, I knew first aid and basic life support, but my knowledge and skills were limited. I came to that sudden realization when I stopped at the scene of a roadside accident one day and found myself completely unprepared to provide the needed care of the victims until paramedics arrived.

But then I took a wilderness medicine course several years ago, and I finally felt that I had taken major step in rounding out my skills at being the kind of doctor that I had originally wanted to be. I learned about trauma and orthopedic care, cardiac care, environmental injuries, and infectious disease maladies in austere and resource-limited environments. I finally felt that I could adequately respond to patients in need of emergency care outside of the cocoon of the emergency department. It was an incredibly rewarding experience, and I cannot wait for the next time I take one of these courses.

For anyone who can relate to my own feelings of inadequacy in resource-limited settings or for anyone that yearns to be the "complete" doctor, this issue of *Emergency Medicine Clinics of North America* is written for you. This issue provides a fantastic course in wilderness medicine for the acute care provider. Guest Editors Drs Eric Weiss and Douglas Sward, both experienced and certified wilderness medicine providers and teachers, have assembled an outstanding group of authors to teach us about emergency care in a potpourri of non–emergency department settings. A large

Emerg Med Clin N Am 35 (2017) xv–xvi
http://dx.doi.org/10.1016/j.emc.2017.02.003
0733-8627/17/© 2017 Published by Elsevier Inc.

number of topics that they address relate to environmental emergencies, including high-altitude illness, accidental hypothermia and frostbite, decompression illness, and envenomations. They also discuss combat injuries and airline emergencies. Additional articles focus on point-of-care ultrasound, which has become a staple of medical evaluation in resource-limited settings. Finally, they address medical-legal issues as well as travel and global medical care.

This issue of *Emergency Medicine Clinics of North America* is one of my all-time favorites. Other issues of *Emergency Medicine Clinics of North America* have certainly helped me during my daily work in the emergency department, but this issue will help me with my life *outside* the department. Kudos to these editors and authors for putting together such a practical and informative issue that will help all of us during our next patient encounter…outside the cocoon.

Amal Mattu, MD
Department of Emergency Medicine
University of Maryland School of Medicine
Baltimore, MD 21201, USA

E-mail address:
amalmattu@comcast.net

Preface

Wilderness and Environmental Medicine

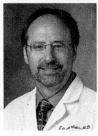 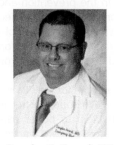

Eric A. Weiss, MD   Douglas G. Sward, MD
Editors

Wilderness medicine is a rapidly growing discipline that is becoming increasingly more significant in today's era of globalization, international travel, and wilderness exploration. The diverse field of wilderness medicine evolved from "mountain medicine," the investigation of the physiology of maladies experienced during man's quest to climb the highest peaks on the planet. Its roots, however, date back many centuries, as the manifestations of high-altitude illness were noted by the Chinese, who described headaches and vomiting in travelers along the high passes of the Silk Road between China and Afghanistan.

Today, wilderness medicine is a dynamic multidisciplinary field. It comprises many of the qualities and characteristics that are inherent in emergency medicine (EM). There is a requisite need to know about other specialties of medicine and the frequent requirement for urgent intervention, stabilization procedures, and expertise with prehospital care and transportation. It also overlaps extensively with environmental, travel, military, disaster, and sports medicine.

Although wilderness medicine generally focuses on medical problems and patient care in remote and austere environments, many of its lessons are essential to mainstream EM, and its application extends into urban communities. Natural and manmade disasters, like the Haiti earthquake, Hurricane Katrina, and the September 11, 2001 attacks may create an environment as limited as the wilderness in the midst of a city by destroying or damaging power, transportation, communication, and health care facilities. With escalating emergency department (ED) crowding and limited resources, improvised care has become a skill that many ED providers practice on a frequent basis. Wilderness medicine will continue to inform the real-life practice of EM as both fields grow and interact.

EM has often been a springboard for pursuing wilderness medicine. In 2003, the first fellowship in wilderness medicine was established at Stanford University to provide EM residency graduates the opportunity to gain advanced knowledge, formal training, and

Emerg Med Clin N Am 35 (2017) xvii–xviii
http://dx.doi.org/10.1016/j.emc.2017.02.002
0733-8627/17/© 2017 Published by Elsevier Inc.

proficiency in research and practice in wilderness and environmental medicine. Currently, there are fifteen wilderness medicine fellowships at academic EM programs throughout the country. These programs are helping develop new leaders in the field and are facilitating vital research to advance our knowledge and improve clinical care.

This issue of *Emergency Medicine Clinics of North America* brings together updates on both the core content of wilderness medicine and additional topic areas that have not been previously addressed. Advances in the prevention and treatment of high-altitude illness, hypothermia, snake envenomation, frostbite, decompression illness, and marine envenomation are juxtaposed with more novel articles that include medical emergencies onboard commercial aircraft, medical-legal topics, the application of ultrasound to austere environments, and lessons learned from the battlefields of Iraq and Afghanistan.

We are indebted to all of the contributing authors for their time and expertise and to Casey Potter and the editorial staff of Elsevier. We hope that the dedicated work of our colleagues will help guide health care providers to better care for patients in all environments, especially in the wildest and most austere places on earth.

Eric A. Weiss, MD, FACEP
Professor of Emergency Medicine
Founder, Wilderness Medicine Fellowship
Department of Emergency Medicine
Stanford University School of Medicine
Stanford, CA 94305, USA

Douglas G. Sward, MD, FACEP
Division of Hyperbaric Medicine
Program in Trauma
Department of Emergency Medicine
University of Maryland School of Medicine
Baltimore, MD 21201, USA

E-mail addresses:
eaweiss@stanford.edu (E.A. Weiss)
dsward@em.umaryland.edu (D.G. Sward)

Erratum

An error was made to a contributor address for the article "Diagnosis and Treatment of Central Nervous System Infections in the Emergency Department" in the November 2016 issue of Emergency Medicine Clinics (34 (2016) 917–942) on page 917.

The correct address for Maia Dorsett, MD, PhD is: Division of Emergency Medicine, Washington University School of Medicine, 660 South Euclid Avenue, Campus Box 8072, St Louis, MO 63110, USA; b Division of Infectious Diseases, Washington University School of Medicine, 660 South Euclid Avenue, Campus Box 8051, St Louis, MO **63110**, USA

In the same article, on page 937, "Streptococcus" should actually be "Staphylococcus".

Emerg Med Clin N Am 35 (2017) xix
http://dx.doi.org/10.1016/j.emc.2017.02.001
0733-8627/17/© 2016 Elsevier Inc. All rights reserved.

emed.theclinics.com

Advances in the Prevention and Treatment of High Altitude Illness

Christopher Davis, MD, DiMM, DTMH[a],*, Peter Hackett, MD[b]

KEYWORDS

- Altitude • Acute mountain sickness • High altitude pulmonary edema
- High altitude cerebral edema • Prevention • Treatment

KEY POINTS

- Acetazolamide remains the best choice for prevention of acute mountain sickness (AMS).
- The best treatment for all high altitude illness is descent or oxygen, or both.
- Dexamethasone is excellent for treating moderate to severe AMS, and for high altitude cerebral edema (HACE).
- Supplemental oxygen is first-line therapy for high altitude pulmonary edema; descent is primary therapy if oxygen is not available.
- Descent is the definitive treatment for HACE and should not be delayed. Dexamethasone and supplemental oxygen are important adjunctive treatments for HACE until descent can be facilitated.

INTRODUCTION

High altitude illness (HAI) comprises a spectrum of conditions that occur at elevation as a result of hypoxia, and includes acute mountain sickness (AMS), high altitude cerebral edema (HACE), and high altitude pulmonary edema (HAPE). Whereas AMS is self-limited, HACE and HAPE represent true emergencies that require timely intervention and stabilization. This review focuses on recent advances in the prevention and treatment of these conditions.

Background

The concentration of oxygen in air remains constant at 21% regardless of the altitude. However, the partial pressure of oxygen decreases with increasing altitude, resulting

Disclosure Statement: The authors have nothing to disclose.
[a] Department of Emergency Medicine, University of Colorado School of Medicine, 12401 East 17th Avenue, Aurora, CO 80045, USA; [b] Institute for Altitude Medicine, PO Box 1229, Telluride, CO 81435, USA
* Corresponding author.
E-mail address: christopher.davis@ucdenver.edu

in alveolar hypoxia, hypoxemia and eventual tissue hypoxia. In the lower Rocky Mountain resorts of Colorado (2500 m/8000 ft), there is one-quarter less available oxygen than at sea level. At Everest Base Camp (5300 m/17,500 feet) there is one-half the available oxygen, and on the summit of Mount Everest there is only one-third. Although a given elevation primarily determines oxygen availability, barometric pressure also decreases with increasing latitude, the winter season, and with low-pressure storm fronts. Accordingly, these effects may combine to raise the effective altitude by hundreds of meters, resulting in an increased risk of HAI.

The high altitude environment is roughly organized into stages according to physiologic stress and resultant pathology.

- *Intermediate altitude* (1520–2440 m/5000–8000 ft): Increased compensatory ventilation occurs along with a decrease in exercise performance. However, blood oxygen saturation is typically preserved at greater than 90%. For most susceptible individuals, AMS will occur above 2100 m.
- *High altitude* (2440–4270 m/8000–14,000 ft): Most HAI occurs in this range owing to the easy availability of overnight tourist facilities at these elevations. In this altitude range, oxygen saturation can be less than 90%, and hypoxemia worsens during exercise and sleep.
- *Very high altitude* (4270–5490 m/14,000–18,000 ft): Abrupt ascent is dangerous. A period of acclimatization is required to prevent HAI. Rates of HAPE and HACE are increased.
- *Extreme altitude* (>5490 m/18,000 ft): Marked hypoxemia and hypocapnia are present. Hypoxic stress leads to progressive physiologic deterioration that eventually overwhelms the body's ability to acclimatize. Long-term human habitation is, therefore, impossible.

Table 1 summarizes the effect of increasing altitude on barometric pressure, blood oxygen saturation, and arterial concentration of Po_2 and Co_2.

Acclimatization

A full discussion of high altitude acclimatization is beyond the scope of this review. Several excellent publications cover this topic in full detail.[1,2] **Table 2** provides a basic summary of the acclimatization process organized by organ system.

Table 1
Effects of increasing altitude on respiratory physiology

Altitude	Equivalent	Pb (mm Hg)	Estimated Pao$_2$ (mm Hg)	Estimated Sao$_2$ (%)	Paco$_2$ (mm Hg)
Sea level	—	760	90–100	97–99	38–42
5280 ft (1610 m)	Denver	623	65–80	93–97	32–42
8000 ft (2440 m)	Machu Pichu	564	45–70	88–95	31–36
12,000 ft (3660 m)	La Paz, Bolivia	483	42–53	80–89	24–34
17,500 ft (5330 m)	Everest Basecamp	388	38–50	65–81	22–30
29,000 ft (8840 m)	Everest Summit	253	28–32	54–62	10–14

Pressures expressed in mm Hg.
Abbreviations: Pb, barometric pressure; Sao$_2$%, arterial oxygen saturation.
Adapted from Roach CR, Lawley JS, Hackett PH. The physiology of high altitude. In: Auerbach PS, editor. Wilderness medicine. Philadelphia: Elsevier; 2016. p. 3.

Table 2		
Acclimatization by organ system		
Organ System	**Effect**	**Onset**
Pulmonary	Increased ventilation modulated by hypoxic ventilatory response and limited by respiratory alkalosis. Pulmonary vascular remodeling	Immediate onset with maximum effect 4–7 d
Renal	Bicarbonate diuresis counteracts alkalosis, increases ventilation	Onset within hours, reaching maximal effect 4–7 d
Cardiovascular	Increased sympathetic tone	Immediate onset, peaks 5 d
	Systemic blood pressure	Response immediate but variable, may remain elevated
	Increased heart rate	Peak effect 3–4 d, then declines
	Decreased stroke volume	Peaks 2–3 d, remains 20% below baseline
	Overall cardiac output	Increases 20% in 2–3 d, then returns to baseline
Hematologic	Hemoconcentration followed by increased red cell mass	First 2 d increased hematocrit from plasma volume loss; erythropoietin levels increase within hours of hypoxic exposure; increased red cell mass peaks in 4–6 wk
Brain	Increased cerebral blood flow	Immediate; lasts 3–5 d, then approximates baseline values

There are limits to an individuals ability to acclimatization to high altitude. Above 5500 m (18,000 ft), weight loss owing to catabolic loss of fat and lean body mass is inevitable. Intestinal malabsorption, impaired renal function, polycythemia leading to microcirculatory sludging, right ventricular strain from excessive pulmonary hypertension, fragmented sleep, and prolonged cerebral hypoxia all combine to limit the human body's ability to adapt to extreme altitude. Even at more modest altitudes, some individuals suboptimally acclimatize owing to genetic or acquired factors.

Pathophysiology

Hypobaric hypoxia resulting in hypoxemia is the pathogenic stressor that leads to all forms of high-altitude illness.[2] Broadly speaking, HAI is the clinical manifestation of inadequate acclimatization. One's susceptibility to illness is largely driven by degree and rate of onset of hypoxemia (altitude and rate of ascent), along with genetic factors; fitness is not protective. Therefore, susceptibility to high-altitude illness varies markedly among both individuals and populations. It is useful to distinguish the pathophysiology of cerebral forms of HAI (AMS and HACE) from the pulmonary form—HAPE.

Cerebral high altitude illness: acute mountain sickness and high altitude cerebral edema

Clinically, AMS and HACE represent a continuum of illness, because AMS usually precedes HACE, although not always. They may share an initial common pathophysiology, with HACE the extreme end result. On ascent to high altitude, cerebral vasodilation in response to hypoxemia leads to increased cerebral blood flow and increased cerebral blood volume, which causes the initial headache. Whether headache is owing to distension of pain-sensitive structures such as arteries, venous sinuses, or meninges, or owing to activation of the trigeminal vascular system, or owing to an increase in intracranial pressure, or a combination of these factors, is unclear. See Lawley and colleagues[3] for a recent comprehensive review. With acclimatization, cerebral blood flow returns toward normal and symptoms resolve. For those who progress beyond a headache and develop AMS, cerebral blood flow and possibly intracranial pressure remain elevated longer, but eventually intracranial dynamics and blood flow are restored to baseline, with eventual resolution of AMS. Although a small amount of vasogenic brain edema is present on MRI after 8 to 12 hours of altitude hypoxia, it is now clear that this edema does not necessarily correlate with AMS.[4] Therefore, mild edema alone is unlikely to be responsible for the clinical manifestations of mild to moderate AMS.[5] In those who go on to develop severe AMS and HACE, edema is apparent on computed tomography scans and MRI. As illness progresses, intracranial pressure progressively increases, and can lead to death. Exactly how AMS progresses to HACE is unclear; possible mechanisms include disruption of the blood–brain barrier from mechanical and biochemical insults, intracellular edema (cytotoxic), and perhaps venous outflow obstruction. **Fig. 1** summarizes current hypotheses of the pathophysiology of AMS and HACE.

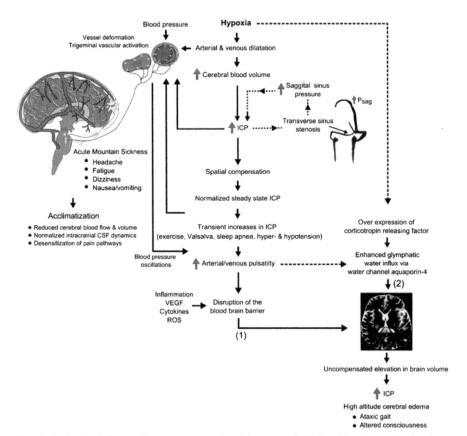

Fig. 1. Pathophysiology of acute mountain sickness and high altitude cerebral edema (HACE). ICP, intracranial pressure; ROS, reactive oxygen species; VEGF, vascular endothelial growth factor.

Pulmonary high altitude illness: high altitude pulmonary edema

HAPE is a noncardiogenic edema in which a leak in the pulmonary blood–gas barrier leads to accumulation of edema fluid in the lung. Left ventricular function is preserved. Pulmonary artery pressure increases in all individuals at high altitude, owing to hypoxic pulmonary vasoconstriction. In those with HAPE, hypoxic pulmonary vasoconstriction is thought to be uneven, such that high microvascular pressure occurs in the pulmonary capillary beds that are not protected by arteriolar vasoconstriction. Capillary hypertension results in fluid shifts via Starling principles, as well as stretching or disruption of cellular junctions and pores. Other factors include inadequate ventilatory response, increased sympathetic tone, inadequate production of endothelial nitric oxide, and impaired clearance of alveolar fluid.[6–8] **Fig. 2** summarizes our current understanding of the pathophysiology of HAPE.

PATIENT EVALUATION OVERVIEW
Acute Mountain Sickness

The diagnosis of AMS is purely clinical. The symptoms are nonspecific, often described as being similar to an ethanol hangover. The setting is rapid ascent of an unacclimatized individual above 2000 m (6560 ft), or ascent to a higher altitude when already at altitude. The classic symptoms develop after several hours, but may be delayed until the next day. For research purposes, the diagnosis of AMS requires a headache in addition to at least 1 of the following symptoms: nausea,

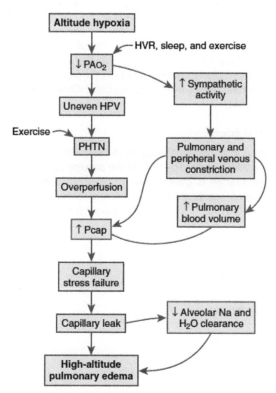

Fig. 2. Pathophysiology of high-altitude pulmonary edema. HPV, hypoxic pulmonary vasoconstriction; HVR, hypoxic ventilatory response; PHTN, pulmonary hypertension.

vomiting or anorexia, general weakness or fatigue, dizziness or lightheadedness, or difficulty sleeping. For clinical purposes, a headache is not a requirement for the diagnosis. Sleep disturbance caused by periodic breathing is common at high altitude, but is exacerbated in those with AMS. These symptoms constitute The Lake Louise Acute Mountain Sickness Scoring System.[9]

The headache of AMS ranges from mild to incapacitating. It is typically bitemporal, dull or throbbing in nature, and is made worse with exertion or with Valsalva maneuvers such as when an individual bends over to lift a backpack. Classically the headache is worst during the night or just after awakening. As the illness progresses the headache becomes more severe and gastrointestinal and constitutional symptoms also worsen. The person with AMS can be irritable and wants to be left alone. Symptoms reach maximum severity in 18 to 24 hours[10] if ascent is halted, followed by gradual resolution. Most individuals become symptom free by the second or third day without further ascent. Symptoms with onset after 3 days of acclimatization should not be attributed to AMS.

Physical findings in AMS are not helpful except to exclude other diagnoses. Heart rate and blood pressure are usually within the normal range. Oxygen saturation is typically normal or slightly low for a given altitude, but overall correlates poorly with the diagnosis of AMS.[11] Facial and peripheral edema may be observed, but are not specifically related to AMS. Central nervous system (CNS) findings indicate HACE, not AMS.

The differential diagnosis of AMS is summarized in **Box 1**. Two conditions deserve special attention. Carbon monoxide poisoning is a risk at high altitude owing to use of heaters or stoves within confined spaces. Carbon monoxide poisoning is easily misdiagnosed as AMS, given the similar symptoms.[12,13] Migraine can also be confused with AMS, and hypoxia is a known trigger for migrainous headache in those with and without a previous history of migraine.[14,15] When there is diagnostic uncertainty, an altitude headache often dissipates within 15 to 20 minutes of supplemental oxygen administration, unlike headaches from other causes. Clinicians may find an oxygen trial useful if it is available.

High Altitude Cerebral Edema

Altered mental status and ataxia are the classic findings in HACE.[16] Individuals usually suffer from preceding AMS and/or HAPE over the previous 24 to 48 hours but isolated HACE can occur. Headache is often present but is not universal. Early symptoms include drowsiness and subtle psychological and behavioral changes, including apathy and social withdrawal.[17,18] Eventually, these more subtle signs lead to overt

---

Box 1
Differential of acute mountain sickness

- Migraine
- Carbon monoxide poisoning
- Dehydration
- Viral syndrome
- Alcohol hangover
- Physical exhaustion
- Heat exhaustion

confusion. Ataxia has been reported in approximately 40% to 60% of cases and papilledema may be present in up to 50%.[16] Gastrointestinal symptoms including anorexia and vomiting may also occur. Visual and auditory hallucinations and seizures are rare. HACE is an encephalopathy; focal CNS findings are unusual and should be investigated thoroughly. Retinal hemorrhages are associated with HACE, but may also be present in those who are asymptomatic. An initially alert patient with HACE may deteriorate rapidly to coma, so initial mental status is a poor predictor of eventual disease severity. It is critical to maintain a broad differential diagnosis for those patients with altered mental status at high altitude, especially in patients with atypical presentations or those who are not responding to conventional therapy. **Box 2** summarizes the differential diagnosis for HACE.

HACE diagnosis is based on the setting, symptoms, and findings. Imaging studies and laboratory analysis are primarily used to rule out an alternative diagnosis. Importantly, the clinician should evaluate for concurrent HAPE. Laboratory tests including electrolytes, complete blood count, glucose, ethanol level, carboxyhemoglobin level, and toxicology screen can be used to exclude other disorders (see **Box 2**).[18] Patients with HACE may mount a mild leukocytosis, so clinical correlation is necessary to exclude infection.[16] A lumbar puncture may be performed if there is sufficient concern for encephalitis or subarachnoid hemorrhage; typical findings in HACE include normal cell counts and elevated opening pressure. Values up to 220 cm water have been reported in the literature.[19] Head computed tomography typically shows white matter signal attenuation with effacement of sulci and flattening of gyri. MRI findings include increased T2 signal observed in the splenium of the corpus callosum.[20] Alternatively, MRI using susceptibility-weighted imaging can show hemosiderin deposition owing to microhemorrhage in the corpus callosum (**Fig. 3**). This finding is detectable by MRI for years after an episode of HACE, making this imaging useful when diagnosis of HACE is historically uncertain.[21] Because imaging findings lag behind clinical recovery, imaging can be used to confirm the diagnosis of HACE even after empiric therapy and clinical improvement.

Box 2
Differential of high altitude cerebral edema

- Hypoglycemia
- Hyponatremia
- Hypothermia
- CNS infection
- Postictal state
- Complex migraine
- Psychosis
- Stroke
- CNS space-occupying lesion
- Intracranial hemorrhage
- Carbon monoxide poisoning
- Drugs, alcohol or toxins

Abbreviation: CNS, central nervous system.

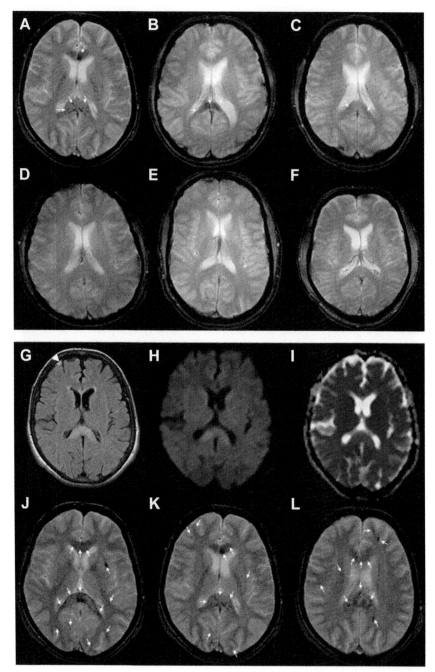

Fig. 3. MRI findings representative of HACE. Susceptibility-weighted T2* images show the differences between the normal MRI of acute mountain sickness patients (*D–F*) and HACE patients (*A–C*), with multiple lesions representing hemosiderin deposits predominantly located in the splenium of the corpus callosum (*arrows*). Fluid-attenuated inversion recovery (FLAIR) (*G*) shows edema in the corpus callosum. The right frontal meningioma (*arrowhead*) is an incidental finding. Areas of edema are confirmed by diffusion-weighted imaging (*H*), with increased values in the apparent diffusion coefficient (*I*), indicating increased water diffusivity compatible with vasogenic edema. Multiple microhemorrhages consistent with hemosiderin deposition (*arrows*) are displayed on the T2* images (*J–L*).

High Altitude Pulmonary Edema

The classic victim of HAPE is a young, healthy person, often male, who is fit enough to rapidly ascend to high altitude. Early recognition is paramount, because in this stage HAPE can be easily treated with descent or low-flow oxygen. Decreased exercise performance and dry cough are the earliest symptoms of HAPE. Whereas AMS is present in one-half of cases, it may notably be absent.[22] Symptoms typically develop on the second night of a new and higher sleeping altitude. Development of HAPE after 4 days at a given altitude is rare and should prompt the consideration of alternative diagnoses (**Box 3**). Without intervention, symptoms quickly progress from dyspnea with exertion to dyspnea at rest. Fever is common and does not preclude a diagnosis of HAPE. Oxygen saturation is often 10 to 20 points lower than asymptomatic individuals at the same altitude. As HAPE progresses, patients experience worsening tachycardia, tachypnea, lassitude, productive cough, and cyanosis. Eventually, altered mental status and coma develop, either from profound hypoxemia or concomitant HACE.

On physical examination, a prominent P_2 and right ventricular heave may be appreciated with auscultation and palpation. Râles are often first appreciated in the right mid-lung field. In a minority of patients, râles absent at rest can be elicited after brief exertion. Electrocardiographic findings of right heart strain may be observed, consistent with acute pulmonary hypertension. Chest radiographs typically show patchy lung infiltrates with normal heart size (**Fig. 4**). The absence of infiltrates on chest radiographs suggest an alternate diagnosis. Arterial blood gas analysis reveals respiratory alkalosis with severe hypoxemia. Partial pressure of arterial oxygen is typically between 30 and 40 mm Hg.[23]

PREVENTION AND TREATMENT OF HIGH ALTITUDE ILLNESS

The overall goals of prophylaxis and treatment of HAI are to optimize acclimatization to prevent illness, and to recognize and manage illness correctly. Three guiding principles hold true for the management of all HAI:

- Never proceed to a higher sleeping altitude with symptoms of HAI.
- Descend if symptoms do not improve despite expectant management or temporizing pharmacologic treatment.
- Descend and/or treat immediately in the presence of confusion, ataxia, or dyspnea at rest with relative hypoxemia.

Descent is the definitive treatment for all forms of altitude illness. However, descent may not always be possible owing to weather or logistic constraints. Nor is descent

---

Box 3
Differential diagnosis of high altitude pulmonary edema

- Asthma
- Bronchitis
- Heart failure
- Mucus plugging
- Myocardial infarction
- Pneumonia
- Pulmonary embolus

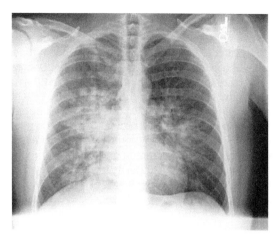

Fig. 4. Chest radiograph showing patchy lung infiltrates with normal heart size.

always necessary. Although prevention and treatment strategies are organized into pharmacologic and nonpharmacologic approaches, in clinical practice these strategies are often combined for best results. **Table 3** summarizes the pharmacologic approach for prevention and treatment of HAI, including newer strategies.

Pharmacologic Strategies

Prevention of acute mountain sickness

Acetazolamide Acetazolamide benefits those with a known history of AMS or those with rapid ascent to sleeping altitude above 2500 m.[24] By inhibiting the enzyme carbonic anhydrase, acetazolamide reduces renal reabsorption of bicarbonate, causing a bicarbonate diuresis and metabolic acidosis that increases one's respiratory rate and enhances (speeds) acclimatization. As a result, the Pa_{O_2} is higher. The recommended regimen is 125 mg orally twice daily, started 8 to 24 hours before the ascent. Using this lower dosage minimizes side effects.[25,26] The drug should be continued for the first 2 days at a stable altitude, or continued for ongoing ascent. It can be restarted safely if symptoms of AMS recur with ascent to a higher altitude. Acetazolamide reduces incidence of AMS by approximately 75% in persons ascending rapidly to sleeping altitudes of greater than 2500 m (>8200 ft).[27] Although several other pharmaceutical options are available, acetazolamide remains the mainstay for AMS prophylaxis.

Benzolamide Acetazolamide can have several side effects, including headache and nausea. It has also been linked with Stevens-Johnson syndrome.[28] More hydrophilic carbonic anhydrase inhibitors such as benzolamide may have fewer CNS side effects. Recently, benzolamide was compared with acetazolamide for the prevention and AMS.[29] In this trial, fewer side effects were noted in the benzolamide cohort. Unfortunately, benzolamide is not currently licensed for use in the United States. However, in the future, alternative carbonic anhydrase inhibitors may represent a viable alternative to acetazolamide once further validation is completed.

Dexamethasone Dexamethasone is an effective prophylactic agent for AMS.[24,30] However, because of more potential side effects, it is usually reserved for treatment. Dexamethasone is an appropriate agent for those with anaphylaxis to sulfonamides or acetazolamide intolerance. The dose for prophylaxis is either 2 mg PO every 6 hours or

Table 3
Pharmacologic strategies for high-altitude illness

Agent	Indication	Dosage	Adverse Effects	Comments
Acetazolamide	Prevention of AMS	125 mg every 12 h. Begin 24 h before ascent. Continue for at least 48 h after arrival at highest altitude.	Common: paresthesiae, polyuria, altered taste of carbonated beverages Less common: nausea, fatigue, headache Rare: Stevens-Johnson or anaphylaxis	Enhances acclimatization; pregnancy category C; avoid if breastfeeding
	Treatment of AMS	250 mg PO every 12 h.		
Dexamethasone	Treatment of AMS HACE	4 mg every 6 h PO, IM, or IV. 8 mg initially, then 4 mg every 6 h PO, IM, or IV.	Common: Mood changes, insomnia, dyspepsia Rare: Adrenal suppression, psychosis, hyperglycemia	Rapidly improves AMS symptoms, beware minor rebound symptoms; life saving in cases of HACE; pregnancy category C
Ibuprofen	Prevention of AMS?	600 mg every 8 h during ascent.	Dyspepsia; exercise-induced kidney injury	Risk of gastrointestinal bleed
Budesonisde	Prevention of AMS	200 µg every 12 h, beginning 3 d before ascent.	Sore throat, myalgias, headache, oral candidiasis	Vastly more expensive than acetazolamide or dexamethasone; optimal regimen needs validation
Tadalafil	Prevention of HAPE	10 mg PO every 12 h starting 24 h before ascent. Continue for 2–4 d at max sleeping altitude,	Common: headache, facial swelling Rare: priapism	BID dosing, compared with TID dosing with sildenafil; fewer side effects, less hypotension when compared with nifedipine; pregnancy category B
Nifedipine	Prevention of HAPE	30 mg extended release, PO every 12 h, starting 24 h before ascent.	Reflex tachycardia, hypotension (uncommon)	Pregnancy category C; Not necessary, if oxygen available
	Treatment of HAPE	30 mg extended-release PO every 12 h.		

Abbreviations: AMS, acute mountain sickness; HACE, high-altitude cerebral edema; HAPE, high-altitude pulmonary edema; IM, intramuscularly; IV, intravenous.

4 mg PO every 12 hours, starting the day of ascent and continuing for the first 2 days at altitude, or for a rapid increase in altitude.

Budesonide In 2 recent studies, inhaled budesonide was shown to be effective in prevention of AMS.[31,32] In these experiments, 200 µg budesonide was inhaled twice daily, starting 3 days before ascent. In a study by Zheng and colleagues,[32] inhaled budesonide reduced the incidence of AMS by 36% relative to placebo, comparable with the reduction observed with oral dexamethasone in the same study. These data raise important as mechanistic question: Why is an inhaled steroid with minimal systemic absorption effective at preventing AMS? Although more study is necessary for external validation and to explore mechanism of action, these data may herald an important shift in the approach to AMS prophylaxis. Nonetheless, it is also important to consider that budesonide is far more expensive compared with acetazolamide and dexamethasone.

Ibuprofen Several recent studies have explored the efficacy of ibuprofen for prevention of AMS, but they did not compare ibuprofen with acetazolamide. In 1 trial, 86 individuals were taken from 1240 to 3810 m and were randomized to receive either ibuprofen or placebo. The ibuprofen cohort had a significantly lower rate of AMS (odds ratio, 0.3; 95% CI, 0.1–0.8).[33] During the ASCENT trial (Altitude Sickness in Climbers and Efficacy of NSAIDs Trial), trekkers in the Himalayas were randomized to placebo or ibuprofen on ascent from approximately 4200 to 4900 m. Using an intent-to-treat analysis, the investigators demonstrated that ibuprofen was somewhat effective for the prevention of AMS, but it was not in those who completed the protocol; nor did it prevent severe AMS.[34] In these studies, a regimen of 600 mg PO was given 3 times per day. More study is necessary, because it is not clear whether ibuprofen reduced headache as an analgesic or had a significant impact on AMS.

Ginkgo biloba Conflicting evidence exists on the efficacy of ginkgo biloba for AMS prophylaxis.[35,36] A lack of consistency between commercially available gingko preparations may explain these differing results. Despite the variable results, ginkgo is a safe option for those individuals who strongly prefer a more natural alternative.

Prevention of high altitude cerebral edema
Based on the pathophysiology, agents that prevent AMS and HAPE will also prevent HACE. However, adequate acclimatization is the best strategy.

Prevention of high altitude pulmonary edema
Nifedipine Nifedipine 30 mg PO every 12 hours while ascending may provide effective prophylaxis in HAPE susceptible individuals.[37] Although controlled data are scarce, nifedipine is used commonly for this purpose.

Phosphodiesterase inhibitors The phosphodiesterase inhibitors sildenafil and tadalafil have shown promise for prevention of HAPE.[38] These agents blunt hypoxic pulmonary vasoconstriction and thereby prevent the pathologic pulmonary hypertension associated with HAPE. Anecdotally, tadalafil is used more frequently than sildenafil because of its longer half-life. It is also important to note that both of these agents can cause headache. In 1 study, tadalafil 10 mg PO twice a day effectively prevented HAPE in HAPE-susceptible individuals started the day before ascent.[39]

Dexamethasone Dexamethasone was effective for preventing HAPE in HAPE-susceptible individuals in a single study.[39] Data are not available comparing efficacy of dexamethasone with nifedipine or other agents, and clinical experience is limited.

However, if an individual who is susceptible to both AMS and HAPE is required to travel to a high altitude, dexamethasone may offer a useful preventive approach.

Salmeterol Using high-dose inhaled salmeterol (125 μg twice daily), investigators were able to demonstrate a 50% reduction in the incidence of HAPE in those persons with known susceptibility, which is less than nifedipine or tadalafil.[40] Clinical experience is limited. Therefore, salmeterol is recommended as an adjunctive treatment in addition to a medication such as nifedipine.[41]

Treatment of acute mountain sickness
Acetazolamide Acetazolamide is not well-established as a treatment for AMS, unlike for prevention. A single small study found that 2 doses of 250 mg given 8 hours apart was superior to placebo and improved gas exchange.[42] Specific data regarding optimal treatment dose are lacking. Side effects are dose related and include peripheral paresthesiae, headache, and nausea. Treatment should be continued until symptoms of AMS have abated.

Dexamethasone Dexamethasone 4 mg every 6 hours is effective for treatment of AMS. Dexamethasone can be administrated PO, intramuscularly, or intravenously depending on available resources and the presence of vomiting. However, dexamethasone is best reserved for cases of moderate or severe AMS because of its side effect profile and small risk of rebound symptoms. A short taper period is not required if used for 5 days or less. In contrast with acetazolamide, dexamethasone does not aid acclimatization. Combination treatment with acetazolamide has not been studied, but acetazolamide to speed acclimatization and dexamethasone to abort illness is rational, and is used in the field.

Symptomatic care (analgesia plus antiemetic)
Symptomatic treatment of AMS is often sufficient. Acetaminophen 650 to 1000 mg or ibuprofen 600 mg are both effective for headache. Ondansetron orally disintegrating tablets dosed at 4 mg every 4 to 6 hours will effectively treat nausea and vomiting associated with AMS. Ultimately, pharmacologic treatment for AMS offers an alternative to descent or oxygen if these options are unavailable, or if symptoms are only mild to moderate in severity.

Treatment of high altitude cerebral edema
Dexamethasone The gold standard for treatment of HACE is descent whenever possible and evacuation to a medical facility (see Nonpharmacologic Approach). However, dexamethasone should also be administered and is given as an 8-mg loading dose, followed by 4 mg every 6 hours. In the patient with HACE, dexamethasone must often be given intramuscularly owing to coma or tenuous mental status.

Other adjunctive treatment There are no data to support the use of hypertonic saline, loop diuretics, or mannitol in HACE patients. Loop diuretics should be avoided because of the danger of hypotension, reduced cerebral perfusion pressure, and ischemia.

Treatment of high altitude pulmonary edema
Nifedipine Controlled studies for the treatment of HAPE are lacking and only 1 study has demonstrated the efficacy of nifedipine for HAPE.[43] Nonetheless, nifedipine has been used extensively in the field, especially when oxygen and descent are not available. The suggested regimen is nifedipine 30 mg (extended release) administered twice daily by mouth until the victim has descended and been evacuated to medical

care. However, recent data suggest that nifedipine is unnecessary if descent and oxygen therapy are available.[44]

Phosphodiesterase inhibitors There are only case reports supporting the use of phosphodiesterase inhibitors for treatment of HAPE.[45] However, their use in the field is relatively common in anecdotal reports, when oxygen and descent are not available. Tadalafil 10 mg twice daily by mouth is the accepted regimen. Importantly, tadalafil should not be used with nifedipine owing to the overlap in mechanism of action. This could result in deleterious hypotension.

Neither of these pharmaceutical regimens are as effective as oxygen or descent for the treatment of HAPE.

Nonpharmacologic Strategies

Prevention of high altitude illness
Graded ascent Graded ascent to allow time for acclimatization is the best prevention for all HAI. For those traveling from sea level to the Rocky Mountains (>2500 m), spending a night at an intermediate elevation such as Denver or Salt Lake City (1500–2000 m) lessens the risk of AMS. Although controlled studies are scare,[46] above 2500 m mountaineers and trekkers should not ascend faster than 500 m/d. Furthermore, for every 1500 m gain in sleeping elevation, an extra night should be budgeted for acclimatization.[41]

Preacclimatization Preacclimatization strategies are now being used by several commercial guiding companies in the Himalaya to reduce "time to summit day" when climbing. These strategies use intermittent exposure either to hypobaric hypoxia or normobaric hypoxia through a commercial hypoxia tent, chamber, or mask. These devices vary considerably in hypoxic "dose" (simulated altitude) and exposure time. Only a few preacclimatization programs are able to demonstrate a meaningful decrease in AMS incidence.[47–49] Intermittent, short-term exposure to hypoxia of less than 6 h/d does not seem to prevent AMS. Sleep quality may also suffer during these preacclimatization programs.[50]

Remote ischemic preconditioning Remote ischemic preconditioning is a technique in which brief, discrete episodes of ischemia–reperfusion are induced in the extremities, typically with an inflated blood pressure cuff. Data suggest that this preexposure may result in resistance to further hypoxemic insults in tissue such as the myocardium.[51] Theoretically, such an approach could have a benefit for the prevention of AMS. Unfortunately, the application of this technique for AMS prevention is not supported currently by the literature.[52]

Oxygen Low-flow oxygen (<2 L/min), delivered via nasal cannula, especially during sleep, is a reasonable strategy for HAI prevention. Oxygen relieves the physiologic stress of hypobaric hypoxia and effectively simulates sea level if below 3000 m. Oxygen concentrators are readily available in mountain resort towns of the Rocky Mountain region and oxygen supplementation may be an appropriate strategy for lowlanders, especially those with chronic medical conditions, or those with second homes at high altitude.

Treatment of acute mountain sickness
Oxygen Oxygen quickly and effectively relieves symptoms of AMS, especially headache and dizziness. Nocturnal administration of low-flow oxygen (0.5–1 L/min) is often sufficient to alleviate mild to moderate AMS.

Descent A decrease in altitude of 300 to 1000 m (980–3280 ft) will resolve AMS.

Treatment of high altitude cerebral edema

Oxygen If available, oxygen should be given for any patient with suspected HACE. Given the high rate of concomitant HAPE, oxygen supplementation becomes even more important in the treatment of critically ill patients with HAI. Oxygen saturation should be titrated to 90% or higher. Care should be given to avoid prolonged hyperoxia given the recent association of increased mortality in critically ill patients.[53] Comatose patients may require oxygen supplementation through an advanced airway.

Body position Keep the patient's head elevated to 30° in the supine position.

Descent Descent is critical for victims of HACE. At a minimum, providers should attempt to evacuate the patient to an altitude where the patient was previously asymptomatic. Descent of at least 1000 m is an alternative goal.

Portable hyperbaric chambers Portable hyperbaric chambers are effective for the treatment of severe HAI (**Fig. 5**).[54] The patient is inserted into a zippered fabric chamber. A rescuer then raises the ambient pressure within the chamber to 0.9 kg/2.5 cm^2 (2 lb/in.^{2}) with a manual or automated pump. This increase in pressures simulates a descent of up to 1500 m (4920 ft), depending on the ambient elevation. A valve system provides sufficient ventilation to avoid carbon dioxide accumulation. Patients must stay in the chamber for several hours to see meaningful effect, and rebound symptoms are possible when the patient is removed from the bag.[55] Clinical care in a chamber can be complicated by vomiting, voiding, suboptimal communication, and claustrophobia. Nonetheless, these devices can be life saving if descent is impossible owing to weather or logistics, and if oxygen is not available. More recent designs have decreased the weight of these portable chambers to less than 4 kg (8.8 lbs).

Treatment of high altitude pulmonary edema

Oxygen Oxygen supplementation immediately lowers pulmonary artery pressure in those with HAPE. Oxygen, even without descent, can resolve mild to moderate HAPE within 2 to 3 days. In resource-rich settings such as Colorado ski resorts, supplemental oxygen is a practical alternative to descent or evacuation. Oxygen flow rates should be titrated to maintain an oxygen saturation of 90% to 92%.

Descent If oxygen is unavailable, all patients with suspected HAPE should be evacuated to an altitude at least 1000 m lower.

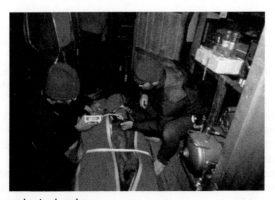

Fig. 5. Portable hyperbaric chamber.

Portable hyperbaric chambers See the description in the section on the treatment of high altitude cerebral edema.

Other management considerations Providers should attempt to mitigate any environmental factors that would lead to further pulmonary hypertension. Because cold stress increases the pulmonary artery pressure, the patient should be kept warm. Patients should also avoid exertion whenever possible.

TREATMENT COMPLICATIONS AND PITFALLS
Pharmacologic

Acetazolamide
There are decades of experience using acetazolamide for AMS. Although acetazolamide is usually a safe drug, there are several considerations worth noting. Acetazolamide does contain a sulfhydryl moiety. Some individuals who are allergic to antimicrobial sulfonamides may also be allergic to nonmicrobial sulfonamide drugs. Therefore, acetazolamide should be avoided in individuals with a history of anaphylaxis to sulfa antibiotics. In those individuals who have experienced rash or less severe reactions to sulfa antibiotics, a test dose of acetazolamide before ascent is a reasonable strategy to test tolerance. The most commonly reported side effects are increased urination, paresthesia, fatigue, and gastrointestinal upset.[56] Stevens-Johnson syndrome is rare, but documented.[28]

Dexamethasone
Dexamethasone is a remarkably effectively drug, with wide applications across the spectrum of HAI. However, its use must be weighed cautiously against the risk of adverse events such as adrenal suppression and steroid psychosis. These adverse events typically occur with use beyond 7 days. Although controlled data are lacking, there are reports of frequent use or abuse among the mountaineering population in the Himalayan Everest with disastrous consequences.[57]

Ibuprofen
Recent data suggest that mountaineers climbing above 4000 m are at risk for hemorrhagic gastritis and duodenitis based on endoscopies performed at extreme altitude.[58] Whether the use of ibuprofen for AMS places individuals at higher risk for gastrointestinal bleed, or whether the risk of altitude gastritis or duodenitis translates to lower altitudes (2000–4000 m) is worthy of further study.

Nonpharmacologic

- Critically ill patients with HACE who progress to coma require an advanced airway and bladder drainage. In these patients, avoid hyperventilation, which may result in cerebral ischemia.
- Avoid rapid depressurization of portable hyperbaric chambers, which may result in middle ear squeeze. Although barotrauma has not been reported, it is theoretically possible.
- Critically ill patients with HAPE are often volume depleted and require intravenous fluid resuscitation. Despite the presence of pulmonary edema, intravenous fluids are not contraindicated to treat dehydration because cardiac function is most often preserved.
- Monitor blood pressure carefully in patients with HACE. Hypotension may lead to a drop in cerebral perfusion pressure, leading to further cerebral ischemia.
- Infection and HAPE may coexist; when in doubt, treat for both.

SUMMARY

- Acetazolamide remains the best choice for prevention of AMS.
- The best treatment for all HAI is descent or oxygen, or both.
- Dexamethasone is excellent for treating moderate to severe AMS, and for HACE.
- Supplemental oxygen is first-line therapy for HAPE; descent is primary therapy if oxygen is not available. Oxygen and descent are more efficacious than pharmacologic therapy such as nifedipine or phosphodiesterase inhibitors.
- Descent is the definitive treatment for HACE and should not be delayed. Dexamethasone and supplemental oxygen are important adjunctive treatments for HACE until descent can be facilitated.

REFERENCES

1. Bartsch P, Swenson ER. Clinical practice: acute high-altitude illnesses. N Engl J Med 2013;368(24):2294–302.
2. Hackett P, Roach RC. High-altitude illness. N Engl J Med 2001;345:107–14.
3. Lawley JS, Levine BD, Williams MA, et al. Cerebral spinal fluid dynamics: effect of hypoxia and implications for high-altitude illness. J Appl Physiol (1985) 2016; 120(2):251–62.
4. Lawley JS, Alperin N, Bagci AM, et al. Normobaric hypoxia and symptoms of acute mountain sickness: elevated brain volume and intracranial hypertension. Ann Neurol 2014;75(6):890–8.
5. Wilson MH, Newman S, Imray CH. The cerebral effects of ascent to high altitudes. Lancet Neurol 2009;8(2):175–91.
6. Stream JO, Grissom CK. Update on high-altitude pulmonary edema: pathogenesis, prevention, and treatment. Wilderness Environ Med 2008;19(4):293–303.
7. Bartsch P, Mairbaurl H, Maggiorini M, et al. Physiological aspects of high-altitude pulmonary edema. J Appl Physiol 2005;98(3):1101–10.
8. Scherrer U, Allemann Y, Rexhaj E, et al. Mechanisms and drug therapy of pulmonary hypertension at high altitude. High Alt Med Biol 2013;14(2):126–33.
9. Roach RC, Bärtsch P, Oelz O, et al. The Lake Louise acute mountain sickness scoring system. In: Sutton JR, Houston CS, Coates G, editors. Hypoxia and molecular medicine. Burlington (VT): Queen City Press; 1993. p. 272–4.
10. Beidleman BA, Tighiouart H, Schmid CH, et al. Predictive models of acute mountain sickness after rapid ascent to various altitudes. Med Sci Sports Exerc 2013; 45(4):792–800.
11. Leichtfried V, Basic D, Burtscher M, et al. Diagnosis and prediction of the occurrence of acute mountain sickness measuring oxygen saturation–independent of absolute altitude? Sleep Breath 2016;20(1):435–42.
12. Foutch RG, Henrichs W. Carbon monoxide poisoning at high altitudes. Am J Emerg Med 1988;6:596–8.
13. Keyes LE, Hamilton RS, Rose JS. Carbon monoxide exposure from cooking in snow caves at high altitude. Wilderness Environ Med 2001;12(3):208–12.
14. Broessner G, Rohregger J, Wille M, et al. Hypoxia triggers high-altitude headache with migraine features: a prospective trial. Cephalalgia 2016;36(8):765–71.
15. Schoonman GG, Sandor PS, Agosti RM, et al. Normobaric hypoxia and nitroglycerin as trigger factors for migraine. Cephalalgia 2006;26(7):816–9.
16. Dickinson JG. High altitude cerebral edema: cerebral acute mountain sickness. Semin Respir Med 1983;5:151–8.
17. Gallagher SA, Hackett PH. High-altitude illness. Emerg Med Clin North Am 2004; 22(2):329–55, viii.

18. Hackett PH, Roach RC. High altitude cerebral edema. High Alt Med Biol 2004; 5(2):136–46.
19. Houston CS, Dickinson JG. Cerebral form of high altitude illness. Lancet 1975;2: 758–61.
20. Hackett PH, Yarnell PR, Hill R, et al. High-altitude cerebral edema evaluated with magnetic resonance imaging: clinical correlation and pathophysiology. J Am Med Assoc 1998;280(22):1920–5.
21. Schommer K, Kallenberg K, Lutz K, et al. Hemosiderin deposition in the brain as footprint of high-altitude cerebral edema. Neurology 2013;81(20):1776–9.
22. Viswanathan R, Subramanian S, Lodi ST, et al. Further studies on pulmonary oedema of high altitude. Respiration 1978;36:216–22.
23. Scherrer U, Vollenweider L, Delabays A, et al. Inhaled nitric oxide for high-altitude pulmonary edema. N Engl J Med 1996;334:624–9.
24. Ellsworth AJ, Larson EB, Strickland D. A randomized trial of dexamethasone and acetazolamide for acute mountain sickness prophylaxis. Am J Med 1987;83(6): 1024–30.
25. van Patot MC, Leadbetter G 3rd, Keyes LE, et al. Prophylactic low-dose acetazolamide reduces the incidence and severity of acute mountain sickness. High Alt Med Biol 2008;9(4):289–93.
26. Basnyat B, Gertsch JH, Johnson EW, et al. Efficacy of low-dose acetazolamide (125 mg BID) for the prophylaxis of acute mountain sickness: a prospective, double-blind, randomized, placebo-controlled trial. High Alt Med Biol 2003; 4(1):45–52.
27. Greene MK, Kerr AM, McIntosh IB, et al. Acetazolamide in prevention of acute mountain sickness: a double-blind controlled cross-over study. Br Med J (Clin Res Ed) 1981;283(6295):811–3.
28. Her Y, Kil MS, Park JH, et al. Stevens-Johnson syndrome induced by acetazolamide. J Dermatol 2011;38(3):272–5.
29. Collier DJ, Wolff CB, Hedges AM, et al. Benzolamide improves oxygenation and reduces acute mountain sickness during a high-altitude trek and has fewer side effects than acetazolamide at sea level. Pharmacol Res Perspect 2016;4(3): e00203.
30. Ellsworth AJ, Meyer EF, Larson EB. Acetazolamide or dexamethasone use versus placebo to prevent acute mountain sickness on Mount Rainier. West J Med 1991; 154(3):289–93.
31. Chen GZ, Zheng CR, Qin J, et al. Inhaled budesonide prevents acute mountain sickness in young Chinese men. J Emerg Med 2015;48(2):197–206.
32. Zheng CR, Chen GZ, Yu J, et al. Inhaled budesonide and oral dexamethasone prevent acute mountain sickness. Am J Med 2014;127(10):1001–9.e2.
33. Lipman GS, Kanaan NC, Holck PS, et al. Ibuprofen prevents altitude illness: a randomized controlled trial for prevention of altitude illness with nonsteroidal anti-inflammatories. Ann Emerg Med 2012;59(6):484–90.
34. Gertsch JH, Corbett B, Holck PS, et al. Altitude Sickness in Climbers and Efficacy of NSAIDs Trial (ASCENT): randomized, controlled trial of ibuprofen versus placebo for prevention of altitude illness. Wilderness Environ Med 2012;23(4): 307–15.
35. Moraga FA, Flores A, Serra J, et al. Ginkgo biloba decreases acute mountain sickness in people ascending to high altitude at Ollague (3696 m) in northern Chile. Wilderness Environ Med 2007;18(4):251–7.
36. Kenrick PA. Altitude sickness: gingko biloba does not prevent altitude sickness. Br Med J 2003;327(7406):106.

37. Bartsch P, Maggiorini M, Ritter M, et al. Prevention of high-altitude pulmonary edema by nifedipine. N Engl J Med 1991;325(18):1284–9.

38. Tsai BM, Turrentine MW, Sheridan BC, et al. Differential effects of phosphodiesterase-5 inhibitors on hypoxic pulmonary vasoconstriction and pulmonary artery cytokine expression. Ann Thorac Surg 2006;81(1):272–8.

39. Maggiorini M, Brunner-La Rocca HP, Peth S, et al. Both tadalafil and dexamethasone may reduce the incidence of high-altitude pulmonary edema: a randomized trial. Ann Intern Med 2006;145(7):497–506.

40. Swenson ER, Maggiorini M. Salmeterol for the prevention of high-altitude pulmonary edema. N Engl J Med 2002;347(16):1282–5 [author reply: 1282–5].

41. Luks AM, McIntosh SE, Grissom CK, et al. Wilderness Medical Society practice guidelines for the prevention and treatment of acute altitude illness: 2014 update. Wilderness Environ Med 2014;25(4 Suppl):S4–14.

42. Grissom CK, Roach RC, Sarnquist FH, et al. Acetazolamide in the treatment of acute mountain sickness: clinical efficacy and effect on gas exchange. Ann Intern Med 1992;116(6):461–5.

43. Oelz O, Maggiorini M, Ritter M, et al. Nifedipine for high altitude pulmonary edema. Lancet 1989;2:1241–4.

44. Deshwal R, Iqbal M, Basnet S. Nifedipine for the treatment of high altitude pulmonary edema. Wilderness Environ Med 2012;23(1):7–10.

45. Fagenholz PJ, Gutman JA, Murray AF, et al. Treatment of high altitude pulmonary edema at 4240 m in Nepal. High Alt Med Biol 2007;8(2):139–46.

46. Bloch KE, Turk AJ, Maggiorini M, et al. Effect of ascent protocol on acute mountain sickness and success at Muztagh Ata, 7546 m. High Alt Med Biol 2009;10(1):25–32.

47. Muza SR, Beidleman BA, Fulco CS. Altitude preexposure recommendations for inducing acclimatization. High Alt Med Biol 2010;11(2):87–92.

48. Fulco CS, Muza SR, Beidleman BA, et al. Effect of repeated normobaric hypoxia exposures during sleep on acute mountain sickness, exercise performance, and sleep during exposure to terrestrial altitude. Am J Physiol Regul Integr Comp Physiol 2011;300(2):R428–36.

49. Fulco CS, Beidleman BA, Muza SR. Effectiveness of preacclimatization strategies for high-altitude exposure. Exerc Sport Sci Rev 2013;41(1):55–63.

50. Dehnert C, Bohm A, Grigoriev I, et al. Sleeping in moderate hypoxia at home for prevention of acute mountain sickness (AMS): a placebo-controlled, randomized double-blind study. Wilderness Environ Med 2014;25(3):263–71.

51. Birnbaum Y, Hale SL, Kloner RA. Ischemic preconditioning at a distance: reduction of myocardial infarct size by partial reduction of blood supply combined with rapid stimulation of the gastrocnemius muscle in the rabbit. Circulation 1997;96(5):1641–6.

52. Berger MM, Kohne H, Hotz L, et al. Remote ischemic preconditioning delays the onset of acute mountain sickness in normobaric hypoxia. Physiol Rep 2015;3(3) [pii:e12325].

53. Damiani E, Adrario E, Girardis M, et al. Arterial hyperoxia and mortality in critically ill patients: a systematic review and meta-analysis. Crit Care 2014;18(6):711.

54. Bärtsch P, Merki B, Hofstetter D, et al. Treatment of acute mountain sickness by simulated descent: a randomised controlled trial. Br Med J 1993;306:1098–101.

55. Taber RL. Protocols for the use of a portable hyperbaric chamber for the treatment of high altitude disorders. J Wilderness Med 1990;1:181–92.

56. Vahedi K, Taupin P, Djomby R, et al. Efficacy and tolerability of acetazolamide in migraine prophylaxis: a randomised placebo-controlled trial. J Neurol 2002; 249(2):206–11.
57. O'Neil D. Climber's Little Helper. Outside Magazine 2013.
58. Fruehauf H, Erb A, Maggiorini M, et al. T1080 Unsedated Transnasal Esophago-Gastroduodenoscopy at 4559 M (14957 Ft) -endoscopic findings in healthy mountaineers after rapid ascent to high altitude. Gastroenterology 138(5):S-483–4.

Out-of-Hospital Evaluation and Treatment of Accidental Hypothermia

Ken Zafren, MD[a,b,c,d],*

KEYWORDS

- Hypothermia • Accidental hypothermia • Afterdrop • Thermoregulation
- Cardiac arrest • Avalanche • Rewarming • Circumrescue collapse

KEY POINTS

- Hypothermia can be life-threatening. Rescuers should attempt to minimize further heat loss and begin rewarming of hypothermic patients in the field while minimizing afterdrop and preventing circumrescue collapse.
- Some patients are cold and dead but other cold patients who are apparently dead can be resuscitated with full neurologic recovery.
- Unless there are definite contraindications, rescuers should do their best to resuscitate hypothermia patients, even if they appear to be beyond hope.

INTRODUCTION
Definition

Accidental hypothermia is an unintentional drop in core temperature, which is the temperature of the heart and central circulation, to 35°C or below. Accidental hypothermia can be caused by environmental exposure and by diseases or conditions that decrease thermoregulatory responses. Iatrogenic accidental hypothermia can occur during resuscitation in emergency settings. Accidental hypothermia is a disease of wars and other disasters, as well as a condition that can affect people who are outdoors for work or recreation or because they are homeless. Accidental hypothermia can occur during any season and in any climate, including subtropical or tropical. Accidental hypothermia can also be caused by trauma, sepsis, or other diseases that decrease metabolic heat production or affect thermoregulation.

The author has nothing to disclose.
[a] Alaska Department of Health and Social Services, State of Alaska, Juneau, AK, USA;
[b] International Commission for Mountain Emergency Medicine (ICAR MEDCOM), Zürich, Switzerland; [c] Department of Emergency Medicine, Stanford University Medical Center, Stanford, CA, USA; [d] Alaska Native Medical Center, Anchorage, AK, USA
* 10181 Curvi Street, Anchorage, AK 99507.
E-mail address: kenzafren@gmail.com

Emerg Med Clin N Am 35 (2017) 261–279
http://dx.doi.org/10.1016/j.emc.2017.01.003
0733-8627/17/© 2017 Elsevier Inc. All rights reserved.

Therapeutic hypothermia, a form of targeted temperature management, can be induced to protect the brain in resuscitated cardiac arrest patients who remain unconscious after return of spontaneous circulation (ROSC). Hypothermia for neuroprotection may also be induced for cardiac surgery. Induced hypothermia is not discussed in this article.

Physiology

In normal conditions, the human body maintains a core temperature of 37° plus or minus 0.5°C. In response to input from peripheral and, to a lesser degree, central thermoreceptors, the hypothalamus regulates autonomic reflexes that increase body cooling or warming.[1] The main physiologic warming responses to defend against hypothermia are shivering and peripheral vasoconstriction. Peripheral vasoconstriction can be triggered centrally or by decreased local skin temperature.

Hypothermia is the result of net heat loss. Heat can be lost by conduction, convection, radiation, and evaporative mechanisms. Heat always flows from a warmer object or medium to a cooler object or medium. Conduction is the direct transfer of heat between objects that are touching each other. Convection is the transfer of heat from an object to a gas or liquid that is in motion. Radiation is the transfer of heat by electromagnetic energy between 2 objects that are exposed to each other; the body can be warmed by the sun or cooled by exposure to the night sky. Evaporation causes heat to be lost by the endothermic reaction of vaporizing water in sweat or wet clothing. Heat loss due to evaporation also accounts for insensible losses from skin and from breathing.

Humans are adapted to tropical climates. Human physiologic responses to cold have limited potential to protect against hypothermia. In a well-nourished person, if conditions are mild or insulation is adequate, exercise and shivering can raise the metabolic rate enough to prevent hypothermia. In colder conditions, humans must depend on behavioral responses to wear insulating clothing and to take shelter.

Pathophysiology

Cooling of the body results in decreased resting metabolism and decreased neurologic function. Shivering is induced by skin cooling, even when the core temperature is normal.[1] Shivering increases metabolism directly by increased muscle activity and indirectly by increased ventilation and cardiac output.[2] Shivering increases as core temperature decreases and is maximal at a core temperature of about 32°C. Shivering decreases below 32°C and ceases by about 30°C.[3] Below 32°C, metabolism generally decreases with decreasing core temperature.

The main clinical effects of hypothermia are due to decreases in brain and cardiorespiratory functions. Brain cooling causes impaired function beginning at about 34°C and worsening with further cooling.[4,5] Clinical signs are irritability, confusion, apathy, poor decision-making, lethargy, somnolence, coma, and finally death. Most of these changes, other than death, are reversible. Even patients in coma often recover neurologically intact. Decreased metabolic requirements of a cold brain can be neuroprotective, especially during anoxic conditions such as drowning.[6] Cold-induced diuresis, plasma leak, and decreased fluid intake decrease circulating blood volume.[7] Cooling of the heart causes decreased cardiac output and, usually, bradycardia. As the heart cools to 30°C and below, atrial dysrhythmias and premature ventricular contractions become common and ventricular fibrillation (VF) can occur.[8] Especially below 28°C, VF can be easily induced by acidosis, hypocarbia, hypoxia, or rough movement.[1] Hypoventilation and respiratory acidosis result from decreased ventilatory sensitivity to carbon dioxide (CO_2).[9]

OUT-OF-HOSPITAL EVALUATION OF HYPOTHERMIA
Classification of Hypothermia Based on Core Temperature

Hypothermia is classified, based on core temperature, as mild, 35°C to 32°C; moderate, 32°C to 28°C; or severe, less than 28°C.[10–12] Some investigators have also included another category, profound hypothermia, less than 24°C[11] or less than 20°C,[1] in which survival is significantly lower. Clinical effects of hypothermia vary greatly among individuals. Some patients are cold but not hypothermic. Because shivering is triggered by skin cooling, a patient can feel cold and be shivering but have a core temperature greater than 35°C. A patient who is cold and shivering but not hypothermic is considered to be cold-stressed.

The classes of hypothermia correlate with the ability of the body to thermoregulate. In mild hypothermia, shivering is effective in increasing metabolic rate and body temperature. Shivering increases in intensity as core temperature declines.[13] A mildly hypothermic patient who is healthy, has sufficient caloric reserves, and is protected from further heat loss, can rewarm to a normal core temperature by shivering. Below about 32°C, the body requires exogenous heat to rewarm to a normal core temperature. Shivering can still be strong in moderate hypothermia at 31°C[3] but becomes progressively weaker until it ceases at about 30°C.

Below 32°C, most patients will have altered mental status and a decreased level of consciousness. Many patients are unconscious at a core temperature of 30°C and most are unconscious by 28°C.[1]

Field Classification of Hypothermia

Standard field classification

When core temperature measurement is not feasible, it is useful to classify a patient using clinical signs as being cold-stressed, or as having mild, moderate, or severe hypothermia, corresponding to the same classifications based on core temperature (**Fig. 1**). Field classification will help to optimize treatment. Patients who are shivering but who are fully alert and functioning normally are likely to be cold-stressed rather than hypothermic. A patient who is alert and shivering but not functioning completely normally is most likely to be mildly hypothermic. A patient with a decreased level of consciousness is likely to be moderately hypothermic. A moderately hypothermic patient may or may not be shivering. Unconscious patients should be considered to be severely hypothermic. Clinical staging of hypothermia serves as a useful guide but is not completely correlated with measured core temperatures. As with any clinical condition, individuals are highly variable in their responses to cold. In addition, a patient whose level of consciousness has been altered by a condition other than hypothermia, such as intoxication or brain injury, may have a higher core temperature than predicted clinically.

The Swiss system

An alternate system of field classification, the Swiss system, correlates clinical signs with the standard core temperature ranges of mild, moderate, and severe hypothermia, as well as with 2 additional stages: profound hypothermia and death due to hypothermia.[11] Hypothermia (HT) stages are HT I, HT II, HT III, HT IV, and HT V, as follows:

- HT I: clear consciousness with shivering: 35° to 32°C
- HT II: impaired consciousness without shivering: 32° to 28°C
- HT III: unconscious: 28° to 24°C
- HT IV: apparent death: 24° to 13.7°C
- HT V: death due to irreversible hypothermia: less than 13.7°C? (<9°C?).

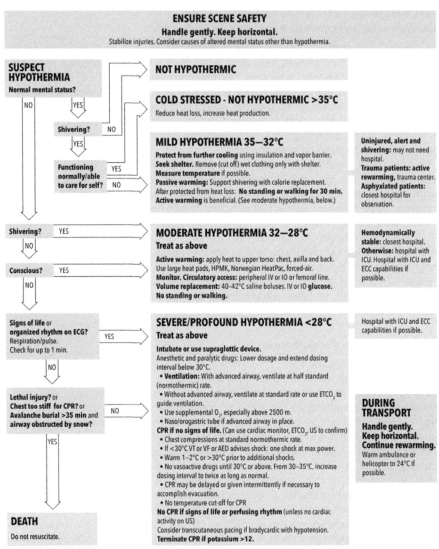

Fig. 1. Out-of-hospital treatment of hypothermia. AED, automated external defibrillator; CPR, cardiopulmonary resuscitation; ECC, extracorporeal circulation; ECG, electrocardiogram; HPMK, Hypothermia Protection and Management Kit; ICU, intensive care unit; O₂, oxygen; US, ultrasound; VF, ventricular fibrillation. (*From* Zafren K, Giesbrecht GG, Danzl DF, et al. Wilderness medical society practice guidelines for the out-of-hospital evaluation and treatment of accidental hypothermia: 2014 update. Wilderness Environ Med 2014;25(4 Suppl):S69; with permission.)

This system is widely used in Europe. The Swiss system shares the limitations of standard field classification but is also limited by inconsistencies. A patient with moderate hypothermia (HT II) is likely to be shivering if the core temperature is above 30° to 31°C. Rescuers who use the Swiss system should focus on level of consciousness rather than the presence or absence of shivering. A second inconsistency in the Swiss system involves patients with core temperature less than 24°C who have vital signs. There are many reports of such patients who may succumb to sudden death by VF.[14] This inconsistency does not affect treatment. Based on the results of a study correlating measured core temperatures of hypothermia victims with staging by the Swiss system, adjustments of the estimated core temperature parameters of the stages have been proposed.[15]

Associated conditions can complicate field assessment and treatment of hypothermia
Traumatic and medical conditions that cause decreased level of consciousness or abnormal vital signs may confuse the classification of hypothermia. These conditions may also suppress or abolish shivering, necessitating much more aggressive rewarming at a given core temperature than would otherwise be necessary.

Measurement of Core Temperature

Esophageal temperature
Esophageal temperature is the most accurate minimally invasive method of measuring core temperature. The probe must be inserted into the lower third of the esophagus,[16] an average of 24 cm below the larynx in adults. For hypothermic patients with decreased level of consciousness, esophageal temperature monitoring is very helpful to guide evaluation and treatment. Before placing an esophageal probe, which may cause vomiting and aspiration, it is usually best to protect the airway with endotracheal intubation or the placement of a supraglottic airway. Heated, humidified oxygen does not affect esophageal temperature if the probe is inserted in the lower third of the esophagus.[17–19] If the probe does not have markings, it can be marked at 24 cm before insertion in an adult or the correct length of insertion can be estimated visually for an adult or child and marked.

Epitympanic temperature
Epitympanic probes are soft probes in which a thermistor is placed near the tympanic membrane. Thermistor probes are more accurate than the common infrared tympanic thermometers. When an epitympanic probe is used properly, the reading correlates well with carotid artery temperature.[20] In patients with normal cardiac output, carotid temperature approximates core temperature. When cardiac output is low, epitympanic temperature is lower than core temperature.[21] Epitympanic temperature is often falsely lower than core temperature in out-of-hospital settings in which it is difficult to insulate the ear canal from a cold environment. For an accurate reading, there should be no cerumen or snow in the canal and the probe must have an insulating cap to block air entry.[20] Epitympanic thermometers designed for use in the operating room are not accurate when used in field settings. An epitympanic probe can be useful to evaluate a patient if an esophageal probe is not available and are generally preferred to an esophageal probe for a patient whose airway is not protected.

Rectal, urinary bladder, and oral temperatures
Placement of a rectal or bladder probe thermometer in the field requires exposing a possibly hypothermic patient causing further heat loss. Rectal or bladder temperature should not be performed until a patient is in a warm environment. The only use for oral temperature is to rule out hypothermia, because oral temperature is lower than core temperature by a variable amount. Thermometers that contain liquid (mercury or alcohol) usually cannot measure temperatures less than 35.6°C. If a nonelectronic thermometer is used it must be a low-reading thermometer.[1]

Although rectal or urinary bladder temperature is often called a core temperature, they can lag behind core temperature changes by up to 1 hour. During rewarming, monitoring of rectal or bladder temperature can give the false impression that the patient is still cooling.[2,7]

Temporal artery temperature
So-called temporal artery thermometers are too inaccurate to be used in the assessment of a possibly hypothermic patient.[22]

Heat flux thermometer
The noninvasive heat flux or double sensor thermometer combines a skin temperature sensor with a heat flux sensor.[23] Readings accurately reflect core temperature in operative and intensive care unit settings.[24] The heat flux thermometer is a promising noninvasive method of core temperature measurement that may be useful for out-of-hospital evaluation and treatment of hypothermia if accuracy is demonstrated in field situations.

Safety of Rescuers and Initial Priorities

The first priority during rescue is the safety of the rescuers. If a potentially hypothermic patient has an obvious fatal injury, it may not be necessary for rescuers to enter the scene. Even after it is safe for rescuers to enter the scene, it may be advisable to move the patient to a safer place before further evaluating the patient and initiating treatment.

Once the safety of the rescuers is assured, rescuers should determine whether the patient is in cardiac arrest. If the patient has vital signs but is not completely alert, rescuers should avoid causing cardiovascular collapse by gentle handling and by keeping the patient horizontal as much as possible. Attempt to minimize further decrease in core temperature and begin rewarming. If the patient is in cardiac arrest, rescuers should start resuscitation, if indicated.

Treatment of a Cold-Stressed Patient Who is Not Hypothermic

A patient who is completely alert and shivering, well-nourished, and not hypothermic is not at risk for significant afterdrop or circumrescue collapse. The patient may remove wet clothing and put on dry clothing without shelter. The patient does not need to be horizontal, may sit up to eat and drink, and may ambulate.[12]

Core Temperature Afterdrop

After a patient is removed from a cold environment, core cooling continues due to conductive heat loss from the warm core to cool peripheral tissue and convective heat loss to blood when increased blood flow to peripheral tissue causes increased cooling of blood that returns to the central circulation.[25,26] Conductive cooling is only minimally affected by treatment. Convective cooling can be increased by movement or rewarming of the extremities that results in an increased rate of blood flow to the periphery. Increased peripheral blood flow allows an increased volume of cooled blood to return to the central circulation. This decreases core temperature and increases the workload on the heart. Afterdrops as high as 5° to 6°C have been reported in hypothermic patients during prehospital care.[27–29] For a patient with moderate or severe hypothermia, afterdrop can contribute to cardiovascular instability.

Circumrescue Collapse

Syncope or sudden death that occurs in victims of cold-water immersion during or after rescue and removal from water is called circumrescue collapse.[30] Circumrescue collapse may be due to sudden hypotension or sudden onset of VF.[2] Removal from the water decreases hydrostatic pressure[2] and allows blood to pool in dependent areas. This decreases blood return, causing hypotension or cardiovascular collapse. Blood returning from the periphery is cooled and contributes to afterdrop. If the victim has to perform work there is an increased risk of circumrescue collapse.[31] Fatal circumrescue collapse was observed in shipwrecked sailors subsequent to climbing ladders to board rescue boats.[30] A combination of mechanical stimulation of the heart, acidosis from blood returning from the extremities, and afterdrop may cause VF.[32] Theoretically, imminent rescue may contribute to mental relaxation of a hypothermia victim, causing a decrease in catecholamine levels that results in hypotension. In the water this could precipitate loss of consciousness and drowning.[32] Fatal circumrescue collapse has been documented in terrestrial rescue, as well as in immersion hypothermia.[33,34]

Handling a Hypothermic Patient During Rescue

A hypothermic patient should be kept horizontal, especially after rescue from water, to minimize the effects of decreased hydrostatic pressure.[30] Rescuers should avoid having the patient make any physical effort,[31] but should encourage the victim to stay alert and focus on survival to minimize the chance of circumrescue collapse.

Movement and rewarming of the extremities should be avoided to prevent increased blood flow to cool peripheral tissue with resultant increase in return of cooled blood to the central circulation. Increased return of blood can stress a heart that is already impaired due to cold or can cause increased cooling that might precipitate VF,[35–37] especially at core temperatures less than 28°C.[1]

Protection from Further Heat Loss

In addition to minimizing afterdrop, rescuers should attempt to maintain core temperature by adding insulation and by providing a vapor barrier. Options for insulation include extra clothing, blankets, quilts, sleeping bags, and insulated pads. Insulated pads can prevent large conductive heat losses to the ground.[38] The vapor barrier protects against heat loss from evaporation and convection. Materials that can be used to make a vapor barrier are bubble wrap, sheets of plastic, reflective blankets, and garbage bags, with a hole cut out for the face. Bubble wrap is a good vapor barrier but has minimal value as insulation.[39,40] The vapor barrier is usually placed as the outermost layer[40,41] but can also be effective if placed between wet clothing and outer dry layers. Extra insulation can make up for the lack of a windproof layer or a vapor barrier.[41] Insulation can be placed inside 2 layers of vapor barrier.[40]

Wet clothes should be cut off, rather than pulled off, to minimize movement of the extremities. The patient should be insulated from the ground. The head and neck do not lose heat faster than the rest of the body but may account for a large percentage of heat loss if they are the only areas not protected by insulation. Insulation should be pulled as tightly around the face as possible without interfering with breathing to decrease heat loss from the head and neck.[38,42] If the patient is being evacuated by helicopter, a windproof layer, ideally a vapor barrier, should be used for protection from wind[39] and from rotor wash.

Field Rewarming

After a hypothermic patient has been protected from further cooling, the patient should be rewarmed as much as possible. The best rewarming methods minimize afterdrop even though other methods might be faster overall.[12] Rewarming is not required for mild hypothermia that is not complicated by other conditions but will make patients more comfortable. Patients with decreased level of consciousness require active rewarming.

Support shivering for a cold-stressed or mildly hypothermic patient

Shivering is the most effective method of rewarming a cold-stressed or mildly hypothermic patient. Because shivering is uncomfortable and can stress the cardiovascular system,[35] active rewarming methods are preferred. If active rewarming is not possible, the patient should be insulated and given high carbohydrate drinks[35] and food. Drinks can be warmed but should not be hot enough to cause burns. The heat content of warm high-carbohydrate drinks is negligible compared with the number of calories in the carbohydrates. Vigorous shivering increases heat production up to 5 to 6 times resting metabolic rate.[3,43] Shivering can increase core temperature 1° to 3°C per hour in a well-insulated patient with adequate caloric reserves.[21,44]

Delay standing or walking

A hypothermic patient who is found sitting or lying down should not be allowed stand right away. Standing and walking increase blood flow to the legs, worsening afterdrop, and may increase the risk of hypotension.[16] The patient should be insulated, given calories, and observed for at least 30 minutes before exercising.[31] A patient who tolerates standing without problems can be allowed to walk, slowly at first, then gradually increasing in speed as tolerated.

Active external rewarming

Active external rewarming is beneficial in an alert, shivering patient and is mandatory in a patient who has a decreased level of consciousness, even if shivering. Effective rewarming may be provided using large electric heat pads or blankets,[45] large chemical heat pads,[46,47] warm water bottles,[48] or a Norwegian charcoal-burning HeatPac (Normeca, Loerenskeg, Norway).[35,45,48] Providing heat to a shivering patient decreases shivering and does not change the rate of core rewarming but is more comfortable, requires fewer calories, and is less stressful for the heart than relying on shivering alone. Shivering or use of rewarming devices should be used in combination with insulation and vapor barriers. The HeatPac should only be used outdoors or with good ventilation to prevent carbon monoxide (CO) poisoning.[19] The Hypothermia Protection and Management Kit (HPMK), developed by the United States Armed Forces, uses a heat blanket with 4 large chemical heat pads and a heat-reflective shell. The HPMK provides effective insulation[49] and rewarming. The HPMK is commercially available. Small chemical heat packs may be helpful to protect hands and feet from frostbite but have insufficient heat content to treat hypothermia.

Body-to-body rewarming of a shivering person in a sleeping bag decreases shivering and does not increase the rate of rewarming.[44,45] Body-to-body rewarming may make a cold patient more comfortable but requires an extra rescuer. Body-to-body rewarming should not be used if it will delay evacuation.

A warm shower or bath should not be used for rewarming. Vasodilation of the skin causes increased afterdrop and decreased blood pressure.[16,26] Rewarming in a shower or bath has the potential to cause cardiovascular collapse.

Protection of cold skin

Cold skin is very susceptible to injury from pressure and heat.[50] Anecdotal reports of skin damage associated with the use of hot water bottles filled with lukewarm water represent pressure injuries rather than burns but can still be devastating. The HPMK may cause burns.[49] A barrier should be used to protect the skin when using chemical or electrical heat pads and precautions should be taken against pressure injuries.

Heated humidified oxygen

Heated-humidified oxygen can prevent respiratory heat loss but has very little heat content. Heated humidified oxygen should not be used alone as a rewarming method[17–19] but can add to the effectiveness of other methods.[17] Caution should be used to prevent burns of the face.

Distal limb warming

Unlike rewarming of the whole body in a hot shower or bath, distal limb rewarming of the arms and legs to the elbows and knees in water at 42° to 45°C works by opening arteriovenous anastomosis in the hands and feet. This causes increased return flow of warmed blood directly to the central circulation, decreasing afterdrop, and providing effective rewarming.[7] This method is the exception to the rule that peripheral rewarming is dangerous in a hypothermic patient. Distal limb rewarming is safe only for a mildly hypothermic patient. The method was developed for use on ships and is not likely to be practical in other out-of-hospital settings.

Rewarming during transport

Large chemical heat pads can provide limited rewarming during transport. Forced air warming is an effective rewarming method[17,51,52] that can limit afterdrop compared with the afterdrop with shivering.[53] Liquid-filled heat blankets are neither effective nor practical for rewarming during transport. The Norwegian HeatPac can be used with CO monitoring[19] in a well-ventilated passenger compartment of a vehicle after the unit is no longer generating an initial small amount of smoke. The HeatPac should never be used in an aircraft. The ideal temperature in the patient compartment of an ambulance is 28°C, the thermoneutral temperature of humans in air.[1] However, 28°C is too hot for normally clothed patient attendants as well as for pilots or drivers. A reasonable compromise is to maintain the temperature of the patient compartment at 24°C or above.[12]

Resuscitation of an Hypothermic Patient

Decision to resuscitate

Hypothermic patients in cardiac arrest have survived with normal neurologic function.[54–57] Fixed, dilated pupils, and apparent rigor mortis are not contraindications to resuscitation in a hypothermic patient.[55,56] However, it is not true that no one is dead until they are warm and dead. Some patients are cold and dead. Rescuers should not attempt to resuscitate a patient with fatal injuries such as decapitation, open head injury with loss of brain matter, truncal transection, or incineration.[12] Attempted resuscitation is also contraindicated when the chest wall is too stiff to allow chest compressions. Rescuers should not attempt to resuscitate an avalanche victim who has been buried for 60 minutes or longer with an airway completely obstructed by snow or ice.[10] This indicates death from asphyxia.

Indications for cardiopulmonary resuscitation

Cardiopulmonary resuscitation (CPR) is indicated for cardiac arrest due to hypothermia. If there are signs of life, CPR should not be performed. In a hypothermic patient, signs of life are often difficult to detect. Pulses can be very slow and faint. Pulses can be difficult to find, especially when a rescuer has cold fingers. Breathing may be slow and shallow but is sometimes easier to detect than pulses.[58] Rescuers should feel for a carotid pulse for 1 minute.[10] If there is no pulse or other sign of life, rescuers should start CPR with ventilation. If possible, rescuers should move the patient to a warm setting, such as a ground or air ambulance in which cardiac monitoring can be used to guide resuscitation.

Cardiac end-tidal carbon dioxide and echocardiographic monitoring

Rescuers should use cardiac monitoring, if available, to diagnose cardiac arrest. If pulses are not found, an organized rhythm on the monitor could represent pulseless electrical activity (PEA) or a perfusing rhythm with very faint pulses. Lack of a waveform on end-tidal CO_2 (ETCO$_2$) monitoring indicates cardiac arrest.[10] Point of care echocardiography can be used to diagnose PEA if there is electrical activity without cardiac contractions.[10] Rescuers should start CPR if a patient has a nonperfusing rhythm such as ventricular tachycardia (VT), VF, or asystole. If the rhythm appears to be asystole, the gain on the cardiac monitor should be set to maximum to detect low amplitude QRS complexes.[8] If there is an organized rhythm other than VT, CPR is only indicated if ETCO$_2$ monitoring shows lack of perfusion or echocardiography confirms absence of contractions.

Automated external defibrillator

An automated external defibrillator (AED) with a cardiac monitor can be used to determine cardiac rhythm. If an AED without a monitor gives the instruction shock advised, the rhythm is VT or VF. If shock is advised, the rescuer should attempt defibrillation and start CPR. If no shock is advised, the rhythm could be asystole or an organized rhythm. If there are no signs of life and no carotid pulse is found after 1 minute, the rescuer should start CPR unless echocardiography shows contractions.

Delayed, intermittent, and prolonged cardiopulmonary resuscitation

Hypothermia protects the brain from hypoxia by reducing brain activity.[6] In severe hypothermia, the brain can tolerate circulatory arrest for over 30 minutes.[10,34] Full neurologic recovery in severe hypothermia has been reported after 8 hours 40 minutes of cardiac arrest,[59] as well as after CPR for as long as 6 hours 30 minutes.[54,59–62] Cases of full neurologic recovery after hypothermic cardiac arrest have also been reported with delays of 15 minutes[54] and 70 minutes[34] before CPR was started. In another case, good neurologic outcome was reported in a hypothermic patient who was treated with alternating 1-minute periods with and without CPR while being carried in a litter.[61] Further evidence comes from cardiac surgery with induced hypothermia.[63] In a rescue situation, immediate, continuous CPR may not be possible. If immediate, continuous CPR is not possible, delay to CPR and interruptions to CPR should be as short as possible. A conservative recommendation is to delay CPR for no longer than 10 minutes to allow rescuers time to move a patient to a safer location.[63] If core temperature is 20° to 28°C, or unknown, rescuers should perform CPR continuously for 5 or more minutes and limit interruptions to CPR to 5 minutes or less. If core temperature is 20°C or below, CPR should be continuous for 5 or more minutes with interruptions 10 minutes or less.[63] There is no known limit for the duration of CPR in a severely hypothermic patient.

Low core temperature should not limit resuscitation

A patient with a core temperature of 13.7°C due to accidental hypothermia was successfully resuscitated.[64] The lowest known core temperature induced for surgery was 9°C.[65] Both patients survived neurologically intact. If there are no contraindications to CPR, rescuers should attempt to resuscitate a patient with severe hypothermia regardless of the measured core temperature.

Defibrillation in hypothermic patients

Patients with core temperatures less than 26°C have been successfully defibrillated.[66–68] Rescuers should make an attempt to defibrillate a patient whose core temperature is 30°C or below. This attempt can be a single shock at maximum power[69,70] or 3 shocks,[10] depending on local protocols. Rescuers should wait until a patient has been rewarmed at least 1° to 2°C before reattempting defibrillation.[12] Above a core temperature of 30°C, rescuers should follow usual defibrillation protocols.[10]

Chest compressions and ventilation in hypothermic patients

Chest compressions in hypothermic patients are relatively ineffective compared with chest compressions in normothermic patients[71] but metabolic demands are also markedly reduced. Rescuers should perform chest compressions at the same rate as in a normothermic patient. Manual chest compressions are more difficult to perform than mechanical compressions, especially during transport. High-quality CPR, using mechanical compressions, can be used as a temporizing measure for a patient with prolonged cardiac arrest who is being transported to a hospital or other facility for extracorporeal circulation (ECC) rewarming.

Ventilations in hypothermic patients are also relatively ineffective[71] unless an advanced airway (endotracheal tube or supraglottic device) is in place. If $ETCO_2$ monitoring is not available and there is no advanced airway, rescuers should administer ventilations to a hypothermic patient at the same rate as for a normothermic patient.[10,69] If there is an advanced airway, ventilation should be at half the usual rate. If $ETCO_2$ is available, ventilations should be given at a rate that keeps $ETCO_2$ in the normal range. This range should be adjusted for altitudes above 1200 m.[12]

It is difficult to measure oxygen saturation in a hypothermic patient but a hypothermic patient being ventilated at sea level is not likely to be hypoxemic.[72] Supplemental oxygen may be helpful at altitudes above 2500 m.[12]

Management of the airway is similar in hypothermic and normothermic patients. Endotracheal intubation or use of a supraglottic airway device may be necessary for adequate ventilation and prevention of aspiration.[10] Although VF can occur during endotracheal intubation, it is uncommon.[73] The risk of VF should not preclude standard airway management with intubation, if indicated. Cold-induced trismus may be resistant to neuromuscular blockade. If trismus prevents laryngoscopy, placement of a supraglottic device is usually a better option than fiberoptic intubation or cricothyroidotomy. Rescuers should not overinflate the cuff of an endotracheal tube or supraglottic device with cold air. Overinflation could cause kinking of the tube or rupture of the cuff as the patient rewarms and the air in the cuff expands.

Anesthetic and neuromuscular blocking agents are likely to be ineffective below 30°C but metabolism is decreased and the effects are likely to be prolonged when the agents become effective as the patient rewarms.[74–76] If drugs are used, dosages should be lowered and dosing intervals extended.[12]

Circulatory access in hypothermia

Intravenous (IV) access in a hypothermic patient is often difficult due to peripheral vasoconstriction. Unless an IV can be placed immediately, rescuers should use intraosseous (IO) access. Placement of central venous catheters can cause VF if the catheter or guidewire comes into contact with the myocardium. Femoral catheters are safer, but are difficult to place in the field.

Volume replacement and fluid management

Blood volume is decreased in moderate and severe hypothermia.[7] As a patient rewarms, peripheral vasoconstriction is reversed, increasing the vascular space. Normal saline should be given to replace volume to prevent hypotension and shock. Because the liver cannot metabolize lactate at cold temperatures, lactated Ringer should not be infused.[1] Fluids should be warmed to 40° to 42°C. Commercial fluid warmers and insulated tubing should be used to avoid infusing cold fluid.

Fluids are best given rapidly as boluses to avoid cooling or freezing of lines. IV lines are ideally saline-locked when not in use but IO lines require continuous flow to remain patent. Sufficient fluid should be given to maintain a blood pressure that supports adequate perfusion. There are no existing guidelines that specify optimum blood pressures.

Administration of glucose and insulin

Either hypoglycemia or hyperglycemia can occur in a hypothermic patient.[67,77] If point-of-care testing is not available, IV or IO glucose should be given to a hypothermic patient with altered mental status. Hyperglycemia has no known adverse effects in hypothermia.[67] Administration of insulin is not necessary if a hypothermic patient is hyperglycemic and may not be effective below 30°C.

Cardiovascular drugs

Most of the evidence regarding drug effects in cardiac arrest due to hypothermia comes from animal studies.[78] Animal studies with the vasopressors epinephrine[78] and vasopressin[79,80] have shown some potential benefits, including improved cardiac perfusion pressure, ROSC, and increased survival. There is 1 human case report in which a patient had ROSC after vasopressin was given[81] but the patient later succumbed to multiple organ system failure. The antidysrhythmic agents amiodarone[78,82,83] and bretylium[83,84] have been studied for treatment of ventricular dysrhythmias in hypothermic animals with mixed results. There are 2 human case reports of ROSC after administration of bretylium for VF.[85,86]

There are insufficient human data to justify recommendations for cardiovascular drugs in hypothermia below 30°C. Metabolism of drugs is decreased and protein binding increased in hypothermia.[1] When a patient rewarms, drugs that were given during hypothermia may become bioavailable at toxic levels. It is prudent not to give vasoactive drugs to a patient with core temperature less than 30°C. Between 30° and 35°C drugs should be given at the normal dose but with twice the usual interval between doses.

Atrial dysrhythmias during rewarming

Atrial dysrhythmias often occur during rewarming and should not be treated in a patient who is hemodynamically stable.[87] Atrial dysrhythmias generally resolve during rewarming.

Transcutaneous pacing

Transcutaneous pacing may be indicated in a bradycardic patient whose blood pressure is too low to allow arteriovenous rewarming.[88] Transvenous pacing is contraindicated in hypothermia due to cardiac irritability.

Transport and Triage

An alert patient who is shivering can be treated in the field unless the patient has an injury or medical condition requiring evacuation. Any patient who had asphyxia from drowning or avalanche burial is at risk for delayed complications and should be evacuated to a facility capable of managing acute respiratory distress syndrome.[89]

A patient with severe trauma is at risk for the lethal triad of acidosis, coagulopathy, and hypothermia.[90] Severely injured patients are unable to shiver and become hypothermic quickly, even during mild weather. A severely injured patient should be treated as soon as possible with active rewarming to prevent hypothermia.[91] Injuries should be stabilized and the patient transported ideally to a trauma center.

A cold-stressed or hypothermic patient with a decreased level of consciousness should be treated with active rewarming even if shivering. A patient with moderate or severe hypothermia who is hemodynamically stable should be transported to the nearest hospital or rural clinic with rewarming capabilities. A hemodynamically unstable patient should be transferred to a hospital that can perform ECC using extracorporeal membrane oxygenation or, less desirably, cardiopulmonary bypass.[89] If transport to a hospital with ECC capabilities is not feasible, due to distance or bad weather, the patient should be transferred to the closest facility capable of rewarming. Hemodynamically unstable patients and patients in cardiac arrest have made full recoveries after resuscitation without ECC.[60,92–94]

Use of serum potassium to determine viability

High serum potassium is a marker of cell lysis and death. The highest known serum potassium in a patient who was successfully resuscitated was 11.8 mmol/L in a 31-month-old child.[95] The true value of serum potassium may have been lower based on a rapid reported drop to 4.8 mmol/L in 25 minutes without specific intervention. A more recent case involved successful resuscitation of a 7-year-old girl who had profound hypothermia, with a nasopharyngeal temperature of 13.8°C, and a serum potassium of 11.3 mmol/L after drowning and submersion for an estimated 83 minutes.[96] There is no report of survival of a hypothermia patient with serum potassium greater than 12 mmol/L. If a hypothermic patient in cardiac arrest has serum potassium greater than 12 mmol/L, CPR should be discontinued and the patient can be declared dead without further rewarming.

Avalanche Burial

The most common cause of death in avalanche burial is asphyxia.[97] A victim who survives an avalanche initially may die from asphyxiation due to hypercapnia and hypoxemia, airway obstruction due to snow or other debris, trauma, or constriction of the chest preventing inspiration. A rapid decrease in survival occurs during the initial 35-minute asphyxial phase. If the airway is not patent, death will occur within 35 minutes.[98] In a victim with a patent airway, an open space in front of the mouth or nose, referred to as an air pocket, can slow asphyxiation, prolonging survival.[99]

Cooling of a victim of avalanche burial can be rapid, especially if the victim is asphyxiated.[100,101] The average cooling rate after avalanche burial is reported be about 3°C per hour.[102] Previous recommendations suggested using standard resuscitation for a victim buried less than 35 minutes or with a core temperature 32°C or above.[103] In 2015, recommendations by the European Resuscitation Council (ERC) were changed to be consistent with other hypothermia recommendations. The current recommendation is to use standard resuscitation if burial was 60 minutes or less or core temperature is 30°C or above.[10] If there is ROSC, the victim should be evacuated to the closest hospital that is able to manage associated injuries.

A victim with vital signs who was buried longer than 60 minutes or with core temperature less than 30°C should be transferred to the nearest facility capable of providing active rewarming. If the victim is in cardiac arrest and has a patent airway, CPR should be started.[97] If the victim is in cardiac arrest and does not have a patent airway, the decision to withhold CPR and resuscitation is reasonable.

A victim of avalanche burial is most likely to be asphyxiated before becoming hypothermic. The highest serum potassium documented in an avalanche victim who was successfully resuscitated was 6.4 mmol/L.[102] In 2015, the ERC proposed serum potassium of 8 mmol/L as the upper limit for attempting resuscitation of an avalanche victim.[10] Resuscitation should be discontinued if serum potassium is 8 mmol/L or more.

SUMMARY

Hypothermia can be life-threatening. Rescuers should attempt to minimize further heat loss and begin rewarming of hypothermic patients in the field while minimizing afterdrop and preventing circumrescue collapse. Some patients are cold and dead but other cold patients who are apparently dead can be resuscitated with full neurologic recovery. Unless there are definite contraindications, rescuers should do their best to resuscitate hypothermia patients, even if they appear to be beyond hope.

REFERENCES

1. Danzl D. Accidental hypothermia. In: Auerbach PS, editor. Wilderness Medicine. 6th edition. Philadelphia: Elsevier; 2012. p. 116–42.
2. Giesbrecht GG. Cold stress, near drowning and accidental hypothermia: a review. Aviat Space Environ Med 2000;71(7):733–52.
3. Bristow GK, Giesbrecht GG. Contribution of exercise and shivering to recovery from induced hypothermia (31.2 degrees C) in one subject. Aviat Space Environ Med 1988;59(6):549–52.
4. Giesbrecht GG, Arnett JL, Vela E, et al. Effect of task complexity on mental performance during immersion hypothermia. Aviat Space Environ Med 1993;64(3 Pt 1):206–11.
5. FitzGibbon T, Hayward JS, Walker D. EEG and visual evoked potentials of conscious man during moderate hypothermia. Electroencephalogr Clin Neurophysiol 1984;58(1):48–54.
6. Michenfelder JD, Milde JH. The relationship among canine brain temperature, metabolism, and function during hypothermia. Anesthesiology 1991;75(1):130–6.
7. Vanggaard L, Eyolfson D, Xu X, et al. Immersion of distal arms and legs in warm water (AVA rewarming) effectively rewarms mildly hypothermic humans. Aviat Space Environ Med 1999;70(11):1081–8.
8. Duguid H, Simpson RG, Stowers JM. Accidental hypothermia. Lancet 1961; 2(7214):1213–9.
9. Giesbrecht GG. The respiratory system in a cold environment. Aviat Space Environ Med 1995;66(9):890–902.
10. Truhlar A, Deakin CD, Soar J, et al. European resuscitation council guidelines for resuscitation 2015: section 4. Cardiac arrest in special circumstances. Resuscitation 2015;95:148–201.
11. Durrer B, Brugger H, Syme D. The medical on-site treatment of hypothermia: ICAR-MEDCOM recommendation. High Alt Med Biol 2003;4(1):99–103.
12. Zafren K, Giesbrecht GG, Danzl DF, et al. Wilderness Medical Society practice guidelines for the out-of-hospital evaluation and treatment of accidental hypothermia: 2014 update. Wilderness Environ Med 2014;25(4 Suppl):S66–85.
13. Tikuisis P, Giesbrecht GG. Prediction of shivering heat production from core and mean skin temperatures. Eur J Appl Physiol Occup Physiol 1999;79(3):221–9.
14. Pasquier M, Zurron N, Weith B, et al. Deep accidental hypothermia with core temperature below 24°c presenting with vital signs. High Alt Med Biol 2014; 15(1):58–63.
15. Deslarzes T, Rousson V, Yersin B, et al. An evaluation of the Swiss staging model for hypothermia using case reports from the literature. Scand J Trauma Resusc Emerg Med 2016;24:16.
16. Hayward JS, Eckerson JD, Kemna D. Thermal and cardiovascular changes during three methods of resuscitation from mild hypothermia. Resuscitation 1984; 11(1–2):21–33.

17. Goheen MS, Ducharme MB, Kenny GP, et al. Efficacy of forced-air and inhalation rewarming by using a human model for severe hypothermia. J Appl Physiol 1997;83(5):1635–40.
18. Mekjavic IB, Eiken O. Inhalation rewarming from hypothermia: an evaluation in -20 degrees C simulated field conditions. Aviat Space Environ Med 1995; 66(5):424–9.
19. Sterba JA. Efficacy and safety of prehospital rewarming techniques to treat accidental hypothermia. Ann Emerg Med 1991;20(8):896–901.
20. Walpoth BH, Galdikas J, Leupi F, et al. Assessment of hypothermia with a new "tympanic" thermometer. J Clin Monit 1994;10(2):91–6.
21. Giesbrecht GG, Goheen MS, Johnston CE, et al. Inhibition of shivering increases core temperature afterdrop and attenuates rewarming in hypothermic humans. J Appl Physiol 1997;83(5):1630–4.
22. Kimberger O, Cohen D, Illievich U, et al. Temporal artery versus bladder thermometry during perioperative and intensive care unit monitoring. Anesth Analg 2007;105(4):1042–7.
23. Gunga HC, Werner A, Stahn A, et al. The double sensor-a non-invasive device to continuously monitor core temperature in humans on earth and in space. Respir Physiol Neurobiol 2009;169(Suppl 1):S63–8.
24. Kimberger O, Thell R, Schuh M, et al. Accuracy and precision of a novel non-invasive core thermometer. Br J Anaesth 2009;103(2):226–31.
25. Giesbrecht GG, Bristow GK. A second postcooling afterdrop: more evidence for a convective mechanism. J Appl Physiol 1992;73(4):1253–8.
26. Romet TT. Mechanism of afterdrop after cold water immersion. J Appl Physiol 1988;65(4):1535–8.
27. Baumgartner FJ, Janusz MT, Jamieson WR, et al. Cardiopulmonary bypass for resuscitation of patients with accidental hypothermia and cardiac arrest. Can J Surg 1992;35(2):184–7.
28. Fox JB, Thomas F, Clemmer TP, et al. A retrospective analysis of air-evacuated hypothermia patients. Aviat Space Environ Med 1988;59(11 Pt 1):1070–5.
29. Stoneham MD, Squires SJ. Prolonged resuscitation in acute deep hypothermia. Anaesthesia 1992;47(9):784–8.
30. Golden FS, Hervey GR, Tipton MJ. Circum-rescue collapse: collapse, sometimes fatal, associated with rescue of immersion victims. J R Nav Med Serv 1991;77(3):139–49.
31. Giesbrecht GG, Bristow GK. The convective afterdrop component during hypothermic exercise decreases with delayed exercise onset. Aviat Space Environ Med 1998;69(1):17–22.
32. Giesbrecht GG, Hayward JS. Problems and complications with cold-water rescue. Wilderness Environ Med 2006;17(1):26–30.
33. Mutschlechner H, Lorenz I, Oberhammer R, et al. Hyperinsulinaemia may impair outcome after hypothermic cardiac arrest. Resuscitation 2009;80(8):959.
34. Althaus U, Aeberhard P, Schupbach P, et al. Management of profound accidental hypothermia with cardiorespiratory arrest. Ann Surg 1982;195(4):492–5.
35. Giesbrecht GG. Emergency treatment of hypothermia. Emerg Med 2001;13(1): 9–16.
36. Osborne L, Kamal El-Din AS, Smith JE. Survival after prolonged cardiac arrest and accidental hypothermia. Br Med J 1984;289(6449):881–2.
37. Lee CH, Van Gelder C, Burns K, et al. Advanced cardiac life support and defibrillation in severe hypothermic cardiac arrest. Prehosp Emerg Care 2009;13(1): 85–9.

38. Hayward JS, Collis M, Eckerson JD. Thermographic evaluation of relative heat loss areas of man during cold water immersion. Aerosp Med 1973;44(7):708–11.

39. Henriksson O, Lundgren JP, Kuklane K, et al. Protection against cold in prehospital care-thermal insulation properties of blankets and rescue bags in different wind conditions. Prehosp Disaster Med 2009;24(5):408–15.

40. Thomassen O, Faerevik H, Osteras O, et al. Comparison of three different prehospital wrapping methods for preventing hypothermia–a crossover study in humans. Scand J Trauma Resusc Emerg Med 2011;19:41.

41. Henriksson O, Lundgren P, Kuklane K, et al. Protection against cold in prehospital care: evaporative heat loss reduction by wet clothing removal or the addition of a vapor barrier - a thermal manikin study. Prehosp Disaster Med 2012;27(1): 53–8.

42. Pretorius T, Bristow GK, Steinman AM, et al. Thermal effects of whole head submersion in cold water on nonshivering humans. J Appl Physiol 2006;101(2): 669–75.

43. Iampietro PF, Vaughan JA, Goldman RF, et al. Heat production from shivering. J Appl Physiol 1960;15:632–4.

44. Giesbrecht GG, Sessler DI, Mekjavic IB, et al. Treatment of mild immersion hypothermia by direct body-to-body contact. J Appl Physiol 1994;76(6):2373–9.

45. Hultzer MV, Xu X, Marrao C, et al. Pre-hospital torso-warming modalities for severe hypothermia: a comparative study using a human model. CJEM 2005;7(6): 378–86.

46. Watts DD, Roche M, Tricarico R, et al. The utility of traditional prehospital interventions in maintaining thermostasis. Prehosp Emerg Care 1999;3(2):115–22.

47. Lundgren JP, Henriksson O, Pretorius T, et al. Field torso-warming modalities: a comparative study using a human model. Prehosp Emerg Care 2009;13(3): 371–8.

48. Giesbrecht GG, Bristow GK, Uin A, et al. Effectiveness of three field treatments for induced mild (33.0 degrees C) hypothermia. J Appl Physiol 1987;63(6): 2375–9.

49. Allen PB, Salyer SW, Dubick MA, et al. Preventing hypothermia: comparison of current devices used by the US Army in an in vitro warmed fluid model. J Trauma 2010;69(Suppl 1):S154–61.

50. Steinman AM. Cardiopulmonary resuscitation and hypothermia. Circulation 1986;74(6 Pt 2):IV29–32.

51. Ducharme MB, Giesbrecht GG, Frim J, et al. Forced-air rewarming in -20 degrees C simulated field conditions. Ann N Y Acad Sci 1997;813:676–81.

52. Steele MT, Nelson MJ, Sessler DI, et al. Forced air speeds rewarming in accidental hypothermia. Ann Emerg Med 1996;27(4):479–84.

53. Giesbrecht GG, Schroeder M, Bristow GK. Treatment of mild immersion hypothermia by forced-air warming. Aviat Space Environ Med 1994;65(9):803–8.

54. Oberhammer R, Beikircher W, Hormann C, et al. Full recovery of an avalanche victim with profound hypothermia and prolonged cardiac arrest treated by extracorporeal re-warming. Resuscitation 2008;76(3):474–80.

55. Leitz KH, Tsilimingas N, Guse HG, et al. Accidental drowning with extreme hypothermia–rewarming with extracorporeal circulation. Chirurg 1989;60(5):352–5 [in German].

56. Ko CS, Alex J, Jeffries S, et al. Dead? Or just cold: profoundly hypothermic patient with no signs of life. Emerg Med J 2002;19(5):478–9.

57. Walpoth BH, Walpoth-Aslan BN, Mattle HP, et al. Outcome of survivors of accidental deep hypothermia and circulatory arrest treated with extracorporeal blood warming. N Engl J Med 1997;337(21):1500–5.

58. Feiss P, Mora C, Devalois B, et al. Accidental deep hypothermia and circulatory arrest. Treatment with extracorporeal circulation. Ann Fr Anesth Reanim 1987; 6(3):217–8 [in French].

59. Meyer M, Pelurson N, Khabiri E, et al. Sequela-free long-term survival of a 65-year-old woman after 8 hours and 40 minutes of cardiac arrest from deep accidental hypothermia. J Thorac Cardiovasc Surg 2014;147(1):e1–2.

60. Lexow K. Severe accidental hypothermia: survival after 6 hours 30 minutes of cardiopulmonary resuscitation. Arctic Med Res 1991;50(Suppl 6):112–4.

61. Boue Y, Lavolaine J, Bouzat P, et al. Neurologic recovery from profound accidental hypothermia after 5 hours of cardiopulmonary resuscitation. Crit Care Med 2014;42(2):e167–70.

62. Hilmo J, Naesheim T, Gilbert M. "Nobody is dead until warm and dead": Prolonged resuscitation is warranted in arrested hypothermic victims also in remote areas - A retrospective study from northern Norway. Resuscitation 2014;85(9): 1204–11.

63. Gordon L, Paal P, Ellerton JA, et al. Delayed and intermittent CPR for severe accidental hypothermia. Resuscitation 2015;90:46–9.

64. Gilbert M, Busund R, Skagseth A, et al. Resuscitation from accidental hypothermia of 13.7 degrees C with circulatory arrest. Lancet 2000;355(9201):375–6.

65. Niazi SA, Lewis FJ. Profound hypothermia in man; report of a case. Ann Surg 1958;147(2):264–6.

66. DaVee TS, Reineberg EJ. Extreme hypothermia and ventricular fibrillation. Ann Emerg Med 1980;9(2):100–2.

67. Koller R, Schnider TW, Neidhart P. Deep accidental hypothermia and cardiac arrest–rewarming with forced air. Acta Anaesthesiol Scand 1997;41(10):1359–64.

68. Thomas R, Cahill CJ. Successful defibrillation in profound hypothermia (core body temperature 25.6 degrees C). Resuscitation 2000;47(3):317–20.

69. Vanden Hoek TL, Morrison LJ, Shuster M, et al. Part 12: cardiac arrest in special situations: 2010 American Heart Association Guidelines for Cardiopulmonary Resuscitation and Emergency Cardiovascular Care. Circulation 2010;122(18 Suppl 3):S829–61.

70. Ujhelyi MR, Sims JJ, Dubin SA, et al. Defibrillation energy requirements and electrical heterogeneity during total body hypothermia. Crit Care Med 2001; 29(5):1006–11.

71. Maningas PA, DeGuzman LR, Hollenbach SJ, et al. Regional blood flow during hypothermic arrest. Ann Emerg Med 1986;15(4):390–6.

72. Kondratiev TV, Flemming K, Myhre ES, et al. Is oxygen supply a limiting factor for survival during rewarming from profound hypothermia? Am J Physiol Heart Circ Physiol 2006;291(1):H441–50.

73. Danzl DF, Pozos RS, Auerbach PS, et al. Multicenter hypothermia survey. Ann Emerg Med 1987;16(9):1042–55.

74. Leslie K, Sessler DI, Bjorksten AR, et al. Mild hypothermia alters propofol pharmacokinetics and increases the duration of action of atracurium. Anesth Analg 1995;80(5):1007–14.

75. Caldwell JE, Heier T, Wright PM, et al. Temperature-dependent pharmacokinetics and pharmacodynamics of vecuronium. Anesthesiology 2000;92(1): 84–93.

76. Heier T, Caldwell JE. Impact of hypothermia on the response to neuromuscular blocking drugs. Anesthesiology 2006;104(5):1070–80.
77. Strapazzon G, Nardin M, Zanon P, et al. Respiratory failure and spontaneous hypoglycemia during noninvasive rewarming from 24.7°C (76.5°F) core body temperature after prolonged avalanche burial. Ann Emerg Med 2011;60(2):193–6.
78. Wira CR, Becker JU, Martin G, et al. Anti-arrhythmic and vasopressor medications for the treatment of ventricular fibrillation in severe hypothermia: a systematic review of the literature. Resuscitation 2008;78(1):21–9.
79. Raedler C, Voelckel WG, Wenzel V, et al. Vasopressor response in a porcine model of hypothermic cardiac arrest is improved with active compression-decompression cardiopulmonary resuscitation using the inspiratory impedance threshold valve. Anesth Analg 2002;95(6):1496–502.
80. Schwarz B, Mair P, Raedler C, et al. Vasopressin improves survival in a pig model of hypothermic cardiopulmonary resuscitation. Crit Care Med 2002; 30(6):1311–4.
81. Sumann G, Krismer AC, Wenzel V, et al. Cardiopulmonary resuscitation after near drowning and hypothermia: restoration of spontaneous circulation after vasopressin. Acta Anaesthesiol Scand 2003;47(3):363–5.
82. Khan JN, Prasad N, Glancy J. Amiodarone use in therapeutic hypothermia following cardiac arrest due to ventricular tachycardia and ventricular fibrillation. Europace 2009;11(11):1566–7.
83. Stoner J, Martin G, O'Mara K, et al. Amiodarone and bretylium in the treatment of hypothermic ventricular fibrillation in a canine model. Acad Emerg Med 2003; 10(3):187–91.
84. Elenbaas RM, Mattson K, Cole H, et al. Bretylium in hypothermia-induced ventricular fibrillation in dogs. Ann Emerg Med 1984;13(11):994–9.
85. Danzl DF, Sowers MB, Vicario SJ, et al. Chemical ventricular defibrillation in severe accidental hypothermia. Ann Emerg Med 1982;11(12):698–9.
86. Lloyd EL. Accidental hypothermia. Resuscitation 1996;32(2):111–24.
87. Rankin AC, Rae AP. Cardiac arrhythmias during rewarming of patients with accidental hypothermia. Br Med J (Clin Res Ed) 1984;289(6449):874–7.
88. Ho JD, Heegaard WG, Brunette DD. Successful transcutaneous pacing in 2 severely hypothermic patients. Ann Emerg Med 2007;49(5):678–81.
89. Ruttmann E, Weissenbacher A, Ulmer H, et al. Prolonged extracorporeal membrane oxygenation-assisted support provides improved survival in hypothermic patients with cardiocirculatory arrest. J Thorac Cardiovasc Surg 2007;134(3): 594–600.
90. Mitra B, Tullio F, Cameron PA, et al. Trauma patients with the 'triad of death'. Emerg Med J 2012;29(8):622–5.
91. Jurkovich GJ, Greiser WB, Luterman A, et al. Hypothermia in trauma victims: an ominous predictor of survival. J Trauma 1987;27(9):1019–24.
92. Gruber E, Beikircher W, Pizzinini R, et al. Non-extracorporeal rewarming at a rate of 6.8°C per hour in a deeply hypothermic arrested patient. Resuscitation 2014; 85(8):e119–20.
93. Turtiainen J, Halonen J, Syvaoja S, et al. Rewarming a patient with accidental hypothermia and cardiac arrest using thoracic lavage. Ann Thorac Surg 2014; 97(6):2165–6.
94. Roggero E, Stricker H, Biegger P. Severe accidental hypothermia with cardiopulmonary arrest: prolonged resuscitation without extracorporeal circulation. Schweiz Med Wochenschr 1992;122(5):161–4.

95. Dobson JA, Burgess JJ. Resuscitation of severe hypothermia by extracorporeal rewarming in a child. J Trauma 1996;40(3):483–5.
96. Romlin BS, Winberg H, Janson M, et al. Excellent outcome with extracorporeal membrane oxygenation after accidental profound hypothermia (13.8°C) and drowning. Crit Care Med 2015;43(11):e521–5.
97. Brugger H, Durrer B, Elsensohn F, et al. Resuscitation of avalanche victims: Evidence-based guidelines of the International Commission for Mountain Emergency Medicine (ICAR MEDCOM): intended for physicians and other advanced life support personnel. Resuscitation 2013;84(5):539–46.
98. Boyd J, Brugger H, Shuster M. Prognostic factors in avalanche resuscitation: a systematic review. Resuscitation 2010;81(6):645–52.
99. Boue Y, Payen JF, Brun J, et al. Survival after avalanche-induced cardiac arrest. Resuscitation 2014;85(9):1192–6.
100. Grissom CK, Radwin MI, Harmston CH. Improving survival during snow burial in avalanches. JAMA 2000;284(10):1242–3.
101. Brugger H, Sumann G, Meister R, et al. Hypoxia and hypercapnia during respiration into an artificial air pocket in snow: implications for avalanche survival. Resuscitation 2003;58(1):81–8.
102. Locher T, Walpoth BH. Differential diagnosis of circulatory failure in hypothermic avalanche victims: retrospective analysis of 32 avalanche accidents. Praxis (Bern 1994) 1996;85(41):1275–82 [in German].
103. Soar J, Perkins GD, Abbas G, et al. European Resuscitation Council Guidelines for Resuscitation 2010 Section 8. Cardiac arrest in special circumstances: electrolyte abnormalities, poisoning, drowning, accidental hypothermia, hyperthermia, asthma, anaphylaxis, cardiac surgery, trauma, pregnancy, electrocution. Resuscitation 2010;81(10):1400–33.

Frostbite

Charles Handford, MBChB (Hons), MRCS, DMCC[a],*,
Owen Thomas, MBChB (Hons), BMedSc (phys), DTM&H[b],
Christopher H.E. Imray, MB BS, DiMM, MSc, PhD, FRCS, FRCP, FRGS[c]

KEYWORDS

- Frostbite • Rewarming • Thrombolysis • Prostacyclin • rTPA • Gangrene
- Amputation • Telemedicine

KEY POINTS

- Frostbite is associated with significant morbidity, and prevention is key.
- Freeze-thaw-freeze cycles must be avoided.
- New therapies, such as parenteral iloprost or thrombolytics, offer significant promise in the management of deep frostbite injury.
- Expert opinion is now readily available via telemedicine.

INTRODUCTION

Frostbite injury can result in debilitating long-term irreversible morbidity. Despite this, frostbite management strategies remained constant and unchanged until recent years, when novel therapies have led to promising, tissue-saving, outcomes. This article gives a background understanding of frostbite and its pathophysiology and reviews the current evidence and latest frostbite management strategies to educate clinicians to maximize the outcomes of their patients.

Epidemiology

The first physical evidence of frostbite injury is in a 5000-year-old pre-Columbian mummy discovered in the Andes.[1] In military medicine, cold injuries, including frostbite, have long been recognized as a significant cause of mortality and morbidity. Examples of this include Hannibal crossing the Alps in 218 BC, when only 19,000 survived out of 38,000, or the American War of Independence, in which cold casualty rates in George Washington's army were described as being as high as 10%.[2,3] Napoleon

Disclaimer: The opinions and/or assertions and/or guidance in this article are the personal understandings of the authors. They are not to be construed as official or as reflecting the views and/or policies of the Army Medical Services, British Armed Forces, or Ministry of Defence.
[a] 2 Medical Regiment, St George's Barracks, North Luffenham, Oakham, Rutland, LE15 8RL, UK; [b] Dept of Anaesthetics, Musgrove Park Hospital, Taunton, Somerset, UK; [c] Department of Vascular Surgery, University Hospital Coventry and Warwickshire NHS Trust, Warwick Medical School and Coventry University, Coventry, UK
* Corresponding author.
E-mail address: charleshandford@hotmail.co.uk

Emerg Med Clin N Am 35 (2017) 281–299
http://dx.doi.org/10.1016/j.emc.2016.12.006
emed.theclinics.com

Bonaparte's Surgeon in Chief, Dominique Jean Larrey,[4] during the failed invasion of Russia in the winter of 1812 to 1813, wrote the first authoritative report on frostbite and cold injury. Frostbite continues to afflict modern militaries.[5–7]

Within the civilian environment, frostbite can affect a myriad of individuals. One civilian subgroup is that of mountaineers. A cross-sectional questionnaire found a mean incidence of 366 per 1000 population per year.[8] The British Antarctic Survey found an incidence for cold injury of 65.6 per 1000 per year; 95% of this was for frostbite, with recreation being a risk factor.[9] On Denali, frostbite was found to be the most common (18.1%) individual diagnosis made at the medical facilities.[10] An epidemiologic review of the first 10 years of the so-called Everest ER (emergency room) found that cold exposure accounted for 18.4% of all trauma visits, of which 83.7% were attributable to frostbite.[11]

In the nonadventurer civilian population, there are certain recognized risk factors for frostbite injury. These risk factors include alcohol consumption, smoking, vagrancy, psychiatric disturbance, unplanned exposure to cold with inadequate protection, previous cold injury, several medications (eg, β-blockers), and working with equipment that uses NO_2 or CO_2.[12–17] Alongside the aforementioned, there seem to be important genetic risk factors that include African American ethnicity and O group blood typing.[6,18] Possession of the angiotensin-converting enzyme DD allele may also increase risk.[19]

Pathophysiology

Frostbite is a freezing cold thermal injury that occurs when tissues are exposed to temperatures below their freezing point. Pathologic changes can be divided into direct cellular injury and indirect cellular injury, also referred to as progressive dermal ischemia.

Direct cellular injury

Direct cellular injury occurs because of a variety of mechanisms. These mechanisms can be summarized as ice crystal formation (intracellular and extracellular), cell dehydration and shrinkage, electrolyte disturbances, denaturation of lipid-protein complexes, and thermal shock.[20] These mechanisms result in cell injury and death.

Indirect cellular injury (progressive dermal ischemia)

Indirect cellular injury is secondary to progressive microvascular insult and is more severe than the direct cellular effect.[20,21] Following thawing, microvascular thrombosis occurs, resulting in continued cell injury and death.[22] Endothelial damage, intravascular sludging, increased levels of inflammatory mediators and free radicals, reperfusion injury, and thrombosis all play a role in contributing to progressive dermal ischemia and positively reinforce each other.[22–30]

Classification

There have been several proposed classifications for frostbite and historically the degrees classification has been favored. This system divided frostbite into frostnip, first-degree, second-degree, third-degree, and fourth-degree frostbite depending on depth of injury. Others clinicians have opted for a simpler classification of superficial (first-degree and second-degree) and deep (third-degree and fourth-degree).[22] Because bone loss is always distal to the observed extent of frostbite, these classifications often fail to predict likely amputation levels, which only become apparent at subsequent mummification.

Over recent years there has been an effort to formulate a reproducible and prognostic classification system rather than the established observational systems. Cauchy and colleagues[31] proposed a classification system of 4 grades for frostbite of the hand or foot based on the appearance of the lesion after rapid rewarming, appearance at day 2, and radioisotope uptake on bone scan at day 2. The advantage of this classification is that it gives an early prognostic indicator of bone and tissue loss and the likely anatomic level of loss. This grading system relies on isotope bone scanning. In the field, Cauchy and colleagues[32] suggest the use of portable Doppler or the clinical stigmata of soft tissue cyanosis as surrogate markers for amputation risk.

PREHOSPITAL MANAGEMENT
Prevention

Prevention of frostbite enables effective and safe functioning within a cold environment and is the responsibility of individuals, team leaders, and companies/employers who place individuals in at-risk areas. The following are areas of prevention to consider; however, it is not an exhaustive list and an individualized risk assessment and plan formation must be taken for every cold exposure.

- Adequate calorie and fluid intake
- Appropriate clothing for environment, using a layering system
- Avoid sweating by reducing exercise intensity if necessary
- Avoid constricting items
- Mittens are preferable to finger gloves and should be attached to the person; spares should be carried
- Appropriate boots for environment/task that fit correctly
- Do not climb in adverse weather conditions
- Daily foot care
- Buddy-buddy check system
- Avoid alcohol and smoking
- Be aware of the risks associated with increased altitude
- Be aware wind-chill effect
- Avoid prolonged immobility
- Avoid fatigue
- Be careful when removing gloves to perform tasks; never directly touch metal in extreme cold or in moderate cold if wet
- Leaders/commanders must ensure all are fit, trained, and capable of operating in proposed location/climate; this should take into account comorbidities and current medications
- A thorough evacuation and medical plan must be in place before departure; this must include communications

Patient Evaluation Overview

Early recognition
Early recognition is vital; paresthesia may be the first symptom and, if present, measures should be taken to prevent any further damage. Recognition of frostnip, hypothermia, and subsequently taking appropriate action to avoid further cold exposure is important for preventing further damage. Note that it may take several hours for an individual to rewarm after excessive cold and reexposure to the cold too soon risks rapid deterioration. If an individual incurs a cold injury, all other team members must be assessed.

Clinical presentation
Complaint of feeling cold, numb, and/or clumsy. Appearance is variable and can be misleading. The affected area may appear a yellow-white color or be a mottled blue. Clinically it may be insensate or obviously frozen. Note that the characteristic edema and blistering does not occur until after rewarming.

Once frostbite has occurred, evaluation and management depend on several factors, including location, accessibility of definitive care, and severity.

Fig. 1 shows grade 2 and 3 frostbite at various time points.
Consider before evaluation:

1. Once boots are removed swelling may occur, preventing redonning of boots.
2. Freeze-thaw-freeze cycles must be avoided; therefore, only consider rewarming if this can be avoided.
3. Is there a better, more sheltered, area to perform evaluation?
4. Will the patient need to walk out? If yes, consider whether removal of boots and potential rewarming is going to prevent this. It may be better to walk out on a frozen foot.

TREATMENT

Hurley[33] described frostbite in a similar manner to how ischemic cerebrovascular events are now described,[34] with some tissue cells killed, some unaffected, and a

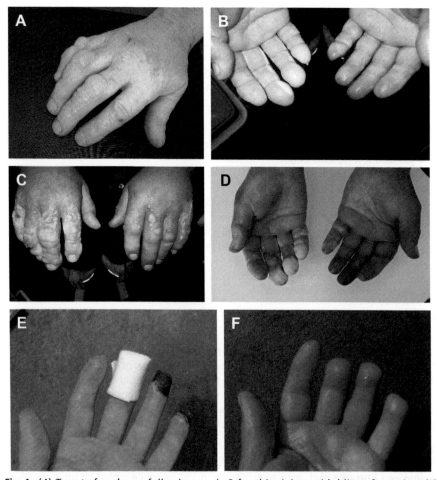

Fig. 1. (*A*) Twenty-four hours following grade 2 frostbite injury with blister formation. (*B*) Grade 2 right hand and grade 3 left hand at 36 hours. (*C*) Grade 2 right hand and grade 3 left hand at 36 hours following soaks in povidone iodine. (*D*) Grade 2 right hand and grade 3 left hand at 5 days. (*E*) Grade 3 at 3 months; note the mummification. (*F*) Grade 3 at 4 months.

large number injured but potentially salvageable with optimum treatment. Treatment is therefore designed to prevent the injured cells from dying, thus minimizing tissue loss.

Nonpharmacologic Options

Open field
Consider turning back, and seek shelter from the elements.[35,36] There is a risk that the casualty may have concurrent hypothermia and if 1 member of a party has cold injury, others are at risk of cold injury so all should be assessed and removed from the elements.

Removal of clothing and jewelry
Ideally, socks and gloves should be replaced for dry pairs and boots removed. Foot swelling may prevent redonning boots, precluding the individual walking any further, so removal should only occur in a stable, sheltered location with the possibility of evacuation. Rings or similar items should be removed because with subsequent swelling this may not be possible.

Rehydration
Adequate hydration with oral (ideally warmed) fluids are warranted; intravenous (IV) fluids are an alternative.

Rewarming
- Hillside:
  - Warming by placing in another person/s armpit or groin can be attempted for up to 10 minutes. With return of sensation, the person can continue with additional improved protective measures, if they have frostnip.[35] If not, the individual needs to get to the nearest warm shelter and seek medical treatment, and a diagnosis of frostbite can be given.
  - Avoid applying dry heat (heat pads) directly on frozen tissue or rubbing, which cause tissue damage via burning and mechanical disruption respectively.
  - Ideally, a frostbitten foot should not be walked on, although this may be required practically for evacuation from remote, cold areas. Efforts should be made with splints and pads to minimize movement if walking is required.[37,38]
  - During transport, there is a risk for partial rewarming and refreezing, and individuals should be protected from indirect heat sources such as engines. The Alaska State Guidelines advocate short transport times (<2 hours) to secondary care sites, because "the risks posed by improper rewarming or refreezing outweigh the risks of delaying treatment for deep frostbite."[36] If transport time is greater than 2 hours, treatment of hypothermia takes precedence, with limb rewarming an unavoidable side effect. However, protecting the limb from refreezing is vital.
- Prehospital medical facility (ie, base camp medical center):
  - Immerse the affected part in water at 37°C to 39°C.[39] The affected limb will have impaired temperature sensation, thus if a thermometer is not available the unaffected limb should be placed in first for at least 30 seconds to ensure that the water is not too hot, which would risk injury.[38]

Once rewarmed, it is highly important that the limb is not refrozen.

Dressing and blisters
- Following rewarming, the limb should be allowed to air dry. Do not rub at any point.
- Apply aloe vera to the area and cover with a dry dressing (avoid circumferential dressings because of risk of continued swelling).

- Blisters indicate thawing[36] and should be left intact, especially if hemorrhagic. Elevation reduces blister size. Blisters are not typically aspirated/deroofed in the field.[38]
- Elevate to minimize swelling.
- Antibacterial daily or twice-daily baths are recommended and redressing every 12 to 24 hours should be performed.[38]
- Splinting and bulky dressings may offer protection to the affected area; attempt to dress between digits.

Smoking
Smoking must be avoided.

Portable recompression bag (Gamow bag)
Hyperbaric pressure bags are widely available and provide a rapid simulated reduction in altitude. Although not practical to rewarm the frostbitten area while in the bag, for 2 reasons it may be beneficial to spend periods of time in the bag following rewarming. First, while in the bag there is increased Spo_2 (peripheral capillary oxygen saturation), and second it is thought that a reduction in altitude helps to minimize cold-induced peripheral vasoconstriction and combat hypothermia.[32,40] This theory requires further evidence; however, as long as it does not interrupt rewarming or delay evacuation it may be a useful in-field adjunct.

Pharmacologic Treatment

Further details on the evidence and mechanism of action for each point discussed here is provided later in the article.

Analgesia
Rewarming can be a painful process and parenteral opioid treatment may be required for adequate analgesia; if given in the prehospital setting, start at a low dose and slowly titrate to pain, and ideally have naloxone available.

Antiinflammatory medications
All patients should be started on ibuprofen because of its dual effect as an analgesic and antiinflammatory (unless contraindicated) at a dose of 12 mg/kg twice a day up to a maximum of 2400 mg/d; 400 mg twice a day is often a practical dose.[41] Aspirin is an alternative; however, it theoretically blocks prostaglandins, which are beneficial to healing, thus ibuprofen is preferred.[42]

Oxygen
Supplementary oxygen to increase Spo_2 theoretically increases oxygen delivery to the tissues; however, this may be limited by peripheral vasoconstriction and/or micro-thrombi. Nevertheless it is thought that, at high altitude, oxygen may be beneficial.[32] Oxygen supplementation at lower altitudes, such as 4000 to 6000 m, is debated, although maintaining saturations greater than 90% is recommended.[38]

Tetanus
Frostbite wounds are not tetanus-prone wounds and thus standard tetanus toxoid guidelines should be followed.

Antibiotics
This area is controversial and prophylactic antibiotics have not been shown to reduce amputation[38]; however, they are often used on clinical judgment in cases of severe/extensive frostbite. If evacuation times are long and signs of infection develop, antibiotic therapy should be started, ideally with swabs taken.

Prehospital novel agents
The in-hospital use of iloprost or thrombolytics (most notable recombinant tissue plasminogen activator [rTPA]) has resulted in reduced amputation rates; however, their use seems to be time dependent, with prolonged evacuation timelines precluding usage.[41] For this reason some clinicians have advocated initiating treatment in the prehospital setting, similar to that of prehospital thrombolysis of myocardial infarction. Supporting this viewpoint is the recent publication of 2 successful case studies describing thrombolysis at K2 basecamp, and iloprost has been used in community hospitals in Canada.[32,43] However, the considerable, potentially life-threatening, side effect/complication profile associated with thrombolysis must be remembered, particularly in patients with trauma. However, iloprost, which has a safer side effect profile, is not licensed for IV usage in the United States. The authors think that the early usage of thrombolysis/iloprost is a positive forward step in frostbite management; however, we advise extreme caution because it is better to have a limb-threatening injury than a life-threatening complication. Practitioners must ensure that they are competent and have the capability to use these medications.

Sympathetic blockade
Current evidence has not shown a positive effect in frostbite management and therefore this is not advised in current guidelines.[38] However, a recent case report describes prehospital blockade to good effect so perhaps early prehospital blockade needs further exploration, but it cannot currently be advised.[44]

Telemedicine
This facilitates access to expert opinion when in austere locations or if evacuation times are long, and it has been successfully used in the past.[45] Details of how to access this can be found later in the article.

HOSPITAL MANAGEMENT
Patient Evaluation Overview

Systematic approach
All patients should be assessed using the <C>ABCDE (Catastrophic bleeding, airway, circulation, disability and exposure) paradigm and injuries treated according to priority. This approach may mean initially ignoring a frostbitten limb.

Hypothermia and frostbite frequently accompany each other. If there is moderate/severe hypothermia, a core temperature of more than 35°C must be achieved before treatment of frostbite commences.[38,46]

Detailed patient history
Areas of specific questioning include time of injury (<24 hours or >24 hours ago), mechanism of injury, climatic conditions at time of injury, freeze-thaw-freeze events, and in-field treatment.

Clinical photography
Undertake on admission and repeat throughout treatment. This photography documents the appearance and prevents the need for repeated dressing removal, which can be painful, damage tissue, and increase infection risk.

Imaging
Bone scanning, magnetic resonance angiography (MRA), and angiography all offer prognostic information and guide management.

Technecium[99] (^{99}Tc) triple-phase bone scanning when used at day 2 postinjury offers prognostic information, accurately predicting amputation level in 84% of cases.[31,47,48] MRA is often easier to access and an attractive alternative. Importantly MRA has been shown to estimate the level of tissue loss and some clinicians suggest that it is advantageous compared with ^{99}Tc triple-phase bone scanning because it allows direct visualization of occluded vessels and surrounding tissue and may show a clearer demarcation of ischemic tissues.[49,50] This argument has yet to be confirmed in larger studies. **Fig. 2** shows an example of ^{99}Tc triple-phase bone scanning in frostbite injury.

Digital subtraction angiography clearly visualizes vessel patency and should be performed on all who are being considered for thrombolysis.[41]

Nonpharmacologic Management

Prevent constriction

Jewelry and other potentially constricting items must be removed because swelling will occur on thawing.

Fluids

Dehydration may have occurred because of cold diuresis, altitude, or extreme activity. Oral hydration is preferred; however, if the patient is hypothermic or severely dehydrated, warmed IV fluids should be used.

Rewarming

Rapid rewarming should be commenced in the presence of fully or partially frozen tissue.[51] A whirlpool bath should be used with the temperature set at 37°C to 39°C and either povidone iodine or chlorhexidine added for antiseptic qualities.[38,39] Rewarming should continue until a red/purple color appears and the extremity tissue becomes pliable; this typically takes up to 30 minutes but may require longer.[38,52] Active motion is encouraged; however, the affected tissue should not touch the side of the bath.

Rewarming may be painful and parenteral analgesia may be required; note that return of sensation is a favorable sign.

Blister management

Blisters can be clear or hemorrhagic and give an indication to the depth of injury. Hemorrhagic blisters indicate injury into the reticular dermis.

Guidelines produced by the Wilderness Medical Society advise selective drainage of clear/cloudy blisters and to leave hemorrhagic blisters alone.[38] However, there is

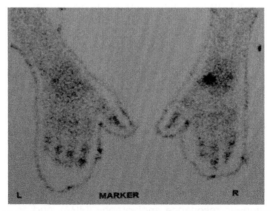

Fig. 2. [99]Tc triple-phase bone scan in frostbite injury. Note the terminal digits have reduced signal, most markedly in the left hand, suggesting that substantial tissue necrosis has occurred.

a limited evidence for this. The authors advocate the drainage and debridement of all blisters when in the hospital setting. This process should be performed in a sterile manner and may require a general anesthetic. The authors believe that this ultimately aids wound care and tissue healing.

Tissue protection and dressings

Protection and prevention of further tissue insult is paramount throughout the patient journey.

Affected areas should be splinted, elevated, and dressed in a loose protective dressing with padding between digits. Topical aloe vera cream/gel (an antiprostaglandin) should be applied to thawed tissue under the dressing.[38]

Later during the demarcation period, tissue protection consists of bespoke protective footwear.

Nutrition

All patients require high-protein, high-calorie, individually tailored diets.[53]

Pharmacologic Options

Analgesia

Rewarming can be intensely painful. Analgesia must be titrated to pain; parenteral opiates may be required.

All patients (unless contraindication) should be commenced on a nonsteroidal anti-inflammatory drug such as ibuprofen[38] because of its dual affect as an analgesic and antiinflammatory. Oral ibuprofen at a dose of 12 mg/kg twice a day provides systemic antiprostaglandin activity that limits the cascade of inflammatory damage.[54] This dosage can be increased to a maximum of 2400 mg/day if the patient is experiencing pain, and can be continued until wounds are healed or amputation occurs. A dose of 400 mg twice a day is a practical regimen on which to start most patients, and this can then be increased to 600 mg 4 times a day as pain dictates. Gut protection, such as a proton pump inhibitor, should be considered.

Aspirin is an alternative to ibuprofen. However, aspirin theoretically blocks some prostaglandins that are beneficial to wound healing.[55] Although aspirin has been shown to be beneficial in a rabbit ear model, even that article advocated ibuprofen rather than aspirin.[42]

Antibiotics

Infection can increase tissue loss and decrease patient outcome, thus systemic antibiotics must be commenced in proven infection and guided by skin swab results. Prophylactic antibiotics are controversial; a retrospective study showed no reduction in amputation with prophylactic antibiotic use.[56] However, some clinicians advocate prophylactic antibiotic use in the presence of edematous tissue, malnutrition, immunosuppression, or severe frostbite over a large surface area. This recommendation is not evidence based.

Tetanus toxoid

Frostbite wounds are not tetanus-prone wounds and thus standard tetanus toxoid guidelines should be followed.

Thrombolytic therapy

The aim is to reverse microvascular thrombosis, restoring blood flow. Endovascular delivery of a thrombolytic agent such as rTPA is used.

In 2005, Twomey and colleagues[57] published their results of an open-labeled study analyzing the effects of tissue plasminogen activator (TPA) in severe frostbite (confirmed by ^{99}Tc triple-phase bone scanning). In cases with no freeze-thaw cycles, cold exposure for less than 24 hours or a warm ischemia time of more than 6 hours TPA resulted in a reduction in expected amputations.[57] In 2007, Bruen and colleagues[17] further added to the literature base with a retrospective comparative study showing that TPA within 24 hours of injury reduced the amputation rate from 41% to 10%. Gonzaga and colleagues[58] undertook a retrospective cohort study within their unit and found that, following thrombolysis, there was an amputation rate of 31.4% for 472 at-risk digits.

Cauchy and colleagues[59] undertook a randomized controlled trial of 44 patients in which 1 arm received rTPA with iloprost and aspirin. The other 2 arms received either aspirin with buflomedil or aspirin with iloprost. rTPA was beneficial (3.1% of digits amputated) compared with the buflomedil arm (39.6%); however, this benefit was inferior to that in the iloprost arm (0%). Individual case reports have also shown positive results with thrombolytic therapy.[46,60,61]

Before delivery of thrombolytic therapy, clinicians must be sure of patient factors, unit ability, and mechanism/technique of delivery, including monitoring.

- The injury must be severe with potential tissue loss and have occurred within the last 24 hours with no freeze-thaw cycles.[57] There must be no contraindications to thrombolysis, including, but not limited to, recent trauma or surgery, bleeding diathesis, and neurologic impairment.
- The unit's staff must be competent in their ability to delivery thrombolysis, which usually requires regular monitoring, blood tests, and imaging, be able to manage complications. Critical care is often required.
- Thrombolysis can be delivered via IV or intra-arterial (IA) routes.[41] IA is our preferred route. A vasodilator such as papaverine may be added to reduce vasospasm. Heparin should be used as an adjunctive therapy in the case of thrombolytic therapy to minimize new clot formation or enlargement of existing clots, and equally heparin should be continued for a period after thrombolytic treatment has concluded.[38,41]
- Monitoring is required to assess efficacy of treatment. This monitoring must include regular patient observations, including assessment of affected area, thromboplastin must be checked (this guides heparin infusion rate), and angiographs repeated as appropriate.

Thrombolysis can be challenging for clinicians with minimal previous exposure to frostbite injury. A recent publication gave a simple stepwise approach for rTPA administration (**Fig. 3**). Nevertheless, contacting a specialist practitioner may be required (discussed later).[41]

Iloprost

Iloprost is a prostacyclin analogue with vasodilatory properties. It also reduces capillary permeability, suppresses platelet aggregation, and activates fibrinolysis.[20] IV iloprost is unavailable in the United States.

Groechenig[62] published his experience of treating severe frostbite with iloprost in 1994 and the results were promising with no amputations. Focus returned to iloprost following a randomized controlled trial published by Cauchy and colleagues[59] that showed a reduced amputation rate among 407 digits that were at risk (47 patients). All received identical initial treatment before being randomized into 1 of 3 arms: buflomedil, iloprost, or iloprost and IV rTPA. The iloprost arm had no amputations.[59] Two recent case reports also showed excellent results in grade 3 frostbite.[43]

Iloprost is administered as an IV infusion at a set rate in a monitored environment; it can be given peripherally or centrally. The infusion should be delivered at an

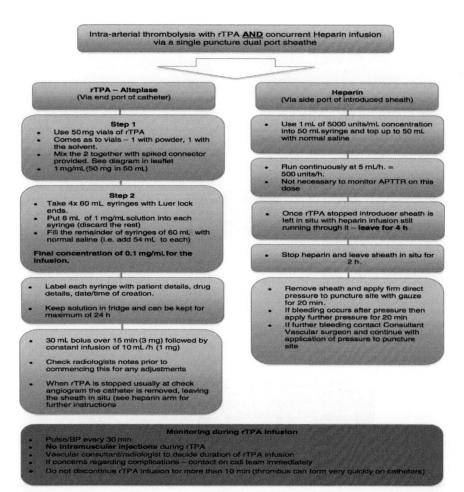

Fig. 3. A stepwise approach to IA thrombolysis and concurrent heparin infusion. APTTR, activated partial thromboplastin time ratio. (*From* Handford C, Buxton P, Russell K, et al. Frostbite: a practical approach to hospital management. Extrem Physiol Med 2014;3:7.)

accurate rate, usually achieved with a syringe driver. Clinicians should start at a rate of 0.5 ng/kg/min and escalate via increments of 0.5 ng/kg/min to a maximum dose of 2 ng/kg/min.[59] Escalation of delivered dose is performed until intolerable side effects develop, such as facial flushing and headache. The dose regimen is usually 6 hours daily for a total of 5 to 8 days.[43,59] A practical guide to aid clinicians in the administration of iloprost was recently published (**Fig. 4**).[41] **Fig. 5** shows a patient following a 5-day course of iloprost.

Iloprost has key advantages compared with rTPA. It does not require radiological intervention for use, can be administered on a general monitored ward, can be used more than 24 hours after injury, and is not contraindicated in trauma.

Surgical Treatment Options

Fasciotomy
On rewarming there is a risk of compartment syndrome if significant swelling occurs on reperfusion. In such a case rapid fasciotomy is indicated.

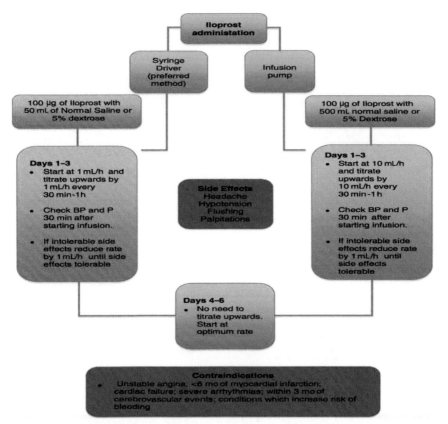

Fig. 4. A stepwise approach to iloprost administration. BP, blood pressure; P, pulse. (*From* Handford C, Buxton P, Russell K, et al. Frostbite: a practical approach to hospital management. Extrem Physiol Med 2014;3:7.)

Amputation

Immediate or early amputation should be avoided and autoamputation/demarcation awaited.

Amputation must be planned to maximize functional outcome. Early amputation may be unavoidable in cases of wet gangrene, liquefaction, overwhelming infection, or spreading sepsis.[63,64] In such cases, planning is still key and using MRA/^{99}Tc triple-phase bone scanning is useful.

Topical negative pressure dressings and tissue reconstruction

Following injury good-quality tissue is wanted after healing. This tissue is key at load-bearing sites and functionally significant areas. Little is published on the best way to achieve this and healing via secondary intention is the usual course of action. Topical negative pressure facilitates wound healing via secondary intention and may be considered as an adjunct to healing.[65–68]

An alternative to healing via secondary intention is skin coverage. An experimental study by Delgado-Martínez and colleagues[69] argues that, in structurally significant areas such as the hands or feet, or areas with a poor vascular bed, which is the case in most significant frostbite injuries, flap coverage should be used. In their

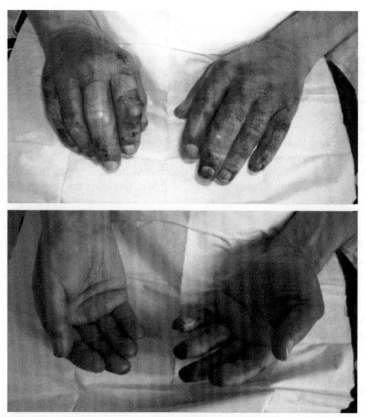

Fig. 5. Appearance following a 5-day iloprost infusion, showing the close correlation between the initial ^{99}Tc triple-phase bone scan (see **Fig. 2**) and the subsequent clinical appearance (day 10 following iloprost).

practice these investigators advocate the use of axial flaps. Skin grafts have a role in areas with limited structural importance; however, their limitations consist of variable take rates, contraction, rigidity, lack of padding, and poor reinnervation, all of which could result in functional problems.[69]

Potential Adjunctive Therapies

The following have been described in case reports and/or animal studies. However, there is insufficient evidence at this time to advocate their use on a routine basis.

Hyperbaric oxygen therapy

Hyperbaric oxygen therapy (HBOT) has been used to aid wound healing.[70] HBOT increases oxygen tension within the blood and thus increases oxygen delivery and may increase the deformability of erythrocytes and decrease bacterial load.[38] However, for the frostbitten tissues to experience increased oxygen tension, there must be a patent microvasculature.

Case reports describe HBOT use in frostbite injury in both immediate and delayed presentations, with no amputations reported.[71,72] Animal studies are contradictory.[73–75] Further investigation is warranted.

Sympathectomy

Surgical or chemical sympathectomy results in reflex vasodilation and increased blood flow but reported outcomes are mixed.[76,77] For this reason, sympathectomy in acute frostbite management is not recommended.[38]

Sympathectomy may have a role in the management of chronic complications such as vasospasm and hyperhidrosis; however, surgical sympathectomy is both invasive and irreversible and further research is warranted.[78,79]

Topical agents

Aloe vera has long been accepted as a topical treatment of frostbite injury. Investigations into other agents, such as poly-l-arginine contained in lotion and ganoderma triterpenids, and nanogel delivery methods have been attempted.[80–82] Trials are limited, small scale, and on animal models, therefore until further data are accumulated these cannot be recommended.

Complications

Functional loss and rehabilitation

Functional loss is variable depending on extent and area affected. All patients with significant injury should be managed by a multidisciplinary team consisting of physicians, occupational therapists, specialist nurses, physiotherapist, and (if needed) a prosthetist/orthotist. Mental health input may also be prudent. The aim should be to return the individual to the optimal function and independence. Many patients will continue to pursue outdoor endeavors and their future risk of cold injury must be discussed with them.

Cold sensitivity

Taylor[78] found that 53% of patients with significant frostbite injury showed subsequent cold hypersensitivity, 40% numbness of the digits, and 33% had reduced sensitivity to touch. Taylor[78] postulated that these may be secondary to a thermophysiologic response with an increased tendency to vasospasm, and others have supported these findings.[83]

Chronic pain

Chronic pain is common and can be troublesome to treat, and early use of chronic pain specialists should be sought. Medications such as amitriptyline or gabapentin may be beneficial.

In major trauma and burns, early commencement of neuropathic pain medication to reduce the risk of chronic neuropathic pain is becoming standard practice.[84,85] Although no trials have been performed in frostbite, the authors advocate consideration of a neuropathy agent as early as possible.

Chronic ulceration

Subsequent poor tissue quality and/or altered biomechanics and pressure areas following lower limb amputations can lead to chronic ulceration in previously frostbitten skin. As is the case in burns, malignant transformation can occur in such areas and must be monitored for.[86]

Arthritis

Arthritis following frostbite is well reported.[87–89] Localized osteoporosis and subchondral bone loss can be seen after injury and likely reflects vascular insult. In the skeletally immature, damage to the epiphysis may occur, leading to growth arrest/deformity.[88,90]

TELEMEDICINE

Increased availability of and reliance on telecommunications, photographic sharing, and video communications have led to a growth in telemedicine, which facilitates access to and use of subject matter experts, optimizing patient outcome.[45,91] Telemedicine can be accessed by those who are in an isolated austere environment, aiding initial management decisions and advising on expedition continuation. Medical practitioners with limited experience or knowledge regarding frostbite can also seek guidance and advice via telemedicine.

Further information can be found on the British Mountaineering Council Web site (https://www.thebmc.co.uk/how-to-get-expert-frostbite-advice). At the time of writing, the University of Utah Health Care Burn Center also provides a frostbite telemedicine service (http://healthcare.utah.edu/burncenter/frostbite.php).

SUMMARY

Management of frostbite is undermined by poor evidence; this is caused by low patient numbers and therefore little economic incentive for drug company/large institutional input. To further progress the understanding and management, large, likely multicenter, trials are warranted. An international patient register would be a positive starting point.

Despite these limitations, new management options in deep frostbite injury offer promise in minimizing the morbidity associated with this significant injury. This article highlights simple and effective treatment steps that all clinicians can perform through every echelon of care. The more complex and specialist treatments, most notably thrombolysis or iloprost infusion, should always be considered and, via telemedicine, expert opinion can be sought, ultimately optimizing patient outcome.

REFERENCES

1. Post PW, Donner DD. Frostbite in a pre-Columbian mummy. Am J Phys Anthropol 1972;37(2):187–91.
2. Robson MC, Krizek TJ, Wray RC. Care of the thermally injured patient. In: Zuidema GD, Rutherford RB, Ballinger WF, editors. Management of trauma. Philadelphia: WB Saunders; 1979. p. 666–730.
3. Golden FS, Francis TJ, Gallimore D, et al. Lessons from history: morbidity of cold injury in the Royal Marines during the Falklands Conflict of 1982. Extrem Physiol Med 2013;2(1):23.
4. Larrey DJ, Hall RW. Memoirs of military surgery. 1st American from the 2d Paris ed, vol. 6. Baltimore (MD): Joseph Cushing; 1814.
5. Heil KM, Oakley EH, Wood AM. British military freezing cold injuries: a 13-year review. J R Army Med Corps 2016;162(6):413–8.
6. DeGroot DW, Castellani JW, Williams JO, et al. Epidemiology of U.S. Army cold weather injuries, 1980-1999. Aviat Space Environ Med 2003;74(5):564–70.
7. Moran DS, Heled Y, Shani Y, et al. Hypothermia and local cold injuries in combat and non-combat situations–the Israeli experience. Aviat Space Environ Med 2003;74(3):281–4.
8. Harirchi I, Arvin A, Vash JH, et al. Frostbite: incidence and predisposing factors in mountaineers. Br J Sports Med 2005;39(12):898–901 [discussion: 901].
9. Cattermole TJ. The epidemiology of cold injury in Antarctica. Aviat Space Environ Med 1999;70(2):135–40.

10. McIntosh SE, Campbell A, Weber D, et al. Mountaineering medical events and trauma on Denali, 1992-2011. High Alt Med Biol 2012;13(4):275–80.

11. Nemethy M, Pressman AB, Freer L, et al. Mt Everest Base Camp Medical Clinic "Everest ER": epidemiology of medical events during the first 10 years of operation. Wilderness Environ Med 2015;26(1):4–10.

12. Mulgrew S, Khoo A, Oxenham T, et al. Cold finger: urban frostbite in the UK. BMJ Case Rep 2013;2013 [pii:bcr1120115167].

13. Sever C, Kulahci Y, Acar A, et al. Unusual hand frostbite caused by refrigerant liquids and gases. Ulus Travma Acil Cerrahi Derg 2010;16(5):433–8.

14. Wegener EE, Barraza KR, Das SK. Severe frostbite caused by freon gas. South Med J 1991;84(9):1143–6.

15. Makinen TM, Jokelainen J, Nayha S, et al. Occurrence of frostbite in the general population–work-related and individual factors. Scand J Work Environ Health 2009;35(5):384–93.

16. Rintamaki H. Predisposing factors and prevention of frostbite. Int J Circumpolar Health 2000;59(2):114–21.

17. Bruen KJ, Ballard JR, Morris SE, et al. Reduction of the incidence of amputation in frostbite injury with thrombolytic therapy. Arch Surg 2007;142(6):546–51.

18. Giesbrecht GG, Wilkerson JA. Hypothermia, frostbite and other cold injuries: prevention, survival, rescue, and treatment. Seattle (Washington): The Mountaineers Books; 2006.

19. Kamikomaki N. A climber with the DD ACE allele developed frostbite despite taking more than adequate measures against cold on Mount Everest. High Alt Med Biol 2007;8(2):167–8.

20. Auerbach PS. Wilderness medicine. 6th edition. Philadelphia: Elsevier/Mosby; 2012.

21. VanGelder CM, Sheridan RL. Freezing soft tissue injury from propane gas. J Trauma 1999;46(2):355–6.

22. Murphy JV, Banwell PE, Roberts AH, et al. Frostbite: pathogenesis and treatment. J Trauma 2000;48(1):171–8.

23. Zacarian SA, Stone D, Clater M. Effects of cryogenic temperatures on microcirculation in the golden hamster cheek pouch. Cryobiology 1970;7(1):27–39.

24. Zacarian SA. Cryogenics: the cryolesion and the pathogenesis of cryonecrosis. Cryosurgery for skin cancer and cutaneous disorders. St Louis (MO): Mosby; 1985. p. 1–30.

25. Mohr WJ, Jenabzadeh K, Ahrenholz DH. Cold injury. Hand Clin 2009;25(4): 481–96.

26. Kulka JP. Histopathologic studies in frostbitten rabbits. Conferences in Cold Injury. New York: Josiah Macy Jr Foundation; 1956.

27. Kulka JP. Microcirculatory impairment as a factor in inflammatory tissue damage. Ann N Y Acad Sci 1964;116:1018–44.

28. Robson MC, Heggers JP. Evaluation of hand frostbite blister fluid as a clue to pathogenesis. J Hand Surg Am 1981;6(1):43–7.

29. Raine TJ. Antiprostaglandins and antithromboxanes for treatment of frostbite. Surg Forum 1980;31:557.

30. Manson PN, Jesudass R, Marzella L, et al. Evidence for an early free radical-mediated reperfusion injury in frostbite. Free Radic Biol Med 1991;10(1):7–11.

31. Cauchy E, Chetaille E, Marchand V, et al. Retrospective study of 70 cases of severe frostbite lesions: a proposed new classification scheme. Wilderness Environ Med 2001;12(4):248–55.

32. Cauchy E, Davis CB, Pasquier M, et al. A new proposal for management of severe frostbite in the austere environment. Wilderness Environ Med 2016;27(1): 92–9.
33. Hurley LA. Angioarchitectural changes associated with rapid rewarming subsequent to freezing injury. Angiology 1957;8(1):19–28.
34. Jivan K, Ranchod K, Modi G. Management of ischaemic stroke in the acute setting: review of the current status. Cardiovasc J Afr 2013;24(3):86–92.
35. Syme D, Commission IM. Position paper: on-site treatment of frostbite for mountaineers. High Alt Med Biol 2002;3(3):297–8.
36. Zafren K, Giesbrecht G. State of Alaska: cold injuries guidelines. Juneau (Alaska): Department of Health and Social Services, Division of Public Health; 2014.
37. McIntosh SE, Hamonko M, Freer L, et al. Wilderness Medical Society practice guidelines for the prevention and treatment of frostbite. Wilderness Environ Med 2011;22(2):156–66.
38. McIntosh SE, Opacic M, Freer L, et al. Wilderness Medical Society practice guidelines for the prevention and treatment of frostbite: 2014 update. Wilderness Environ Med 2014;25(4 Suppl):S43–54.
39. Malhotra MS, Mathew L. Effect of rewarming at various water bath temperatures in experimental frostbite. Aviat Space Environ Med 1978;49(7):874–6.
40. Cauchy E, Leal S, Magnan MA, et al. Portable hyperbaric chamber and management of hypothermia and frostbite: an evident utilization. High Alt Med Biol 2014; 15(1):95–6.
41. Handford C, Buxton P, Russell K, et al. Frostbite: a practical approach to hospital management. Extrem Physiol Med 2014;3:7.
42. Heggers JP, Robson MC, Manavalen K, et al. Experimental and clinical observations on frostbite. Ann Emerg Med 1987;16(9):1056–62.
43. Poole A, Gauthier J. Treatment of severe frostbite with iloprost in northern Canada. CMAJ 2016;188(17–18):1255–8.
44. Pasquier M, Ruffinen GZ, Brugger H, et al. Pre-hospital wrist block for digital frostbite injuries. High Alt Med Biol 2012;13(1):65–6.
45. Russell KW, Imray CH, McIntosh SE, et al. Kite skier's toe: an unusual case of frostbite. Wilderness Environ Med 2013;24(2):136–40.
46. Sheridan RL, Goldstein MA, Stoddard FJ Jr, et al. Case records of the Massachusetts General Hospital. Case 41-2009. A 16-year-old boy with hypothermia and frostbite. N Engl J Med 2009;361(27):2654–62.
47. Cauchy E, Marsigny B, Allamel G, et al. The value of technetium 99 scintigraphy in the prognosis of amputation in severe frostbite injuries of the extremities: a retrospective study of 92 severe frostbite injuries. J Hand Surg Am 2000;25(5): 969–78.
48. Cauchy E, Chetaille E, Lefevre M, et al. The role of bone scanning in severe frostbite of the extremities: a retrospective study of 88 cases. Eur J Nucl Med 2000; 27(5):497–502.
49. Barker JR, Haws MJ, Brown RE, et al. Magnetic resonance imaging of severe frostbite injuries. Ann Plast Surg 1997;38(3):275–9.
50. Raman SR, Jamil Z, Cosgrove J. Magnetic resonance angiography unmasks frostbite injury. Emerg Med J 2011;28(5):450.
51. Mills WJ, Whaley R. Frostbite: experience with rapid rewarming and ultrasonic therapy. 1960-1. Wilderness Environ Med 1998;9(4):226–47.
52. McCauley RL, Hing DN, Robson MC, et al. Frostbite injuries: a rational approach based on the pathophysiology. J Trauma 1983;23(2):143–7.

53. Kiss TL. Critical care for frostbite. Crit Care Nurs Clin North Am 2012;24(4): 581–91.
54. Rainsford KD. Ibuprofen: pharmacology, efficacy and safety. Inflammopharmacology 2009;17(6):275–342.
55. Robson MC, DelBeccaro EJ, Heggers JP, et al. Increasing dermal perfusion after burning by decreasing thromboxane production. J Trauma 1980;20(9):722–5.
56. Valnicek SM, Chasmar LR, Clapson JB. Frostbite in the prairies: a 12-year review. Plast Reconstr Surg 1993;92(4):633–41.
57. Twomey JA, Peltier GL, Zera RT. An open-label study to evaluate the safety and efficacy of tissue plasminogen activator in treatment of severe frostbite. J Trauma 2005;59(6):1350–4 [discussion: 1354–5].
58. Gonzaga T, Jenabzadeh K, Anderson CP, et al. Use of intraarterial thrombolytic therapy for acute treatment of frostbite in 62 patients with review of thrombolytic therapy in frostbite. J Burn Care Res 2015;37(4):e323–34.
59. Cauchy E, Cheguillaume B, Chetaille E. A controlled trial of a prostacyclin and rt-PA in the treatment of severe frostbite. N Engl J Med 2011;364(2):189–90.
60. Wagner C, Pannucci CJ. Thrombolytic therapy in the acute management of frostbite injuries. Air Med J 2011;30(1):39–44.
61. Saemi AM, Johnson JM, Morris CS. Treatment of bilateral hand frostbite using transcatheter arterial thrombolysis after papaverine infusion. Cardiovasc Intervent Radiol 2009;32(6):1280–3.
62. Groechenig E. Treatment of frostbite with iloprost. Lancet 1994;344(8930): 1152–3.
63. Andrew J. Life and limb: a true story of tragedy and survival. London: Portrait; 2005. p. 2003.
64. Mills WJ Jr. Frostbite. A discussion of the problem and a review of the Alaskan experience. 1973. Alaska Med 1993;35(1):29–40.
65. Poulakidas S, Cologne K, Kowal-Vern A. Treatment of frostbite with subatmospheric pressure therapy. J Burn Care Res 2008;29(6):1012–4.
66. Orgill DP, Bayer LR. Negative pressure wound therapy: past, present and future. Int Wound J 2013;10(Suppl 1):15–9.
67. Wolvos T. The evolution of negative pressure wound therapy: negative pressure wound therapy with instillation. J Wound Care 2015;24(4 Suppl):15–20.
68. Sandy-Hodgetts K, Watts R. Effectiveness of negative pressure wound therapy/ closed incision management in the prevention of post-surgical wound complications: a systematic review and meta-analysis. JBI Database Syst Rev Implement Rep 2015;13(1):253–303.
69. Delgado-Martínez J, Martinez-Villen G, Morandeira JR, et al. Skin coverage in frostbite injuries: experimental study. J Plast Reconstr Aesthet Surg 2010; 63(10):e713–9.
70. Thom SR. Hyperbaric oxygen: its mechanisms and efficacy. Plast Reconstr Surg 2011;127(Suppl 1):131S–41S.
71. Kemper TC, de Jong VM, Anema HA, et al. Frostbite of both first digits of the foot treated with delayed hyperbaric oxygen: a case report and review of literature. Undersea Hyperb Med 2014;41(1):65–70.
72. Dwivedi DA, Alasinga S, Singhal S, et al. Successful treatment of frostbite with hyperbaric oxygen treatment. Indian J Occup Environ Med 2015;19(2):121–2.
73. Gage AA, Ishikawa H, Winter PM. Experimental frostbite. The effect of hyperbaric oxygenation on tissue survival. Cryobiology 1970;7(1):1–8.
74. Hardenbergh E. Hyperbaric oxygen treatment of experimental frostbite in the mouse. J Surg Res 1972;12(1):34–40.

75. Uygur F, Noyan N, Sever C, et al. The current analysis of the effect of hyperbaric oxygen therapy on the frostbitten tissue: experimental study in rabbits. Open Med 2009;4(2):198–202.
76. Engkvist O. The effect of regional intravenous guanethidine block in acute frostbite. Case report. Scand J Plast Reconstr Surg 1986;20(2):243–5.
77. Kaplan R, Thomas P, Tepper H, et al. Treatment of frostbite with guanethidine. Lancet 1981;2(8252):940–1.
78. Taylor MS. Lumbar epidural sympathectomy for frostbite injuries of the feet. Mil Med 1999;164(8):566–7.
79. Khan MI, Tariq M, Rehman A, et al. Efficacy of cervicothoracic sympathectomy versus conservative management in patients suffering from incapacitating Raynaud's syndrome after frost bite. J Ayub Med Coll Abbottabad 2008;20(2):21–4.
80. Shen CY, Xu PH, Shen BD, et al. Nanogel for dermal application of the triterpenoids isolated from *Ganoderma lucidum* (GLT) for frostbite treatment. Drug Deliv 2016;23(2):610–8.
81. Shen CY, Dai L, Shen BD, et al. Nanostructured lipid carrier based topical gel of *Ganoderma* triterpenoids for frostbite treatment. Chin J Nat Med 2015;13(6): 454–60.
82. Auerbach LJ, DeClerk BK, Fathman CG, et al. Poly-L-arginine topical lotion tested in a mouse model for frostbite injury. Wilderness Environ Med 2014;25(2):160–5.
83. Ervasti O, Hassi J, Rintamaki H, et al. Sequelae of moderate finger frostbite as assessed by subjective sensations, clinical signs, and thermophysiological responses. Int J Circumpolar Health 2000;59(2):137–45.
84. Aldington DJ, McQuay HJ, Moore RA. End-to-end military pain management. Philos Trans R Soc Lond B Biol Sci 2011;366(1562):268–75.
85. McGreevy K, Bottros MM, Raja SN. Preventing chronic pain following acute pain: risk factors, preventive strategies, and their efficacy. Eur J Pain Suppl 2011;5(2): 365–72.
86. Rossis CG, Yiacoumettis AM, Elemenoglou J. Squamous cell carcinoma of the heel developing at site of previous frostbite. J R Soc Med 1982;75(9):715–8.
87. Kahn JE, Lidove O, Laredo JD, et al. Frostbite arthritis. Ann Rheum Dis 2005; 64(6):966–7.
88. Pettit MT, Finger DR. Frostbite arthropathy. J Clin Rheumatol 1998;4(6):316–8.
89. Wang Y, Saad E, Bonife T, et al. Frostbite arthritis. Am J Phys Med Rehabil 2016; 95(2):e28.
90. Carrera GF, Kozin F, Flaherty L, et al. Radiographic changes in the hands following childhood frostbite injury. Skeletal Radiol 1981;6(1):33–7.
91. Imray CHE, Hillebrandt D. Telemedicine and frostbite injuries. BMJ 2004;328: 1210.

Updates in Decompression Illness

Neal W. Pollock, PhD[a,b,c],*, Dominique Buteau, MD[c,d]

KEYWORDS

- Decompression sickness • Arterial gas embolism • High-fraction oxygen
- Hyperbaric

KEY POINTS

- Decompression sickness (DCS) is a disease resulting from an ascent profile not allowing the orderly elimination of excess gas that was accumulated in tissues during exposure to elevated pressure.
- Decompression sickness (DCS) can present idiosyncratically, affecting a wide range of systems with a variable degree of insult. Masking of important symptoms by chief complaint is possible.
- Arterial gas embolism (AGE) is a disease of frank gas in the arterial systemic circulation following a reduction of ambient pressure so rapid that expanding gases cause pulmonary tissue rupture.
- The first aid for decompression illness (collectively, DCS and AGE) is high fraction oxygen; the definitive treatment is hyperbaric oxygen therapy.
- There are currently no diagnostic tests to confirm decompression sickness.

INTRODUCTION

Diving is a popular recreational pastime, as well as an activity with numerous applications in the scientific, commercial, military, and exploration realms. Although diving can be done safely, the underwater environment is unforgiving. Problems may arise during a dive due to insufficient medical or physical fitness, improper use of equipment, or inadequate management of the high-pressure environment.

The authors have nothing to disclose.
^a Department of Kinesiology, Université Laval, PEPS Building, 2300 rue de la Terrasse, Quebec City, Quebec G1V 0A6, Canada; ^b Department of Medical Research, Divers Alert Network, 6 West colony place, Durham, NC 27705, USA; ^c CISSS Chaudière-Appalaches (CHAU-Hôtel-Dieu de Lévis), Hyperbaric Medicine Unit, Emergency Department, 143 rue Wolfe, Lévis, Quebec G6V 3Z1, Canada; ^d Family Medicine and Emergency Medicine Department, School of Medicine, Université Laval, Quebec City, Quebec, G1V 0A6 Canada
* Corresponding author. Université Laval, Quebec City, Quebec G1V 0A6, Canada.
E-mail address: neal.pollock@kin.ulaval.ca

Emerg Med Clin N Am 35 (2017) 301–319
http://dx.doi.org/10.1016/j.emc.2016.12.002
0733-8627/17/© 2016 Elsevier Inc. All rights reserved.

Decompression illness (DCI) is a term used to encompass injuries due to arterial gas embolism (AGE) and decompression sickness (DCS). AGE typically results from pulmonary barotrauma-induced damage to the alveolar wall and introduction of gas into the systemic arterial circulation. DCS, colloquially known as the bends, results from the uncontrolled release of gas from tissues during or after surfacing with inadequate time for equilibration (decompression).

DIVING PHYSICS

The concentration, or tension, of dissolved inert gas within body tissues is a function of ambient pressure. Inert gases normally exist in equilibrium with the ambient environment, effectively a saturated state. When pressure differences (gradients) are created, molecules flow from the area of higher to lower concentration until equilibrium is re-established.

The pressure range of the diving environment is much greater than the pressure range of the air environment. The pressure exerted at sea level by the entire 100 km (62 mi) atmospheric column of gas is 1 atm absolute (ATA), equal to 101.3 kPa or 14.7 psi. In contrast, water pressure increases by 1 atm for every 10 m (33 ft) of seawater and for every 10.4 m (34 ft) of freshwater (**Fig. 1**).

The lungs play a primary role in gas uptake and elimination and, ultimately, decompression stress. When exposed to increased pressure underwater, the gas in the lungs is compressed. This creates an inflow gradient from concentrated lung gas to the bloodstream and, subsequently, from the bloodstream into tissues as they are perfused. Tissues take up inert gas until saturation is achieved. At the point of saturation, staying longer does not further increase the subsequent decompression obligation.

PREDICTING GAS UPTAKE AND ELIMINATION

Gas uptake and elimination generally follows roughly exponential patterns. The technology is not yet available to measure tissue status directly, so the norm is to rely on

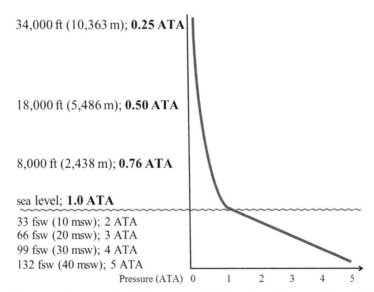

Fig. 1. Air pressure increases slowly from zero at the boundary of space to 1 atm (14.7 psi) at sea level. Water pressure increases much more dramatically, adding 1 atm of pressure for every 10 m of seawater. fsw, feet of seawater; msw, meters of seawater.

mathematical algorithms to predict gas exchange. A range of half-times are used to represent different tissue characteristics; not as exact referents but as mathematical constructs to collectively estimate what happens throughout the body.

The fastest tissues are the lungs, which achieve equilibrium almost instantly. Blood is another extremely fast tissue, followed by the brain. The slowest tissues are those that are relatively poorly perfused, such as ligaments and cartilage, or those that have a high capacity for inert gas uptake, such as fat in poorly perfused areas.

Consider a diver instantly displaced from the surface to a fixed depth as an example. A 5-minute half-time would represent a fast tissue, computed to take up sufficient inert gas uptake to eliminate half of the difference produced by the pressure gradient (50%) in the first 5 minutes. This would be the steepest portion of the uptake curve. The second 5-minute period would eliminate half of the remaining difference (25%). The third 5-minute period would eliminate half of the remaining difference (12.5%) and so on. At the other extreme, a 500-minute half-time could be computed to represent an extremely slow tissue. With no additional influences on the process, equilibration is expected to be nearly achieved after a period equal to about 6 half-times for any given tissue (**Fig. 2**).

Most dives do not last long enough for the diver to reach saturation; these are known as bounce dives. During such exposures, the inflow gradient exists at least through the descent and bottom phase of the dive, which causes continued uptake of inert gases, certainly in slow compartments and probably in intermediate compartments. When the diver ascends, the ambient pressure starts to drop and the gradient begins to reverse, first in fast compartments and then in progressively slower compartments.

When the tissue tension of a gas exceeds the ambient partial pressure of that gas, the tissue is supersaturated. This will be the case of most tissues during and after surfacing. If the degree of supersaturation is modest, equilibrium from peripheral tissues into the blood, then lungs, and then atmosphere, will be orderly. If the degree of supersaturation is too great, the elimination of inert gases becomes disorderly, gas phase (bubbles) can form, and DCS may develop.

Bubble formation does not always cause problems but the greater the supersaturation the greater the likelihood that symptomatic DCS will occur. It is a misconception

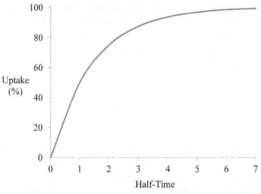

Fig. 2. The half-time concept describes how an undersaturated tissue takes up inert gas. When held at a fixed pressure, enough gas is taken up to eliminate half of the difference in gas pressures in each half-time period. For a hypothetical tissue with a half-time of 10 minutes (and no other influences), 50% of the difference is eliminated in the first 10 minutes, then 25% in the next 10 minutes (half of the remaining 50%), then 12.5%, 6.25%, 3.125%, and 1.56%, and so forth.

that bubbles forming after a dive are of no importance; however, it is also a misconception that bubbles equate to DCS. The formation of gas bubbles during decompression represents a stress greater than is optimal and may lead to DCS.

CONTROLLING DIVE EXPOSURES

Dive computers have supplanted printed dive tables as the primary means of regulating dive profiles over the last 20 years. Dive computers provide more flexible guidance because they continuously assess the pressure-time profile and compute the status of a variety of hypothetical tissue compartments. Exposure limits or decompression obligations are adjusted based on whatever compartment is deemed most critical (effectively the controlling half-time) at any point in the ascent. This is useful because modern divers frequently follow complex descent-ascent profiles, relying on the dive computer to keep track of their state.

Dive computers provide guidance based on the primary determinants of decompression risk: the pressure-time profile and breathing gas. However, gas exchange is also influenced by the timing and intensity of exercise and thermal stressors during a dive, as well as by individual predispositions, none of which are assessed by dive computers in a meaningful way.

Symptoms of DCS may develop after dives conducted within decompression algorithm limits. Decompression algorithms predict outcomes but they do not guarantee them. That a dive is conducted within the limits does not make a DCS hit undeserved.

DEVELOPING DECOMPRESSION SICKNESS

Although DCS is commonly thought of as a bubble disease, bubbles are probably only the gateway to a complex array of consequences. Bubbles can form in or reach a wide variety of tissues, and initiate biochemical cascades to produce secondary insults and effects. Vascular obstruction or interactions may stimulate platelet aggregation, leukocytes activation and aggregation, and fibrin deposition. Intravascular bubbles may also damage the capillary endothelium, possibly leading to increased permeability and tissue edema exacerbating the ischemia process. An increased release of cytokines and/or complement activation has also been demonstrated as possible contributing agents. The inflammatory cascade could play an important role in the pathophysiology of DCI. The variability in activation threshold of this inflammatory cascade might explain the differences between individuals in susceptibility to DCS. The inflammatory and coagulation cascades might also explain the failure of recompression treatment in some cases because, once activated, the resolution of bubbles will not immediately stop the response.

THE MECHANICS OF ARTERIAL GAS EMBOLISM

Unlike DCS, which requires a period of gas uptake, AGE results from an acute decrease in ambient pressure in a tissue unable to accommodate. For example, a diver ascending rapidly from 10 m (2 ATA) to the surface (1 ATA) is faced with a 50% reduction from the bottom pressure. In accordance with Boyle's law ($P_1V_1 = P_2V_2$; assuming constant temperature), an unventilated volume of gas would double during this excursion. Normally, the diver would breathe freely during a slow ascent and constantly re-equilibrate lung volume. If ventilation is not adequate, either due to breath-holding or a localized bronchial obstruction (eg, bronchospasm or mucus plug), an overexpansion injury (pulmonary barotrauma) can result. The maximum sustainable tissue elastic pressure in the alveoli is around 100 to 150 mm Hg (0.13–0.2 atm) over ambient. A pressure of 0.13 atm is found at a depth of 1.3 m (4 ft) in seawater. A rapid ascent with full lungs and an obstructed airway from this very shallow depth could result in pulmonary baro-trauma. Tissue rupture will allow gas from the alveolar space to enter the pleural space (pneumothorax), the pulmonary interstitium, the mediastinum (pneumomediastinum), and/or the pulmonary capillaries. Bubbles entering the pulmonary capillaries can be transported into the systemic arterial circulation and may reach critical tissues, such as the brain or the spinal cord, to produce serious symptoms. The symptoms of AGE can be very similar to those of DCS, sometimes making them difficult to separate.

INCIDENCE OF DECOMPRESSION ILLNESS

The lowest DCI incidence rates have been reported in the scientific diving community at 0.324 per 10,000 person-dives.[1] Divers Alert Network (DAN) estimates of DCI inci-dence rates in the recreational community range from 2.0 to 4.0 per 10,000 person-dives.[2–4] The DCS incidence rate in commercial decompression diving has been reported to be as high as 35.3 per 10,000 person-dives.[5] A more recent study of com-mercial diving DCS described incidence rates ranging from 1.4 to 10.3 per 10,000 person-dives, depending largely on the depth of dive operations.[6]

SIGNS AND SYMPTOMS

A variety of classification systems have been established for DCS. One common approach is to describe cases as type 1 or type 2.

Type 1 DCS is usually characterized by musculoskeletal pain and mild cutaneous symptoms. Common type 1 skin manifestations include itching and mild rashes (as distinct from a clear, mottled or marbled, and sometimes raised discoloration of the skin known as cutis marmorata [**Fig. 3**] that may presage the development of the more serious type 2 symptoms). Less common but still associated with type 1 DCS is obstruction of the lymphatic system, which can result in swelling and localized pain in the tissues surrounding the lymph nodes.

Musculoskeletal manifestations of type 1 DCS are articular or periarticular pain. The joint pain usually has a gradual onset and presents as a deep dull ache. Pain intensity

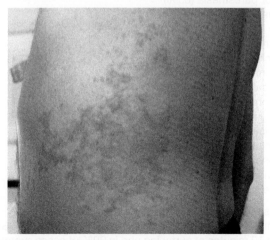

Fig. 3. Skin mottling like this is characteristic of cutis marmorata, a condition that can warn of likely development of more serious type 2 symptoms. (*Courtesy of* N.W. Pollock, PhD, Durham.)

may range from mild to severe. The pain will typically be present at rest and may or may not be exacerbated by movement. Common locations include shoulders, elbows, wrists, hips, knees, and ankles.

Type 2 symptoms are considered more serious. They typically fall into 3 categories: neurologic, inner ear, and cardiopulmonary. Neurologic symptoms include numbness; paresthesia or tingling; muscle weakness; impaired gait, physical coordination or bladder control; paralysis; or change in mental status. Some neurologic symptoms are commonly described as constitutional, such as headache, lightheadedness, unexplained fatigue, malaise, nausea and/or vomiting, or anorexia. Inner ear symptoms include tinnitus, hearing loss, vertigo or dizziness, nausea, vomiting, and impaired balance. Cardiopulmonary symptoms, known as the chokes, include a dry cough, retrosternal pain, dyspnea, and sometimes pink-stained, frothy sputum. Cardiopulmonary involvement occurs when massive bubble loads obstruct a substantial proportion of the pulmonary vascular bed. Cardiopulmonary DCS usually follows highly provocative dive profiles with a significant omitted decompression. It is important to rule out immersion pulmonary edema, which can present like cardiopulmonary DCS.

Type 2 symptoms can develop slowly or quickly. A slow build can obscure the seriousness of the situation, allowing denial to persist. For example, fatigue and weakness may initially be easy to ignore. Less common symptoms, such as difficulty walking, urinating, hearing, or seeing (especially with quick onset) are more difficult to deny.

Other types of classification exist for DCS. For the first-line physician, differentiation between type 1 or type 2 DCS is somewhat unnecessary because DCS is a systemic disease that often involves multiple organs and, in any case, the final treatment approach will not differ that much.

The presentation of DCS is frequently idiosyncratic; that is, its typical pattern can be atypical. In some cases, an affected diver's chief complaint may draw attention away from subtler but potentially more important symptoms. The following list ranks the initial manifestations of DCS, with frequency estimates for each[7]:

- Pain, particularly near the joints (68%)
- Numbness or paresthesia (63%)
- Constitutional symptoms (41%)
- Dizziness or vertigo (19%)
- Motor weakness (19%)
- Cutaneous changes (10%)
- Impaired mental status (8%)
- Impaired coordination (8%)
- Muscle discomfort (7%)
- Pulmonary symptoms (6%)
- Bladder or bowel dysfunction (3%)
- Auditory symptoms (2%)
- Impaired consciousness (2%)
- Lymphatic involvement (2%)
- Compromised cardiovascular function (<1%).

Clinical manifestations are described by system in **Table 1**.

Symptoms might present with some delay. Severe neurologic DCS symptoms usually appear within 10 minutes of surfacing and in 90% of cases symptoms will be present within the first 3 hours.[8] In some cases, it can take up to 24 hours for symptoms to be noticed by the diver.

Table 1
Clinical manifestations of decompression sickness

System involved	Symptoms	Signs
Skin	Itching	Nonspecific skin rash, urticarial rash, well-organized mottling (cutis marmorata)
Lymphatics	Localized pain in the region of lymph nodes	Localized skin and soft tissue swelling (lymphedema)
Musculoskeletal	Articular or periarticular pain, muscular pain	Usually no joint swelling, no redness
Venous blood (pulmonary circulation)	Dyspnea, cough, respiratory distress, retrosternal pain worsened on inspiration	Tachypnea, tachycardia, hypotension, frothy bloody sputum, low oxygen saturation
Central nervous system	Headache, unexplained fatigue, malaise, dizziness, impaired cognitive processes, paresthesias, limb weakness, speech difficulty, visual loss, ataxia, nausea, vomiting, convulsions	Altered state of consciousness, confusion, visual field deficit, unusual distribution of sensory deficits, motor deficits, coordination deficit, gait and walking disturbance, ataxia, positive Romberg sign
Spinal cord	Back pain, girdling abdominal pain, numbness, paresthesias, limb weakness, urinary or fecal dysfunction (with urinary issues being more common)	Motor and/or sensory deficits, anal sphincter weakness, urinary retention, loss of bulbocavernosus reflex, loss of deep tendon reflexes
Peripheral nervous system	Numbness or paresthesias in a peripheral nerve distribution	Patchy sensory deficits
Inner ear	Deafness, vertigo, nausea, vomiting, ataxia, tinnitus	Acute sensorineural hearing loss, nystagmus

MEDICAL ASSESSMENT OF THE INJURED DIVER

The history and physical examination remain the essential tools for the management of suspected DCS. In addition to the usual medical questionnaire, the emergency physician should seek the following information:

- Time of onset and evolution of symptoms and signs: Onset of symptoms less than 10 minutes after surfacing could indicate AGE. Onset of symptoms more than 10 minutes after surfacing are more likely associated with DCS. An exception may appear with the extreme decompression violation possible with technical diving, potentially resulting in symptoms during or immediately after surfacing.
- Profiles of the recent dives: Depth-time exposure, ascent rate, ascent stops (obligatory decompression stops or nonobligatory safety stops), and patterns of repetitive dives. Greater depth and duration imply a larger inert gas burden but using maximum depth alone to assess severity can be misleading given the common use of multilevel dive profiles.
- Breathing gas: The use of oxygen-enriched mixtures (nitrox) is increasingly mainstream, and the use of helium-oxygen and helium-oxygen-nitrogen mixtures

(trimix) is increasingly common. Using nitrox within air exposure limits can substantially reduce decompression stress. Using nitrox to the limits of equivalent air depth tables extends bottom time with a similar risk as using air to the limits of air tables. The other mixed gases are generally used for deeper dives with an intent to limit narcotic effects and optimize decompression.

- Thermal stress: Being warm during the descent and/or bottom phase of a dive will increase inert gas uptake, increasing the subsequent decompression stress. Being cold during the ascent and/or stop phase inhibits inert gas elimination, increasing the decompression stress.[9] Excessive heating during the ascent and/or stop phase can reduce solubility in the peripheral tissues, promoting bubble formation, increasing decompression stress. (Note: physical thermal status is more important than water or air temperatures.)
- Exercise stress: Exercise during the descent and/or bottom phase of a dive will increase inert gas uptake, increasing the subsequent decompression stress. Light exercise during the ascent and/or stop phase promotes inert gas elimination, reducing the decompression stress. Higher levels of exercise during the ascent and/or stop phase can promote bubble formation and increase risk. After-dive exercise, particularly with high joint forces, can promote bubble formation and increase risk.
- Altitude exposure and diving: Flying to a destination near sea level before diving creates no risk (outside the possibility of mild dehydration or impairment due to long periods of relative immobility). Because flights end with compression, the tissues of plane passengers will be undersaturated on landing and subsequently accumulate inert gases to re-establish equilibrium with the ambient pressure. Flying after diving, however, increases decompression stress because the pressure in an aircraft cabin is below that of ground-level atmospheric pressure. Commercial pressurized aircraft must have the capability of maintaining cabin pressure at an equivalent 2438 m (8000 ft), approximately 0.76 ATA. To illustrate, a dive to 20 m (66 ft) at sea level produces an exposure pressure of 3.0 ATA. Returning to the surface at 1.0 ATA produces a 3-fold reduction in pressure (3.0:1.0). Immediately getting on a plane or driving to an altitude of 2438 m would produce a 4-fold reduction (3.0:0.76), a much greater decompression stress.
- State of hydration: Dehydration is often overstated as a risk factor by divers looking for something to blame but a relative state of dehydration can elevate the decompression stress of a given exposure.[10]
- Contributing factors: These include physical and medical fitness (chronic or current), health history (including DCS), and medication use (generally with no research data relative to diving).

A practical likelihood assessment for DCS is summarized in **Table 2**.
The physical examination should focus on the following:

- Vital signs: Shock could be present and may originate from a cardiopulmonary DCS, tension pneumothorax, hypovolemia due to physical trauma, or from a neurogenic shock due to spinal cord DCS. Any abnormality in vital signs should be rapidly identified and managed properly. Vital signs should include rectal temperature to detect hypothermia or heat exhaustion. As with any patient presenting with altered state of consciousness or neurologic symptoms, a blood glucose level should be measured at the bedside to exclude hypoglycemia.
- Cardiac and lung auscultation: Evaluate for diminished sounds on one side, subcutaneous emphysema, displaced trachea, and Hamman's sign (potentially indicating pneumothorax or mediastinal emphysema from a pulmonary barotrauma).

Table 2
Practical likelihood assessment for decompression sickness

	High Likelihood	Low Likelihood[a]
Symptom onset after dive	>10 min–6 h[b]	>12 h
Quality of pain	Unusual[c]	Not unusual
Response to subsequent dive	Symptoms improve at depth	Symptoms unchanged at depth
Dive profile	Difficult without critical examination[d]	—

[a] Symptoms developing at depth, before decompression, will exclude DCS.
[b] Less than 10-minute onset could indicate AGE or an extreme decompression violation possible with technical diving.
[c] Symptoms associated with DCS are commonly described as different from normal pains.
[d] Consultation with subject matter expert is aided by the availability of downloadable dive computers.

- Ear examination: Look for signs of middle-ear barotrauma that could be associated with inner-ear damage. Round window rupture is not easy to differentiate from inner ear DCS.
- Neurologic examination: Access mental status, cognitive function, assessment of gait and walking, cranial nerves, sensory function, limbs strength, cerebellar function, and osteotendinous reflexes. Anal sphincter tone and bulbocavernosus reflex are essential to verify in patients with suspected spinal cord DCS and possible spinal shock. Sensory deficits are often patchy and may not follow the cortical distributions usually seen in patients with acute thrombotic cerebral stroke, or will not conform to dermatomes as seen in patients with traumatic spinal cord injury. Bubbles can cause vascular occlusions at many different locations in the nervous system. The neurologic examination can show very unusual distribution of deficits and can be confusing for the physician. Strange neurologic complaints or findings should not be dismissed as imaginary.
- Skin examination: Look for any rash or swelling.
- Articular examination: Joint examination is often unrevealing in pain-only DCS because there are usually no signs of joint inflammation and joint movement rarely alters the pain. It is commonly recounted that a relief of pain produced by the inflation of a sphygmomanometer cuff over a painful joint could support a diagnosis of musculoskeletal DCS over other strain conditions. This test has poor sensitivity and unknown specificity.[11]
- Abdominal examination: Evaluate for bladder distension that can be present with spinal cord DCS. If present, urinary catheterization will be mandatory.

DIAGNOSTIC WORK-UP

There are no specific diagnostic investigations that can establish the diagnosis of DCS. Research to identify useful diagnostic indicators is ongoing. The following considers some of the available avenues.

Hemoglobin-hematocrit might be useful. In some severe DCS, hemoconcentration can be seen, resulting from increased vascular permeability mediated by endothelial damage and kinin release.[12]

Chest radiographs are essential in the evaluation of the injured divers. Most importantly to exclude pneumothorax and pneumomediastinum in cases in which pulmonary barotrauma is suspected.[13] An untreated pneumothorax is a contraindication for recompression in a hyperbaric chamber. It may also be crucial to recognize and treat a pneumothorax before any medical evacuation to the hyperbaric center. DCS might not kill the patient but a tension pneumothorax could easily produce a life threat during air transportation. Secondarily, chest radiographs may be diagnostic in cases in which the differential diagnosis includes drowning and immersion pulmonary edema.

Computerized tomography (CT) and MRI have been used to delineate cerebral and spinal cord lesions in patients suffering from neurologic DCS. Although these imaging techniques may detect such lesions, and despite MRI seeming to be more useful than CT,[14] both modalities are surprisingly insensitive and often fail to detect lesions in divers with obvious neurologic deficits.[15–17] MRI seems to have a much better sensitivity to show anomalies in spinal cord DCS than in central nervous system DCS.[18] MRI may also be helpful in predicting clinical outcome in divers with spinal cord DCS.[19] CT scanning might prove useful in excluding other causes of neurologic symptoms, such as subarachnoid hemorrhage or cerebrovascular accident. In obvious cases of neurologic DCS, it should be clearly stated that these imaging techniques are not the priority and they should not cause a delay to recompression therapy.

Limb radiographs have occasionally revealed evidence of gas in the soft tissue and periarticular spaces but the absence of such a finding does not exclude DCS. Limb radiographs have very little diagnostic value and, therefore, are not recommended as part of the routine evaluation for DCS.

Research is ongoing to identify diagnostic tests to confirm DCI. It has been demonstrated that coagulation activation can be present in DCI. A relationship has been found between the plasma D-dimers level and the presence of sequelae in neurologic DCS.[20] The accumulation of microparticles in the blood has also received attention as a possible indicator of decompression stress.[21,22] Although all such work is valid, there is no current clinical relevance.

DIFFERENTIAL DIAGNOSIS OF DECOMPRESSION ILLNESS

Some of the other conditions with similar symptom spectra include inner ear barotrauma; middle ear or maxillary sinus barotrauma; contaminated breathing gas (the effects of which can be concentrated when breathing under pressure); oxygen toxicity; musculoskeletal strains or trauma sustained before, during, or after a dive; seafood toxin ingestion; immersion pulmonary edema; water aspiration; and coincidental neurologic disorders, such as stroke.[7] Additional conditions to consider are hypoglycemia, thermal stress, and age-related conditions. Medical or event history can provide important insights. For example, symptoms of immersion pulmonary edema often develop at depth. This occurrence would rule out DCS, which can only develop during or following ascent.

TREATING DECOMPRESSION ILLNESS

There are several elements in DCI management: on-the-scene evaluation and first aid, transport, and definitive medical evaluation and treatment.

FIRST AID

High partial pressure oxygen is the primary first aid measure for DCI.[23,24] High oxygen concentration in the lungs will accelerate inert gas elimination. High oxygen partial pressure in the bloodstream can also alleviate ischemic insults produced by bubble blockages. Sustained oxygen delivery can reduce or even eliminate symptoms.

Continuous-flow oxygen systems, using nonrebreather or pocket masks, are frequently available in diving environments; however, such equipment delivers modest oxygen fractions. Much higher fractions can be achieved for spontaneously breathing patients with demand masks.

First aid oxygen rebreather systems can provide the highest fractions with minimal gas use, especially helpful in remote settings with limited oxygen supplies.[25]

Chemical oxygen generating systems may be the only option available in some remote locations. Problematically, such devices typically provide extremely limited flow rates and volumes.[26]

Medical evaluation is advised even if a diver's symptoms improve or disappear with the administration of oxygen because subtle issues can be missed or signs and symptoms can return once oxygen delivery is stopped.

SPECIALIZED RESOURCES

Following patient stabilization, consultation with subject matter experts may be helpful for diagnosis and management plans. DAN may be able to provide consult support. DAN is a not-for-profit organization created to promote diving safety and support divers in need. Services include and emergency hotline (1-919-684-9111), evacuation logistics, nonemergency information, insurance, and education or training, including continuing medical education programs in diving and hyperbaric medicine.

HYPERBARIC OXYGEN THERAPY

The definitive treatment of DCI is hyperbaric oxygen therapy (HBOT), the delivery of oxygen at a partial pressure substantially higher than that achievable at normal atmospheric pressure.

Recompression in a hyperbaric chamber reduces the volume of bubbles. HBOT promotes the elimination of both bubbles and dissolved gas, increases delivery of oxygen to ischemic tissues, reduces tissue edema, reduces blood vessel permeability, counteracts the adherence of leukocytes to brain vessels, and partially blocks lipid peroxidation in reperfused tissues.

The HBOT regimen most commonly used to treat DCS is the US Navy Treatment Table (USN TT) 6.[27] The initial pressurization is to 2.8 ATA, equivalent to the pressure found at 18 m (60 ft) of seawater (**Fig. 4**). Patients breathe pure oxygen, with scheduled air breathing breaks to reduce the risk of central nervous system oxygen toxicity. The usual duration of the USN TT6 treatment is just under 5 hours but extensions can be added at both step pressures if warranted by the patient's response. The table is almost identical to the Royal Navy Treatment Table 62.

HBOT can be conducted in monoplace chambers, often acrylic tubes that hold just 1 patient (**Fig. 5**), or in multiplace chambers that accommodate 1 or more patients plus 1 or more tenders (**Fig. 6**). Multilock chambers allow patients, tenders, or equipment to be transferred into and out of or between chambers while treatment is ongoing.

TREATMENT EFFICACY

Although definitive data are limited, it seems that the best prognosis is achieved with rapid HBOT. This is logical for an acute ischemic event. Although there is an inverse relationship between delay to treatment and complete resolution of symptoms, the current data available have not established a maximum time after which recompression is ineffective. Many anecdotal reports describe clinical improvement in DCS cases treated many days after the onset, even with neurologic involvement. It could be reasonable to offer this therapy even up to several days after the first symptoms.

Treatment Table 6

1. Descent rate - 20 ft/min.

2. Ascent rate - Not to exceed 1 ft/min. Do not compensate for slower ascent rates. Compensate for faster rates by halting the ascent.

3. Time on oxygen begins on arrival at 60 feet.

4. If oxygen breathing must be interrupted because of CNS Oxygen Toxicity, allow 15 min after the reaction has entirely subsided and resume schedule at point of interruption (see paragraph 20-7.11.1.1).

5. Table 6 can be lengthened up to 2 additional 25-min periods at 60 feet (20 min on oxygen and 5 min on air), or up to 2 additional 75-min periods at 30 feet (15 min on air and 60 min on oxygen), or both.

6. Tender breathes 100 percent O_2 during the last 30 min. at 30 fsw and during ascent to the surface for an unmodified table or where there has been only a single extension at 30 or 60 feet. If there has been more than one extension, the O_2 breathing at 30 feet is increased to 60 min. If the tender had a hyperbaric exposure within the past 18 h an additional 60-min O_2 period is taken at 30 feet.

Treatment Table 6 Depth/Time Profile

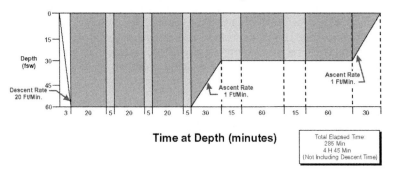

Time at Depth (minutes)

Total Elapsed Time:
285 Min
4 H 45 Min
(Not Including Descent Time)

Fig. 4. The USN TT 6 is probably the most widely used protocol to treat DCS. (*From* US Navy Diving Manual, Volume 2, Revision 6. NAVSEA 0910-LP-106-0957. Naval Sea Systems Command: Washington, DC, 2008.)

The course of HBOT will vary according to the particulars of each case. Full resolution of DCS symptoms can often be achieved with 1 or sometimes multiple HBOT treatments. In some cases, resolution will be incomplete, even after many treatments. The normal clinical approach is to continue treatments until no further improvement is

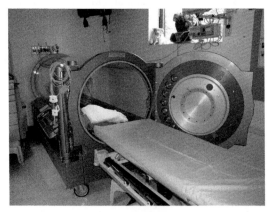

Fig. 5. A monoplace hyperbaric chamber holds a single patient, without any inside support personnel. (*Courtesy of* N.W. Pollock, PhD, Durham.)

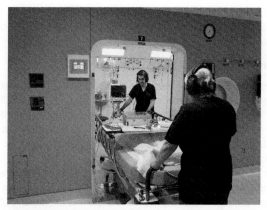

Fig. 6. Critical care can be provided within properly equipped, multiplace, multilock hyperbaric chambers. (*Courtesy of* D. Buteau, MD, Quebec City.)

seen in the patient's symptoms. Modest residual symptoms will then often resolve slowly, after the treatment series is ended. Full resolution of symptoms can sometimes take months to achieve and in some instances may never be realized.

UNUSUAL CIRCUMSTANCES

Two of the rapidly growing subdisciplines in diving are freediving and technical diving. Breath-hold diving that was once used for casual snorkeling is now used for a wide range of activities from spearfishing to competitive freediving. Although the equipment requirement is minimal, the range of activity has advanced massively, with current record resting breath-hold times of 11 minutes and 35 seconds, and maximum excursion depths of 214 m (702 ft). The conventional wisdom that DCS cannot develop from breath-hold exposures is being challenged by a substantial number of anecdotal reports in which primarily transient neurologic symptoms have developed. It is important to determine the scope of activity of an individual rather than assuming that all breath-hold diving is benign.

Technical diving represents the other end of the equipment continuum, often using multiple different gas mixtures in different cylinders or, increasingly, closed-circuit rebreathers that dynamically maintain breathing gases at selected setpoints.[28,29] Rebreathers have dramatically expanded the range of recreational and scientific diving. Technical diving relies on decompression algorithms, many that have not been tested beyond the traditional recreational zone of less than 40 m. It is increasingly common to see recreational use in the 100 m range, with many pushing much deeper. The long runtimes associated with technical diving can produce prolonged exposure to high Po_2 and a complex patterns of gas breathing. The relatively extreme exposures can also produce decompression insults far beyond what is normally seen in traditional scuba diving. Despite the complexity of exposures and insult, standard HBOT typically produces good therapeutic outcomes and is not contraindicated.

ADJUNCTIVE THERAPIES
Fluid Administration

Fluid resuscitation is advocated for the treatment of divers with DCS. Isotonic fluids are preferable to hypotonic fluids to prevent an osmolar gradient that may contribute to tissue edema and to prevent electrolyte imbalance. The goal is to maintain a good urinary output (1–2 mL/kg/h) for the patient with a urinary catheter, or clear urine for the patient who is voiding naturally.

Anticoagulants and Antiplatelet Agents

Inert gas bubbles induce platelet accumulation, adherence, and thrombus formation.[12,30] Consequently, a variety of antiplatelet agents, especially aspirin, have been extensively tried but without success. This failure is probably because bubble-induced platelet accumulation is not as rheologically important as the concurrent accumulation of leukocytes.[31] Aspirin is commonly administered to divers suffering from DCI in France.[32]

Animal models of DCS failed to demonstrate any beneficial therapeutic effect of heparin.[33] Heparin may also pose a significant risk as an anticoagulant, potentially inducing tissue hemorrhage in both spinal cord DCS and inner ear DCS. The opposing concern is the thromboembolic risk in bedridden patients with severe neurologic DCS. Administration of subcutaneous low-molecular-weight heparin for thromboembolic prophylaxis is recommended for those cases.

Corticosteroids

Corticosteroids have been used in the past for the treatment of neurologic DCS. The evidence was based mainly on case reports or retrospective studies in which numerous variables were simultaneously evaluated. It is unclear if corticosteroid administration has meaningful impact on the outcome. Evidence from studies on acute traumatic spinal cord injuries showing that high-dose corticosteroids may have limited benefit and can result in invasive infections and avascular necrosis must also be considered.[34–36] Finally, it should be noted that corticosteroids may predispose to central nervous system oxygen toxicity. Currently, the efficacy of corticosteroids in DCI treatment remains unproven.

Nonsteroidal Anti-inflammatory Drugs

A randomized trial examining adjunctive administration of the nonsteroidal anti-inflammatory drug (NSAID), tenoxicam, to divers suffering with DCI showed no difference on the residual symptoms at the completion of HBOT; however, there was a significant reduction in the number of treatments required and no evidence of complications with this adjunctive treatment.[37] One other NSAID for which there is some evidence is indomethacin but only in combination with prostaglandin PgI$_2$ and heparin.[38,39] NSAIDs are not recommended in the initial first-line treatment of DCS because they can confound the clinical evaluation by masking the pain. They could have some utility for residual pain after the decision has been made to stop HBOT.

Lidocaine

Lidocaine at therapeutic levels has been shown in animal models of cerebral AGE to have the following effects: reduction of intracranial pressure, preservation of cerebral blood flow, reduction of brain edema, preservation of neuroelectrical function, and reduction in infarct size. Possible mechanisms for this cerebral protection include modulation of leukocyte activity, reduction of ischemic excitotoxin release (eg, glutamate), reduction in cerebral metabolic rate and deceleration of ischemic transmembrane ion shifts. A review of the literature[40] identified 1 randomized, double-blind study that demonstrated improved neuropsychological outcomes in cardiac surgery patients receiving lidocaine. Clinical evidence of efficacy in DCI is limited to anecdotal reports. Some case studies of patients suffering from neurologic DCS have shown recovery even when the patient was recompressed with significant delay or had been refractory to recompression therapy.[41–43] A first retrospective cohort study has been published and found no effect of lidocaine on outcome.[44] Lidocaine is not considered part of the routine therapy for DCS but may be considered as an adjunctive agent for severe cerebral DCS or cerebral AGE.

MEDICAL EVACUATION TO THE HYPERBARIC CHAMBER

If aircraft medical evacuation is used to transfer the patient to the hyperbaric chamber, care should be taken to expose the patient to the least possible reduction in atmospheric pressure. Depressurization would cause further inert gas bubbles expansion and can worsen the condition. Recommendations include flying as low as safely possible for unpressurized aircraft or helicopter (preferably lower than 300 m [1000 ft]) or pressurizing the aircraft to sea level pressure, if possible.

Portable hyperbaric chambers (or hyperbaric stretchers) are sometimes available for recompression treatment in remote locations or for transport (**Figs. 7** and **8**). These devices are generally made of Kevlar and can be pressurized up to 3 ATA. Pressurized air and oxygen are provided via portable gas cylinders. The use of these devices is most appropriate for stable patients with mild to moderate symptoms. They do introduce serious limitations in monitoring and access of patients.

ALTERNATIVE TREATMENT TECHNIQUE: IN-WATER RECOMPRESSION

In-water recompression may be an alternative to chamber recompression in remote locations, if there is neither a nearby chamber nor the means to quickly transport the patient to a chamber elsewhere. The technique involves bringing the diver underwater again, to drive gas bubbles back into solution to reduce symptoms and then slowly decompress in a way that maintains an orderly elimination of the excess gas.

Although in-water recompression is simple in concept, it is practical only with a substantial amount of planning, support, equipment, and personnel; appropriate water conditions; and suitable patient status. Critical challenges can arise due to changes in the patient's consciousness, oxygen toxicity, gas supply, and even thermal stress. An unsuccessful in-water recompression may leave the patient in worse shape than had the attempt not been made. The medical and research communities are divided

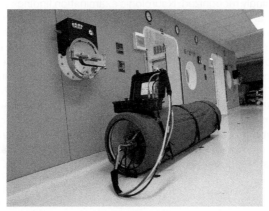

Fig. 7. A hyperbaric stretcher set up in front of a multiplace, multilock hyperbaric chamber. (*Courtesy of* D. Buteau, MD, Quebec City.)

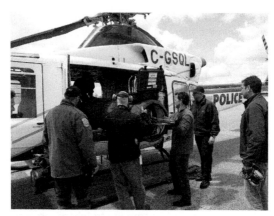

Fig. 8. A hyperbaric stretcher being loaded onto a helicopter. (*Courtesy of* D. Buteau, MD, Quebec City.)

on the utility of in-water recompression. It is beyond the scope of this article to consider all of the relevant factors but it is fair to say that there are probably more situations when in-water recompression should not be undertaken than situations when it would be a reasonable choice.

As a general rule, a diver who develops symptoms consistent with DCS should be removed from the water and receive oxygen first aid on the surface, even if there is likely to be a delay before definitive medical care can be reached.

SUMMARY

DCI represents a relatively rare affliction but a major concern for divers because of the potential severity of the insult and risk of sequelae. Decompression risk is primarily determined by the pressure-time profile and breathing gas but it is also influenced by the timing, intensity, and nature of thermal stressors during a dive, and by individual predispositions.

Signs and symptoms can vary substantially, causing insult to many systems. They frequently involve much more than the classic description of joint pain, with neurologic symptoms increasingly recognized. Neurologic examination findings can be confusing. History and physical examination are critical to evaluation. Symptoms will not develop during the bottom phase of a dive, before decompression. Symptoms of AGE typically present soon after surfacing, normally within 10 minutes. Symptoms of DCS normally appear within 6 hours after surfacing but they may not become apparent for more than 24 hours. Many other medical conditions need to be considered in the differential diagnosis.

High-concentration oxygen is the best first aid for both DCS and AGE. HBOT is the normal definitive medical treatment. The most commonly used and highly effective hyperbaric treatment protocol is the USN TT 6. The search for adjunctive therapies continues but none have been convincingly supported. Early consultation with diving medicine specialists is recommended.

REFERENCES

1. Dardeau MR, Pollock NW, McDonald CM, et al. The incidence rate of decompression illness in 10 years of scientific diving. Diving Hyperb Med 2012;42:195–200.

2. Vann RD, Denoble PJ, Uguccioni DM, et al. Report on decompression illness, diving fatalities and project dive exploration. Durham (NC): Divers Alert Network; 2004. p. 149.

3. Vann RD, Freiberger JJ, Caruso JL, et al. Report on decompression illness, diving fatalities and project dive exploration. Durham (NC): Divers Alert Network; 2005. p. 138.

4. Pollock NW, Dunford RG, Denoble PJ, et al. Annual diving report - 2008 edition. Durham (NC): Divers Alert Network; 2008. p. 139.

5. Imbert JP, Fructus X, Montbarbon S. Short and repetitive decompressions in air diving procedure: the commercial diving experience. In: Lang MA, Vann RD, editors. Proceedings of repetitive diving workshop. Costa Mesa (CA): American Academy of Underwater Sciences; 1992. p. 63–72.

6. Luby J. A study of decompression sickness after commercial air diving in the Northern Arabian Gulf: 1993-95. Occup Med (Lond) 1999;49:279–83.

7. Vann RD, Butler FK, Mitchell SJ, et al. Decompression illness. Lancet 2011;377: 153–64.

8. Elliott DH, Moon RE. Manifestations of the decompression disorders. In: Bennett PB, Elliott DH, editors. The physiology and medicine of diving. 4th edition. London: WB Saunders; 1993. p. 481–505.

9. Gerth WA, Ruterbusch VL, Long ET. The influence of thermal exposure on diver susceptibility to decompression sickness. Panama City (FL): Navy Experimental Diving Unit; 2007. p. 70. NEDU Report TR 06-07.

10. Fahlman A, Dromsky DM. Dehydration effects on the risk of severe decompression sickness in a swine model. Aviat Space Environ Med 2006;77:102–6.

11. Rudge FW, Stone JA. The use of the pressure cuff test in the diagnosis of decompression sickness. Aviat Space Environ Med 1991;62:266–7.

12. Boussuges A. Hemoconcentration in neurological decompression illness. Int J Sports Med 1996;17:351–5.

13. Koch GH, Weisbrod GL, Lepawsky M, et al. Chest radiographs can assist in the diagnosis of pulmonary barotrauma. Undersea Biomed Res 1991;18(Suppl):100.

14. Warren LP, Djang WT, Moon RE, et al. Neuroimaging of scuba diving injuries to the CNS. Am J Roentgenol 1988;151:1003–8.

15. Levin HS, Goldstein FC, Norcross K, et al. Neurobehavorial and magnetic resonance findings in in two cases of decompression sickness. Aviat Space Environ Med 1989;60:1204–10.

16. Moon RE, Massey EW, Debatin JF, et al. Radiographic imaging in neurological decompression illness. Undersea Biomed Res 1992;19(Suppl):42.

17. Reuter M, Tetzlaff K, Hutzelmann A, et al. MR imaging of the central nervous system in diving-related decompression illness. Acta Radiol 1997;38:940–4.

18. Grønning M, Risberg J, Skeidsvoll H, et al. Electroencephalography and magnetic resonance imaging in neurological decompression sickness. Undersea Hyperb Med 2005;32:397–402.

19. Gempp E, Blatteau JE, Stephant E, et al. MRI findings and clinical outcome in 45 divers with spinal cord decompression sickness. Aviat Space Environ Med 2008; 79:1112–6.

20. Gempp E, Morin J, Louge P, et al. Reliability of plasma D-dimers for predicting severe neurological decompression sickness in scuba divers. Aviat Space Environ Med 2012;83:771–5.

21. Thom SR, Milovanova TN, Bogush M, et al. Microparticle production, neutrophil activation and intravascular bubbles following open-water scuba diving. J Appl Physiol 2012;112:1268–78.

22. Thom SR, Milovanova TN, Bogush M, et al. Bubbles, microparticles and neutrophil activation: changes with exercise level and breathing gas during open-water scuba diving. J Appl Physiol 2013;114:1396–405.

23. Longphre JM, Denoble PJ, Moon RE, et al. First aid normobaric oxygen for the treatment of recreational diving injuries. Undersea Hyperb Med 2007;34:43–9.

24. Loveman GAM, Seddon FM, Jurd KM, et al. First aid oxygen treatment for decompression illness in the goat after simulated submarine escape. Aerosp Med Hum Perform 2015;86:1020–7.

25. Pollock NW, Natoli MJ. Performance characteristics of the second-generation remote emergency medical oxygen closed-circuit rebreather. Wilderness Environ Med 2007;18:86–92.

26. Pollock NW, Natoli MJ. Chemical oxygen generation: evaluation of the Green Dot Systems, Inc. portable non-pressurized emOx device. Wilderness Environ Med 2010;21:244–9.

27. US Navy Diving Manual, Volume 2, Revision 6. NAVSEA 0910-LP-106–0957. Washington, DC: Naval Sea Systems Command; 2008. Available at: http://www.scribd.com/doc/8162578/US-Navy-Diving-Manual-Revision-6-PDF#scribd.

28. Doolette DJ, Mitchell SJ. Recreational technical diving part 2: decompression from deep technical dives. Diving Hyperb Med 2013;43:96–104.

29. Mitchell SJ, Doolette DJ. Recreational technical diving part 1: an introduction to technical diving methods and activities. Diving Hyperb Med 2013;43:86–93.

30. Warren BA, Philip PB, Inwood MJ. The ultrastructural morphology of air embolism: platelet adhesion to the interface and endothelial damage. Br J Exp Pathol 1973; 54:163–72.

31. Hallenbeck JM, Dutka AJ, Tanishima T, et al. Polymorphonuclear leukocyte accumulation in brain regions with low blood flow during the early postischemic period. Stroke 1986;17:246–53.

32. Bessereau J, Genotelle N, Brun PM, et al. Decompression sickness in urban divers in France. Int Marit Health 2012;63:170–3.

33. Reeves E, Workman RD. Use of heparin for therapeutic/prophylactic treatment of decompression sickness. Aerosp Med 1971;42:20–3.

34. Evaniew N, Noonan VK, Fallah N, et al. RHSCIR Network. Methylprednisolone for the treatment of patients with acute spinal cord injuries: a propensity score-matched cohort study from a Canadian multi-center spinal cord injury registry. J Neurotrauma 2015;32:1674–83.

35. Bracken MB. Steroids for acute spinal cord injury. Cochrane Database Syst Rev 2012;(1):CD001046.

36. Bowers CA, Kundu B, Hawryluk GW. Methylprednisolone for acute spinal cord injury: an increasingly philosophical debate. Neural Regen Res 2016;11:882–5.

37. Bennett M, Mitchell SJ, Dominguez A. Adjunctive treatment of decompression illness with a non-steroidal anti-inflammatory drug (Tenoxicam) reduces compression requirement. Undersea Hyperb Med 2003;30:195–205.

38. Hallenbeck JM, Leitch DR, Dutka AJ, et al. Prostaglandin I2, indomethacin, and heparin promote postischemic neuronal recovery in dogs. Ann Neurol 1982;12: 145–56.

39. Kochanek PM, Dutka AJ, Kumaroo KK, et al. Effects of prostacyclin, indomethacin, and heparin on cerebral blood flow and platelet adhesion after multifocal ischemia of canine brain. Stroke 1988;19:693–9.

40. Mitchell SJ. Lidocaine in the treatment of decompression illness: a review of the literature. Undersea Hyperb Med 2001;28:165–74.

41. Drewry A, Gorman DF. Lidocaine as an adjunct to hyperbaric therapy in decompression illness: a case-report. Undersea Biomed Res 1992;19:187–90.
42. Cogar WB. Intravenous lidocaine as adjunctive therapy in the treatment of decompression illness. Ann Emerg Med 1997;29:284–6.
43. Mutzbauer TS, Ermisch J, Tetzlaff K, et al. Low dose lidocaine as adjunct for treatment of decompression illness. Undersea Hyperb Med 1999;26(suppl):15.
44. Weenink RP, Hollmann MW, Zomervrucht A, et al. A retrospective cohort study of lidocaine in divers with neurological decompression illness. Undersea Hyperb Med 2014;41:119–26.

Marine Envenomation

Kirsten B. Hornbeak, MD[a],*, Paul S. Auerbach, MD, MS[b]

KEYWORDS

- Marine envenomation • Marine antivenom • Jellyfish • Sea urchin • Sea snake
- Seabather's eruption • Crown-of-thorns • Stingray

KEY POINTS

- Know the marine organisms in your clinical practice area.
- Be prepared to treat anaphylaxis and acute life-threatening envenomations from box jellyfish, irukandji jellyfish, stonefish, cone snail, blue-ringed octopus, or sea snake.
- Know where and how to obtain antivenom.
- Decontamination is species specific and includes removing tentacles, embedded spines, and foreign bodies.
- Attempt pain control with species-specific treatments, including 5% acetic acid (vinegar), hot water immersion, and saline rinse.

INTRODUCTION

Venomous aquatic animals are hazardous to swimmers, surfers, divers, and fishermen. Most marine exposures are mild, so victims may not seek medical care. These exposures include mild stings, bites, abrasions, and lacerations. Severe envenomations from box jellyfish, irukandji jellyfish, cone snails, blue-ringed octopus, stonefish, or sea snakes can be life threatening. In these cases, rapid effective treatment improves immediate outcomes (decrease pain, stabilize systemic symptoms, treat anaphylaxis) and minimizes secondary complications (local allergic response, infection, wound complications). Treatment recommendations evolve in response to acquisition of data, clinical observations, and expert opinion. This article outlines recent management and treatment recommendations for marine envenomations. For the treatment of all envenomations, apply appropriate tetanus immunization. Consider prophylactic or therapeutic antibiotics.

Disclosure Statement: The authors have nothing to disclose.
[a] Department of Emergency Medicine, Stanford Kaiser Emergency Medicine Residency, 300 Pasteur Drive, Alway Building M121, MC 5119, Stanford, CA 94305-2200, USA; [b] Department of Emergency Medicine, Stanford University School of Medicine, 300 Pasteur Drive, Alway Building M121, MC 5119, Stanford, CA 94305-2200, USA
* Corresponding author.
E-mail address: khornbeak@gmail.com

Emerg Med Clin N Am 35 (2017) 321–337
http://dx.doi.org/10.1016/j.emc.2016.12.004
0733-8627/17/© 2016 Elsevier Inc. All rights reserved.

emed.theclinics.com

SPONGES
Epidemiology

Sponges (phylum Porifera) are acellular creatures that attach to the ocean floor. They carry spicules of silicon dioxide or calcium carbonate. Many produce dermal irritants known as crinotoxins.[1] Typical offenders include the fire sponge (*Tedania ignis*), poison bun sponge (*Fibularia nolitangere*), and red moss sponge (*Mammillaria prolifera*).[2]

Presentation

Spicules and crinotoxins enter the skin, causing edema, vesiculation, joint swelling, and stiffness. Mild reactions subside within 7 days. Extensive exposure may induce fever, chills, malaise, dizziness, nausea, muscle cramps, and formication. Retained spicules can result in persistent bullae that take months to heal. Delayed systemic erythema multiforme or dyshidrotic eczema may develop. In severe cases, surface desquamation may follow.[3]

Treatment

Remove spicules using adhesive tape, a thin layer of rubber cement, or facial peel. Apply 5% acetic acid (vinegar) soaks. Steroid cream or an oral antihistamine may provide symptomatic relief. Consider systemic corticosteroids for severe allergy, erythema multiforme, or dyshidrotic eczema. Arrange wound checks because infections may develop requiring antibiotic therapy (**Table 1**).[4]

CNIDARIA

The phylum Cnidaria is divided into four main groups: (1) hydrozoans, including feather hydroids, fire corals, and Portuguese man-of-war; (2) scyphozoans, such as true jellyfish; (3) anthozoans, such as soft corals and anemones; and (4) cubozoans, such as box jellyfish and irukandji.[5]

Hydroids and Fire Coral

Epidemiology
Hydrozoans are multiorganism colonies of diverse configurations. Feather hydroids are plumelike species found in tropical waters. Fire coral has an appearance similar to hard coral. An example is *Millepora*, distributed in shallow tropical waters and dangling tiny nematocyst-bearing tentacles.[6] The stinging tentacle-bearing Portuguese man-of-war (*Physalia physalis*) and blue bottle (*Physalia utriculus*) are widely distributed.

Presentation
Feather hydroids and fire coral cause immediate pain and urticaria, sometimes progressing to hemorrhagic or ulcerating lesions. Pain usually resolves by 90 minutes and inflammation resolves by 1 week, with occasional residual hyperpigmentation.[7] Portuguese man-of-war and bluebottle envenomations cause immediate intense pain and linear rashes, with vesiculation and necrosis. Pain improves within hours, and local symptoms resolve within 72 hours.[8] More severe systemic symptoms include nausea, vomiting, muscle cramps, dyspnea, anxiety, abdominal pain, and headache.

Treatment
For feather hydroid and fire coral envenomations, apply acetic acid 5% (vinegar) to the skin.[9] Consider steroid cream or an oral antihistamine for symptomatic relief; if the

Table 1
Presentation and treatment of envenomation by dermal contact

Species	Presentation	Treatment
Portuguese man-of-war; blue bottle	Local pain, skin blisters, nausea, vomiting, abdominal pain, muscle cramps, dyspnea	Remove tentacles Hot water (upper limit 45°C) immersion
Box jellyfish	Excruciating pain, hypotension, paralysis, respiratory failure, cardiac arrest, skin blisters and necrosis	Apply acetic acid 5% then remove tentacles Support airway and breathing Antivenom if severe symptoms *Avoid hot water immersion or pressure immobilization*
Irukandji jellyfish	Catecholamine release, muscle pain, abdominal pain, hypertension, troponin leak, heart failure, pulmonary edema	Remove tentacles Apply acetic acid 5% Cardiac monitoring Blood pressure control (*avoid β-adrenergic blockers*) Respiratory support
Jellyfish	Mild pain, irritant dermatitis	Remove tentacles Apply acetic acid 5%, lidocaine-containing product, or hot water (upper limit 45°C) immersion
Seabather's eruption	Pruritic papules resembling insect bites in distribution of swim suit	Treat skin with acetic acid 5%, or lidocaine-containing first aid remedy Wash swim suit with hot water and detergent, then machine or sun dry
Sea anemone	Erythema and pruritus Petechiae, blisters, and ulceration	Acetic acid 5% May require prolonged wound care
Feather hydroid; fire coral	Stinging pain, urticaria, petechiae, ulceration, residual hyperpigmentation	Acetic acid 5% May require prolonged wound care
Sponge	Pruritic irritant dermatitis, blisters, delayed desquamation	Remove spicules with tape, rubber cement, or facial peel Acetic acid 5%
Bristle worm	Painful urticarial rash	Remove bristles with tape, rubber cement, or facial peel Acetic acid 5%

reaction is eczematous or indolent, administer systemic corticosteroids. Portuguese man-of-war and bluebottle envenomation treatment is controversial. Acetic acid 5% is shown to worsen cnidocyst discharge in vitro, although some patients report symptomatic relief. A lidocaine-containing product may be equally effective. Recent research supports rinsing with seawater or saline followed by hot water (45°C) immersion.[10] Consider topical steroid cream or ointment; an antihistamine; and for severe reactions, a systemic corticosteroid taper over 14 days (see **Table 1**).[11]

Jellyfish

Epidemiology
Scyphozoans are single-organism jellyfish that range in size from 2 cm to 2 m across the bell and have different forms, including free-floating larva, sessile polyp, and large swimming medusa (**Fig. 1**).[12] Mauve stingers (*Pelagia*) are common in US Pacific

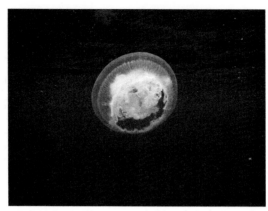

Fig. 1. Medusa form of the moon jellyfish (*Aurelia aurita*). (*Courtesy of* Kirsten B. Hornbeak, MD, Stanford, CA.)

Ocean coastal waters.[13] The large lion's mane jellyfish (*Cyanea capillata*) inhabits cold Arctic and Pacific waters. Stinging larval forms of multiple species are found in warm waters; these notably include pinhead-sized larvae of the thimble jellyfish (*Linuche unguiculata*).[14]

Presentation
Contact with tentacles causes stinging pain and localized erythema that resolve in hours to days. Contact with the larval forms can cause seabather's eruption; pruritic papules resembling bug bites in a bathing suit distribution (within which larvae are trapped) itch and annoy for 2 to 14 days.[15] Other symptoms include fever, headache, chills, malaise, vomiting, conjunctivitis, and urethritis.

Treatment
Management of scyphozoan stings is identical to that for any cnidarian sting, namely, topical acetic acid 5%, hot water immersion, and corticosteroid or antihistamine cream, and in severe cases a systemic corticosteroid.[16] A lidocaine-containing product may be effective as a topical decontaminant. To minimize or prevent seabather's eruption, change swimwear on leaving the water. Use a hot water laundering scrub with detergent and full drying before reuse (see **Table 1**).[2]

Sea Anemones

Epidemiology
Sea anemones and soft corals have tentacles loaded with stinging cnidocytes and secrete mucus that may contain cytolytic and hemolytic toxins, neurotoxins, cardiotoxins, and proteinase inhibitors.[17,18]

Presentation
Victims experience painful skin lesions with central pallor and a halo of erythema and petechial hemorrhage, sometimes progressing to vesiculation and necrosis. Rare systemic reactions include fever, chills, malaise, weakness, nausea, vomiting, muscle spasm, and syncope. Mild envenomations resolve within 48 hours. Severe reactions may become indolent, leading to hyperpigmentation, hypopigmentation, or keloid formation.[17]

Treatment

Treatment of anemone envenomation is similar to that for cnidarian sting (discussed previously). Severe dermatitis may require prolonged wound care with debridement and antibiotics for secondary infection (see **Table 1**).

Box-Shaped Jellyfish

Epidemiology

Some highly venomous box-shaped jellyfish inhabit tropical waters. These include the Hawaiian box jellyfish (*Carybdea alata*), Japanese box jellyfish (*Chironex yamaguchi*), and Australian box jellyfish (*Chironex fleckeri*).[19] Each delivers potentially deadly venom.[20]

Irukandji jellyfish are 1 cm to 2.5 cm box jellyfish and include *Carukia barnesii* and *Malo* species.[21] The "irukandji syndrome" is local vasoconstriction and high blood pressure attributed to sympathetic nervous system stimulation.[22]

Presentation

Box jellyfish stings are excruciating with rapid blistering, muscle spasm, hypotension, and sometimes paralysis. Victims collapse in 1 to 2 minutes from respiratory failure and cardiac arrest. Most deaths occur 5 to 20 minutes after the sting.[23] Skin necrosis is common.

Irukandji envenomation symptoms begin 20 to 30 minutes post sting with muscle pain, abdominal and chest pain, nausea, vomiting, and respiratory failure. Massive catecholamine release causes severe hypertension and tachycardia, leading to cardiomyopathy, pulmonary edema, cerebral edema, troponin leak, and hypokinetic heart failure.[24] Two deaths have occurred because of intracerebral hemorrhage.[25] Symptoms resolve in 6 to 24 hours.

Treatment

If box jellyfish sting is suspected, support the airway and provide artificial ventilation. Immediately flood sting sites with 5% acetic acid (vinegar) for at least 30 seconds before removing adherent tentacles. Avoid contamination of rescue personnel.[16] Administer specific antivenom one vial intravenous (IV) or introsseous 5 minutes, or three vials intramuscular (IM) at three different sites.[8] Repeat as needed every 10 minutes up to three times immediately and then once or twice every 2 to 4 hours until there is no further progression of systemic symptoms. Antivenom use is under scrutiny because of poor efficacy noted during in vitro studies.[26] However, until further notice it remains recommended.

For irukandji envenomation, in addition to standard cnidarian envenomation treatment measures and supportive therapy, serum troponin and cardiac monitoring should be obtained. β-Adrenergic blockers should not be used because these might contribute to unopposed α-adrenergic stimulation and myocardial ischemia (see **Table 1**).[27]

ANNELID WORMS
Epidemiology

Bristle worms (phylum Annelida, class Polychaeta) are covered with chitinous bristles that easily penetrate skin.

Presentation

Human contact causes bristles to break off into the skin, causing pricking sensation and urticarial rash with rare necrosis. Pain remits with a few hours, but urticaria may last for 2 to 3 days and skin discoloration for up to 10 days. Secondary infection and cellulitis may occur.[28]

Treatment

Bristles should be removed with tape, facial peel, or a thin layer of rubber cement. Next, apply acetic acid 5% soaks. If the inflammatory reaction is severe, consider an oral antihistamine or corticosteroid (see **Table 1**).

STARFISH AND SEA URCHINS
Epidemiology

The phylum Echinodermata includes starfish and sea urchins. The crown-of-thorns starfish (*Acanthaster planci*) is particularly venomous and produces a toxic slime that coats the spines (**Fig. 2**). Venom is hemolytic, myonecrotic, hepatotoxic, and anticoagulant.[29]

Sea urchins have globular bodies covered by calcified spines either rounded at the tip or hollow and venom-bearing (**Fig. 3**).[30] They may have pedicellariae (modified spines with flexible heads) that grasp to envenom. Various urchin venoms have been found to contain steroid glycosides, hemolysins, proteases, serotonin, and cholinergic substances.[31]

Presentation

Crown-of-thorns starfish cause puncture wounds with immediate pain, bleeding, and edema. Wounds become dusky and tenosynovitis may develop. Multiple punctures can cause systemic reactions with paresthesias, nausea, vomiting, lymphadenopathy, and paralysis. Pain resolves in 30 minutes to 3 hours. Retained spines can cause granulomas.[32]

Sea urchins cause painful puncture wounds with severe local muscle aching lasting up to 24 hours.[33] Frequently, spines break off into the victim. A spine in a joint can cause synovitis.[30] Systemic symptoms include nausea, vomiting, paresthesias,

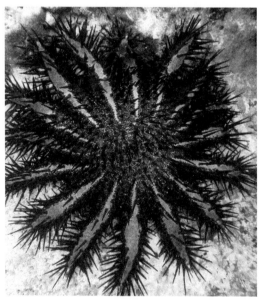

Fig. 2. Spines on the crown-of-thorns sea star (*Acanthaster planci*). (*Courtesy of* Kirsten B. Hornbeak, MD, Stanford, CA.)

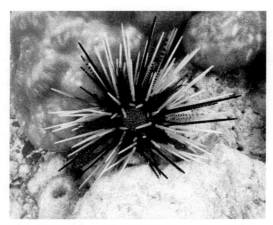

Fig. 3. Spines of the banded sea urchin (*Echinothrix calamaris*). (*Courtesy of* Kirsten B. Hornbeak, MD, Stanford, CA.)

weakness, abdominal pain, syncope, hypotension, and respiratory distress. Secondary infections are common. Granulomas may develop.[34]

Treatment

The puncture wounds should immediately be immersed in hot water to tolerance (upper limit 45°C) for 30 to 90 minutes or until there is significant pain relief. Local anesthetic infiltration or a nerve block may be required. Wounds should be irrigated and explored and spines removed if they are easily reached. Dark discoloration may indicate dye in the tissues in the absence of a spine. If this is the case, the discoloration disappears in 24 to 48 hours. If spines have entered a joint or are close to neurovascular structures a surgeon should be consulted and the joint splinted.[35] Radiography, ultrasound, computed tomography, or MRI may be helpful in spine localization and removal.[30] Reactive neuropathy may respond to a systemic corticosteroid. Secondary infections are common. Granulomas from retained spine fragments may require excision or ablation, and arthritis from retained spines may require synovectomy (**Table 2**).[36]

MOLLUSKS
Epidemiology

Cone snails (genus *Conus*) are shelled mollusks.[37] Envenomation occurs when the proboscis extends to allow a venom-containing radular tooth to stab the victim. Conotoxins target receptors and channels that mediate neuromuscular blockade.[38]

Blue-ringed octopuses have iridescent blue rings, measure less than 20 cm, and are found in shallow waters throughout Indo-Pacific oceans. A parrot-like beak injects venom that causes paralysis.[39]

Presentation

Cone snails cause a bee sting–like puncture wound with local cyanosis. Local paresthesias are followed by spreading paralysis that can lead to respiratory failure within 1 hour. Mild stings cause nausea, blurred vision, malaise, and weakness for a few hours. Paralysis from severe envenomation lasts 12 to 36 hours, with symptom resolution sometimes taking weeks.[40]

Blue-ringed octopus bites create one or two small puncture wounds that often go unnoticed. Within 15 minutes, oral and facial numbness begin that may rapidly

Table 2
Presentation and treatment of envenomation by puncture or laceration

Species	Presentation	Treatment
Crown-of-thorns starfish	Dusky puncture wound, pain, bleeding, edema Multiple punctures cause nausea, vomiting, paresthesias	Hot water to tolerance (maximum 45°C) for 30–90 min Local anesthetic Locate retained spines Surgical removal if spines near nerve, tendon, or joint
Sea urchin	Red, purple, or black puncture wounds; local muscle aching; edema Multiple punctures cause nausea, vomiting, paresthesias	Hot water to tolerance (maximum 45°C) for 30–90 min Local anesthetic Locate retained spines Surgical removal if spines near nerve, tendon, or joint
Cone snail	Puncture wound resembling bee sting, local cyanosis, limb paresthesias, paralysis, respiratory failure, cerebral edema, coma	Pressure immobilization Support breathing Consider edrophonium, 10 mg IV, for paralysis Consider naloxone, 2–4 mg, for severe hypotension Hot water to tolerance (maximum 45°C) for 30–90 min Local anesthetic Remove retained radula
Blue-ringed octopus	Painless small puncture wounds, facial numbness, paralysis, respiratory failure	Support breathing Supportive care
Lionfish and scorpionfish	Painful puncture wound, blistering, nausea, vomiting	Hot water to tolerance (maximum 45°C) for 30–90 min Local anesthetic or nerve block Locate retained spines Surgical removal if spines near nerve, tendon, or joint
Stonefish	Severely painful cyanotic puncture wound, necrotic ulceration, altered mentation, fever, nausea, vomiting, seizures, paralysis, heart block, heart failure, pulmonary edema	Antivenom for severe envenomation Hot water to tolerance (maximum 45°C) for 30–90 min Local anesthetic or nerve block Locate retained spines Surgical removal if spines near nerve, tendon, or joint Debride necrotic tissue
Stingray	Dusky painful laceration, local hemorrhage and necrosis, barb lodged in victim Large envenomation: nausea, vomiting, muscle cramps, syncope, arrhythmias	Hot water to tolerance (maximum 45°C) for 30–90 min Local anesthetic or nerve block Locate retained barb Surgical removal of barb Treat retained barb as stab wound if barb in thorax, abdomen, groin, or neck Serial debridement of necrotic tissue

(continued on next page)

Table 2 (continued)		
Species	**Presentation**	**Treatment**
Sea snake	Painless pinhead-sized fang marks, muscle pain and stiffness, nausea, vomiting, ascending paralysis, respiratory failure, muscle necrosis, renal failure	Pressure immobilization Maintain airway and breathing Antivenom if any symptom Monitor electrolytes and urine output Alkalinize urine if myoglobinuria Dialysis as needed for renal failure and hyperkalemia

progress to paralysis and respiratory failure.[41] Cardiac arrest may follow. Other symptoms include numbness and discomfort of the affected limb, nausea, vomiting, and chest tightness.[42]

Treatment

For cone snail envenomation, cardiovascular and respiratory support take priority. Pressure immobilization is recommended during transport. Edrophonium (10 mg IV adult dose) has been suggested for paralysis. Adverse reactions to edrophonium are treated with atropine, 0.6 mg IV. Naloxone, 2 to 4 mg, has been suggested to treat hypotension. The wound should be soaked in hot water to tolerance (upper limit 45°C) for 30 to 90 minutes. Consider local anesthetic injection. The wound should be irrigated and foreign bodies (radula) removed.

Treatment of blue-ringed octopus bite centers on cardiovascular and respiratory support. Be prepared to provide artificial ventilation. Paralysis lasts 4 to 10 hours, after which the victim who has not suffered significant hypoxia improves rapidly, with complete recovery in 2 to 4 days (see **Table 2**).[41]

SCORPIONFISH
Epidemiology

The family Scorpaenidae has members with spines and associated venom glands covered by integumentary sheaths. Lionfish (*Pterois*) are the least toxic, followed by scorpionfish (*Scorpaena*) with moderate toxicity, and stonefish (*Synanceja*) with potent toxicity.[43] Lionfish (*Pterois*) are beautiful, with long slender spines (**Fig. 4**). Venom may induce local paresthesias and paralysis.[44] Scorpionfish are camouflaged against their surroundings (ocean bottom and rocks) and have medium-length spines. In experimental animals, venom degrades connective tissue, leads to hypotension and pulmonary edema, and can cause paralysis.[45] Stonefish hide motionless and possess short stout spines. Their venom is highly toxic.[46]

Presentation

Pain is immediate and peaks at 60 to 90 minutes. With serious envenomation, pain may cause delirium and persist for hours (scorpionfish) or days (stonefish).[47] The puncture wound is initially ischemic and cyanotic with progressive vesiculation, tissue sloughing, cellulitis, and necrotic ulceration.[48] Systemic effects include anxiety, headache, skin rash, fever, nausea and vomiting, diarrhea, abdominal pain, seizures, paralysis, pericarditis, atrioventricular block, congestive heart failure, and pulmonary edema.[49] Death from a stonefish sting can occur within the first 6 to 8 hours. Wounds are often indolent and may require months to heal.

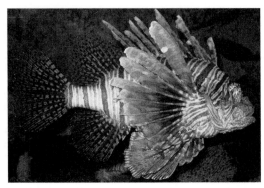

Fig. 4. Spines of the common lionfish (*Pterois miles*). (*Courtesy of* Kirsten B. Hornbeak, MD, Stanford, CA.)

Treatment

The wound should be immersed in hot water to tolerance (upper limit 45°C) for at least 30 to 90 minutes. Consider local anesthetic infiltration or regional nerve block. The wound should be thoroughly cleansed. If the spine has penetrated deeply into the sole of the foot or hand, surgical exploration should be performed. In a case of severe systemic reaction, stonefish antivenom may be administered IV or IM.[50] As a rough estimate, one vial of antivenom should neutralize one or two significant punctures, with additional vials administered for recurrent severe pain or systemic manifestations (see **Table 2**).[51]

STINGRAYS
Epidemiology

Stingrays are flat cartilaginous fish with caudal appendages harboring bilaterally retroserrate barbs and associated venom glands (**Fig. 5**). Venom contains serotonin, 5'-nucleotidase, and phosphodiesterase.[52] Toxin may induce peripheral vasoconstriction, bradycardia, tachycardia, atrioventricular block, and seizure activity.[53]

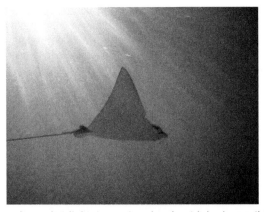

Fig. 5. Australian eagle ray (*Myliobatis tenuicaudatus*), with barb at tail base. (*Courtesy of* Kirsten B. Hornbeak, MD, Stanford, CA.)

Presentation

Stingray envenomations can cause large lacerations, most often on lower extremities. In rare cases the heart is punctured.[54] There is intense pain, edema, and bleeding peaking at 30 to 60 minutes and lasting up to 48 hours. The wound is initially dusky and may progress to hemorrhagic necrosis.[55] Systemic manifestations include weakness, nausea, vomiting, diarrhea, diaphoresis, muscle cramps, headache, syncope, seizures, and arrhythmias.[56]

Treatment

For pain relief, soak in hot water to tolerance (upper limit 45°C) for 30 to 90 minutes.[57] Narcotics, local anesthetic infiltration, or a nerve block may be needed. The wound should be irrigated and debrided, and imaging obtained to rule out a retained spine.[58] If a spine is lodged in the chest, abdomen, or other vital structure it should be secured until surgical removal in the operating room.[59] Wounds are preferably treated with delayed primary closure and should be observed closely because ulceration, necrosis, and secondary infection are common (see **Table 2**).[60]

SEA SNAKES
Epidemiology

Sea snakes (family Hydrophiidae) inhabit tropical Pacific and Indian oceans.[61] Venom is similar across species. It contains peripheral neurotoxins acting at the acetylcholine receptor, and hemolytic and myotoxic compounds that cause muscle necrosis, hemolysis, and renal tubular damage.[62] Species implicated in serious envenomations include *Astrotia stokesii, Enhydrina schistosa, Hydrophis ornatus, Hydrophis cyanocinctus, Lapemis hardwickii, Thalassophina viperina*, and *Pelamis platurus*.[63] Because fangs are short and easily dislodged, approximately 80% of bites do not result in envenomation.[61]

Presentation

Sea snake bites cause minimal pain and may resemble mere pinpricks. In 30 to 60 minutes, nausea, muscle stiffness, swallowing dysfunction, blurry vision, and paralysis occur. Respiratory distress, paralysis, electrolyte disturbances, and myoglobinuria with acute renal failure contribute to the ultimate demise. If symptoms do not develop within 6 to 8 hours, there has rarely been envenomation. Mortality is 25% in victims who do not receive antivenom and 3% overall.[64]

Treatment

Apply pressure immobilization during transport. Administer sea snake antivenom IV as soon as possible.[50] Anticipate respiratory failure and provide mechanical ventilation. Monitor serum electrolytes and renal function because hyperkalemia, rhabdomyolysis, and renal dysfunction are common. If myoglobinuria is detected, alkalinize urine with sodium bicarbonate and administer diuretics. Acute renal failure may require dialysis[61] (see **Table 2**).

TREATMENT RESISTANCE AND COMPLICATIONS
Antivenom and Anaphylaxis

An envenomation or antivenom administration can cause anaphylaxis. Signs include hypotension, bronchospasm, facial and airway swelling, pruritus, urticaria, nausea, vomiting, and diarrhea. Most reactions occur within 15 to 30 minutes and nearly all occur within 6 hours.[65]

A recipient of antivenom should be pretreated with 50 to 100 mg of IV diphenhydramine (1 mg/kg in children). The initial dose of antivenom should be administered no faster than one vial over 5 minutes. If anaphylaxis develops, 0.1- to 0.2-mL aliquots of antivenom should be alternated with 0.03- to 0.1-mg IV doses of epinephrine, or an epinephrine drip administered, titrating to maintain heart rate less than 150 beats/min.

Serum Sickness

Formation of IgG antibodies in response to antigens in antivenom causes deposition of immune complexes that induce vascular permeability, activate complement, degranulate mast cells, and trigger release of proteolytic enzymes. Symptoms present within 8 to 24 days and include fever, arthralgias, malaise, urticaria, lymphadenopathy, rashes, peripheral neuritis, and swollen joints. Serum sickness is managed with systemic corticosteroids until symptoms resolve, followed by a 2-week taper.[66]

Patient evaluation overview

1. ABCs

2. Attempt to identify causative agent
   - Consider the geographic location where the injury took place
   - Wheal and flare reactions are nonspecific
   - Bug bite–type reaction located in areas of a swimsuit is classic for seabather's eruption
   - A gaping laceration, particularly of the lower extremity, with cyanotic edges suggests a stingray wound
   - Multiple punctures in an erratic pattern with or without purple discoloration or retained fragments are typical of a sea urchin sting
   - Fang marks with weakness, respiratory paralysis, myalgias, blurred vision, and vomiting indicate a sea snake bite
   - An ischemic puncture wound with a red halo and rapid swelling and pain not relieved by hot water immersion suggests scorpionfish envenomation
   - Blisters often accompany a lionfish sting
   - Painless punctures with rapid neuromuscular paralysis suggest a blue-ringed octopus bite
   - The site of a cone snail sting is punctate, painful, and ischemic
   - Rapid (within 24 hours) onset of skin necrosis suggests an anemone sting
   - "Tentacle prints" with cross-hatching suggest a box-jellyfish envenomation
   - Hypertension, muscle aches, and vomiting suggests irukandji syndrome
   - Ocular, intraoral, or genital lesions may come from fragmented hydroids, coelenterate tentacles, or scyphozoan larvae

3. Decontaminate (specific to causative organism)

4. Stabilize and treat

Surgical treatment options

- Debridement
- Spine extraction or laser ablation
- Tendon repair, synovectomy, or granuloma removal

Evaluation of outcome and long-term recommendations

1. Prevention
   - Do not touch marine life when snorkeling, diving, or swimming. Avoid touching the bottom or grasping ledges or overhangs.
   - Wear protective gear that covers all exposed skin.
   - Shuffle feet when walking in shallow sandy areas.
   - Do not stand or walk on reefs.
2. Life-threatening envenomations benefit from rapid decontamination and cardiopulmonary support, and may benefit from antivenom administration.
3. Provide tetanus prophylaxis in all cases and have a low threshold for initiating antibiotics.
4. Marine envenomations often heal slowly and poorly, so arrange for follow-up.

Special pharmacologic treatment options

Drug	Indications	Dosage
Acetic acid 5% (vinegar)	All-purpose skin sting decontaminant	Apply topically
Lidocaine or bupivicaine without epinephrine	Local anesthetic infiltration or nerve block for pain control	Lidocaine, max dose 3 mg/kg Bupivicaine, max dose 2.5 mg/kg
Prednisone (or equivalent corticosteroid)	Severe local inflammation or allergic reaction	60–100 mg PO QD adults 2–5 mg/kg (max dose 50 mg) children PO QD Tapered over 10–14 d
Hydrocortisone 1% cream	For local inflammation and symptomatic relief	Apply BID
Antibiotics	Prophylaxis for puncture wounds and at first sign of infection Should cover *Staphylococcus*, *Streptococcus*, and microbes of marine origin, such as *Vibrio*	Ciprofloxacin, 500 mg PO BID Trimethoprim/ sulfamethoazole, 160/ 800 mg PO BID Doxycycline, 100 mg PO BID
Stonefish antivenom	Hyperimmune horse globulin preparation used to neutralize stings of stonefish	Initial dose: 1 vial per two puncture wounds Repeat for recurrent pain
Box jellyfish antivenom	Hyperimmune sheep globulin preparation used to neutralize the stings of *Chironex fleckeri* and *Chiropsalmus*	Initial dose: 1 vial IV or 3 vials IM Repeat up to 3 times every 10 min as needed, and then every 2–4 h until no further worsening
Sea snake antivenom	Hyperimmune horse globulin preparation used to neutralize the bites of most sea snakes	Initial dose: 1–3 vials Up to 10 vials may be required

From Currie BJ. Marine antivenoms: antivenoms. J Toxicol 2003;41(3):301–8.

Nonpharmacologic treatment options		
Treatment	**Indication**	
Hot water immersion	Jellyfish Stingrays Venomous spined fish	Hot water to tolerance (maximum 45°C); immerse for 30–90 min or until pain relief; check water temperature frequently
Adhesive tape, rubber cement, facial peel	Sponge Bristle worm	Apply gently over wound and peel to remove spicules or bristles
Pressure immobilization	Cone snail Sea snake	Wrap an elastic bandage with a wide margin over the envenomation site at venous-lymphatic occlusive pressure; keep the limb immobile
Scrape with razor	Jellyfish, fire coral, hydroid, anemone	Apply a layer of shaving cream and scrape with a razor to remove nematocysts

SUMMARY

Know the marine creatures in your clinical practice area. Be prepared to act in cases of anaphylaxis or acute life-threatening envenomations from box jellyfish, irukandji jellyfish, stonefish, cone snail, blue-ringed octopus, or sea snake. Know where to obtain antivenom. Prompt topical decontamination (if available) should precede removal of tentacles. Provide adequate pain control. Secondary infection is common, so maintain a low threshold for initiating appropriate antibiotics applicable to marine bacteria.

REFERENCES

1. Abdel-Lateff A, Alarif WM, Asfour HZ, et al. Cytotoxic effects of three new metabolites from Red Sea marine sponge, Petrosia sp. Environ Toxicol Pharmacol 2014; 37(3):928–35.
2. Schwartz S, Meinking T. Venomous marine animals of Florida: morphology, behavior, health hazards. J Fla Med Assoc 1997;84(7):433–40.
3. Isbister GK, Hooper JNA. Clinical effects of stings by sponges of the genus Tedania and a review of sponge stings worldwide. Toxicon 2005;46(7):782–5.
4. Auerbach PS, Yajko DM, Nassos PS, et al. Bacteriology of the marine environment: implications for clinical therapy. Ann Emerg Med 1987;16(6):643–9.
5. Fautin DG. Structural diversity, systematics, and evolution of cnidae. Toxicon 2009;54(8):1054–64.
6. Labadie M, Aldabe B, Ong N, et al. Portuguese man-of-war (Physalia physalis) envenomation on the Aquitaine Coast of France: an emerging health risk. Clin Toxicol (Phila) 2012;50(7):567–70.
7. Brown CK, Shepherd SM. Marine trauma, envenomations, and intoxications. Emerg Med Clin North Am 1992;10(2):385–408.
8. Tibballs J. Australian venomous jellyfish, envenomation syndromes, toxins and therapy. Toxicon 2006;48(7):830–59.
9. Rifkin JF, Fenner PJ, Williamson JAH. First aid treatment of the sting from the hydroid Lytocarpus philippinus: the structure of, and in vitro discharge experiments with its nematocysts. Wilderness Environ Med 1993;4(3):252–60.
10. Li L, McGee RG, Webster AC. Pain from bluebottle jellyfish stings. J Paediatr Child Health 2015;51(7):734–7.

11. Ostermayer DG, Koyfman A. What is the most effective treatment for relieving the pain of a jellyfish sting? Ann Emerg Med 2015;65(4):432–3.
12. Daly M, Brugler MR, Cartwright P, et al. The phylum Cnidaria: a review of phylogenetic patterns and diversity 300 years after Linnaeus. Zootaxa 2007;1668: 127–82.
13. Mariottini GL, Giacco E, Pane L. The Mauve Stinger Pelagia noctiluca (Forsskål, 1775). Distribution, ecology, toxicity and epidemiology of stings. A Review. Mar Drugs 2008;6(3):496–513.
14. Rossetto AL, JeM Mora, Correa PR, et al. Seabathers eruption: report of the six cases in southern Brazil. Rev Soc Bras Med Trop 2007;40(1):78–81 [in Portuguese].
15. Tomchik RS, Russell MT, Szmant AM, et al. Clinical perspectives on seabather's eruption, also known as' sea lice'. JAMA 1993;269(13):1669–72.
16. Li L, McGee RG, Isbister G, et al. Interventions for the symptoms and signs resulting from jellyfish stings. Cochrane Database Syst Rev 2013;(12):CD009688.
17. Fraz√£o B, Vasconcelos V, Antunes A. Sea anemone (Cnidaria, Anthozoa, Actiniaria) toxins: an overview. Mar Drugs 2012;10(8):1812–51.
18. Suput D. In vivo effects of cnidarian toxins and venoms. Toxicon 2009;54(8): 1190–200.
19. Bentlage B, Peterson AT, Cartwright P. Inferring distributions of chirodropid box-jellyfishes (Cnidaria: Cubozoa) in geographic and ecological space using ecological niche modeling. Marine Ecology Progress Series 2009;384:121–33.
20. Brinkman DL, Konstantakopoulos N, McInerney BV, et al. Chironex fleckeri (Box Jellyfish) venom proteins expansion of a Cnidarian toxin family that elicits variable cytolytic and cardiovascular effects. J Biol Chem 2014;289(8):4798–812.
21. Little M, Mulcahy RF. A year's experience of Irukandji envenomation in far north Queensland. Med J Aust 1998;169:638–40.
22. Chaousis S, Smout M, Wilson D, et al. Rapid short term and gradual permanent cardiotoxic effects of vertebrate toxins from Chironex fleckeri (Australian box jellyfish) venom. Toxicon 2014;80:17–26.
23. Sutherland SK. Australian animal toxins: the creatures, their toxins and care of the poisoned patient. Melbourne (Australia): Oxford University Press; 1983.
24. Nickson CP, Waugh EB, Jacups SP, et al. Irukandji syndrome case series from Australia's tropical Northern Territory. Ann Emerg Med 2009;54(3):395–403.
25. Fenner PJ, Hadok JC. Fatal envenomation by jellyfish causing Irukandji syndrome. Med J Aust 2002;177(7):362–3.
26. Winter KL, Isbister GK, Jacoby T, et al. An in vivo comparison of the efficacy of CSL box jellyfish antivenom with antibodies raised against nematocyst-derived Chironex fleckeri venom. Toxicol Lett 2009;187(2):94–8.
27. Fenner P, Carney I. The Irukandji syndrome. A devastating syndrome caused by a north Australian jellyfish. Aust Fam Physician 1999;28(11):1131–7.
28. Kay M, Bak R, Kay D. Tropical aquarium aquatic dermatoses: bristle worm envenomation. Skinmed 2009;8(5):303–4.
29. azuo Shiomi K, Kazama A, Shimakura K, et al. Purification and properties of phospholipases A 2 from the crown-of-thorns starfish (Acanthaster planci) venom. Toxicon 1998;36(4):589–99.
30. Liram N, Gomori M, Perouansky M. Sea urchin puncture resulting in PIP joint synovial arthritis: case report and MRI study. J Travel Med 2000;7(1):43–5.
31. Nakagawa H, Tanigawa T, Tomita K, et al. Recent studies on the pathological effects of purified sea urchin toxins. J Toxicol 2003;22(4):633–49.

32. Adler M, Kaul A, Jawad A. Foreign body synovitis induced by a crown-of-thorns starfish. Rheumatology 2002;41(2):230–1.
33. Laird P. Sea-urchin injuries. Lancet 1995;346(8984):1240.
34. Kabigting FD, Kempiak S, Alexandrescu D, et al. Sea urchin granuloma secondary to *Strongylocentrotus purpuratus* and *Strongylocentrotus franciscanus*. Dermatol Online J 2008;15(5):9.
35. Nassab R, Rayatt S, Peart F. The management of hand injuries caused by sea urchin spines. J Hand Surg 2005;30(4):432–3.
36. Wada T, Soma T, Gaman K, et al. Sea urchin spine arthritis of the hand. J Hand Surg 2008;33(3):398–401.
37. Terlau H, Olivera BM. Conus venoms: a rich source of novel ion channel-targeted peptides. Physiol Rev 2004;84(1):41–68.
38. Espiritu DJD, Watkins M, Dia-Monje V, et al. Venomous cone snails: molecular phylogeny and the generation of toxin diversity. Toxicon 2001;39(12):1899–916.
39. Sheumack D, Howden M, Spence I, et al. Maculotoxin: a neurotoxin from the venom glands of the octopus Hapalochlaena maculosa identified as tetrodotoxin. Science 1978;199(4325):188–9.
40. Halford ZA, Yu PY, Likeman RK, et al. Cone shell envenomation: epidemiology, pharmacology and medical care. Diving Hyperb Med 2015;45(3):200–7.
41. Williamson JA. 18 The blue-ringed octopus bite and envenomation syndrome. Clin Dermatol 1987;5(3):127–33.
42. Cavazzoni E, Lister B, Sargent P, et al. Blue-ringed octopus (Hapalochlaena sp.) envenomation of a 4-year-old boy: a case report. Clin Toxicol (Phila) 2008;46(8):760–1.
43. Diaz JH. Marine scorpaenidae envenomation in travelers: epidemiology, management, and prevention. J Travel Med 2015;22(4):251–8.
44. Church JE, Hodgson WC. Adrenergic and cholinergic activity contributes to the cardiovascular effects of lionfish (Pterois volitans) venom. Toxicon 2002;40(6):787–96.
45. Boletini-Santos D, Komegae EN, Figueiredo SG, et al. Systemic response induced by Scorpaena plumieri fish venom initiates acute lung injury in mice. Toxicon 2008;51(4):585–96.
46. Khoo HE. Bioactive proteins from stonefish venom. Clin Exp Pharmacol Physiol 2002;29(9):802–6.
47. Haddad V, Martins IA, Makyama HM. Injuries caused by scorpionfishes (Scorpaena plumieri Bloch, 1789 and Scorpaena brasiliensis Cuvier, 1829) in the Southwestern Atlantic Ocean (Brazilian coast): epidemiologic, clinic and therapeutic aspects of 23 stings in humans. Toxicon 2003;42(1):79–83.
48. Patel M, Wells S. Lionfish envenomation of the hand. J Hand Surg 1993;18(3):523–5.
49. Brenneke F, Hatz C. Stonefish envenomation—a lucky outcome. Trav Med Infect Dis 2006;4(5):281–5.
50. Currie BJ. Marine antivenoms: antivenoms. J Toxicol 2003;41(3):301–8.
51. Kizer KW, McKinney HE, Auerbach PS. Scorpaenidae envenomation: a five-year poison center experience. JAMA 1985;253(6):807–10.
52. Dehghani H, Sajjadi MM, Rajaian H, et al. Study of patient's injuries by stingrays, lethal activity determination and cardiac effects induced by Himantura gerrardi venom. Toxicon 2009;54(6):881–6.
53. Kumar KR, Vennila R, Kanchana S, et al. Fibrinogenolytic and anticoagulant activities in the tissue covering the stingers of marine stingrays Dasyatis sephen and Aetobatis narinari. J Thromb Thrombolysis 2011;31(4):464–71.

54. Parra MW, Costantini EN, Rodas EB, et al. Surviving a transfixing cardiac injury caused by a stingray barb. J Thorac Cardiovasc Surg 2010;139(5):e115–6.
55. Barss P. Wound necrosis caused by the venom of stingrays. Pathological findings and surgical management. Med J Aust 1983;141(12–13):854–5.
56. Grainger C. Occupational injuries due to sting-rays. Trans R Soc Trop Med Hyg 1980;74(3):408.
57. Clark AT, Clark RF, Cantrell FL. A retrospective review of the presentation and treatment of stingray stings reported to a poison control system. Am J Ther 2016. [Epub ahead of print].
58. Diaz JH. The evaluation, management, and prevention of stingray injuries in travelers. J Travel Med 2008;15(2):102–9.
59. Jhamb S, Corsetti RL. Management of penetrating thoracoabdominal stingray trauma. Am Surg 2013;79(2):E54–5.
60. Flint D, Sugrue W. Stingray injuries: a lesson in debridement. N Z Med J 1999; 112(1086):137–8.
61. McGoldrick J, Marx JA. Marine envenomations. Part 1: vertebrates. J Emerg Med 1991;9(6):497–502.
62. Walker MJ, Yeoh PN. The in vitro neuromuscular blocking properties of sea snake (Enhydrina schistosa) venom. Eur J Pharmacol 1974;28(1):199–208.
63. Tan CH, Tan NH, Tan KY, et al. Antivenom cross-neutralization of the venoms of Hydrophis schistosus and Hydrophis curtus, two common sea snakes in Malaysian waters. Toxins (Basel) 2015;7(2):572–81.
64. Fenner P. Marine envenomation: an update. A presentation on the current status of marine envenomation first aid and medical treatments. Emerg Med 2000;12(4): 295–302.
65. Barsan WG, Hedges JR, Syverud SA, et al. A hemodynamic model for anaphylactic shock. Ann Emerg Med 1985;14(9):834–9.
66. Ryan NM, Downes MA, Isbister GK. Clinical features of serum sickness after Australian snake antivenom. Toxicon 2015;108:181–3.

North American Snake Envenomation

Bryan Corbett, MD*, Richard F. Clark, MD

KEYWORDS

- Crotalid • Elapid • Rattlesnake • Copperhead • Cottonmouth • Coral snake

KEY POINTS

- Native North American venomous snakes fall into 3 categories: crotalids, elapids, and colubrids.
- Crotalids include the rattlesnakes, copperheads, and cottonmouths, and their envenomations are characterized primarily by local tissue destruction and hematologic toxicity.
- All native North American members of the elapid family are coral snakes and their envenomation can be characterized by neuromuscular blockade and subsequent muscular weakness.
- Colubrids are generally considered medically inconsequential.
- Treatment of envenomation of all types of snakes includes good supportive care with antivenom administration when indicated.

INTRODUCTION

It is important to have a general understanding of snake taxonomy to help organize venomous snake species and to some extent predict clinical effects. All life is categorized taxonomically under 7 increasingly specific categories. These categories include, in descending order; kingdom, phylum, class, order, family, genus, and species. In addition to these 7 main groups there are subdivisions and superdivisions between them. With regard to snakes and their medical significance, this further classification is most important as it relates to superfamilies and subfamilies. Snakes fall under the order Ophidia or Serpentes. Most modern snakes fall under the superfamily Colubridae, which includes all venomous snakes of medical significance.[1] Within this superfamily, medically significant North American snakes can be classified into 2 main families and to a lesser clinically significant third family. The 2 main families are Viperidae and Elapidae. The third less significant family from a medical standpoint is the Colubridae family.[2,3]

Disclosures: The authors have no financial or commercial affiliations to disclose.
Division of Medical Toxicology, Department of Emergency Medicine, UC San Diego Health, 200 West Arbor Drive # 8676, San Diego, CA 92103, USA
* Corresponding author.
E-mail address: bcorbett1982@gmail.com

A majority of venomous North American snakes belong to the subfamily Crotalinae (often referred to as crotalids), which falls under the Viperidae family. These snakes include the rattlesnakes (genus *Crotalus* and *Sistrurus*) as well as the cottonmouths and copperheads (genus *Agkistrodon*). These snakes are also referred to as pit vipers due to heat-sensing pits behind their nostrils and can be differentiated from nonvenomous native US snakes by their triangular heads and elliptical pupils.[4,5] An exception is the coral snake (discussed later). In addition, this rule does not necessarily hold true outside the United States.[4] Rattlesnakes geographically cover much of the contiguous United States; however, a majority of the bites occur in Southwestern states, such as California, Arizona, New Mexico, and Texas, although there are a significant number reported in Florida as well.[4,6] Copperheads and cottonmouths are found primarily in the Eastern and Southern United States, with a majority of envenomations occurring in the South.[4,6] An average of 4735 native US venomous snakebites are reported every year and approximately half of these are from crotalids (the true fraction is likely higher given several unidentified snakes in this study).[6] A majority of individuals bitten are male and older than 19 years of age but this is not specific for crotalid envenomations and is true across all US native venomous species.[6] Deaths are rare, with an average of 5 to 6 reported a year, and usually occur in children, the elderly, or those with some delay in antivenom treatment.[5] Deaths are almost always from crotalid envenomation and usually from a rattlesnake.[6]

Elapidae snakes are frequently referred to as elapids. Two genera and 3 species of coral snakes make up the North American elapid population: the Arizona or Sonoran coral snake (*Micruroides euryxanthus*), the eastern coral snake (*Micrurus fulvius*), and the Texas coral snake (*Micrurus tener*).[7,8] The eastern coral snake can be found in much of the South whereas the Texas coral snake resides west of the Mississippi river in Louisiana, Arkansas, and Texas. The Arizona coral snake can be found in Arizona and New Mexico.[7] Despite this multistate distribution, 344 of 399 identified coral snake bites from 2001 to 2005 occurred in Florida and Texas.[6] Coral snake bites comprise only approximately 2% of all US venomous snake bites annually, and up until 2006 no deaths had been reported to the American Association of Poison Control Centers since 1983.[6,7] Coral snakes do not have elliptical pupils, triangular heads, or heat-sensing pits like the crotalids but are venomous. US coral snakes can be identified by their circumferential red, yellow, and black banding with red bands abutting yellow bands.[4] This distinction is important to differentiate coral snakes from other similar appearing nonvenomous US snake species with noncircumferential banding (the shovel-nosed snake) or red bands abutting black bands (the king snake). These rules do not necessarily hold true outside the United States.[4]

The oft-ignored Colubridae family of snakes, often referred to as colubrids, are generally not considered poisonous. This is in contrast to being venomous because all snakes produce venom but snakes considered poisonous (such as the crotalids and elapids) are able to puncture human skin and deliver enough venom to produce a clinically significant envenomation. Colubrid snakes are rear-fanged and lack an efficient venom delivery system. If specialized venom glands are present, they do not have significant associated musculature to forcefully expel venom.[1] Clinically significant envenomations from these snakes have been reported, but they are generally mild and of such little clinical significance that this family is not discussed further.[3]

PATIENT EVALUATION OVERVIEW
Crotalid Envenomation

Crotalid venom is a complex mixture of multiple proteins, other macromolecules, and metals with diverse activity (**Box 1**).[9] More than 50 components have been identified.[10]

Box 1 **Various components of crotalid venom**
Arginine ester hydrolase
Thrombin-like enzyme
Collagenase
Hyaluronidase
Phospholipase A2
Phospholipase B
Phosphomonoesterase
Phosphodiesterase
Acetylcholinesterase
RNase
DNase
5′-Nucleotidase
NAD nucleotidase
L-Amino acid oxidase
Data from Gold BS, Dart RC, Barish RA. Bites of venomous snakes. N Engl J Med 2002;347(5):347–56.

Many of these components have enzymatic activity and the specific components can vary between species and even among the same species depending on geography, diet, and time of year.[5,9] The venom is primarily cytotoxic and hemotoxic, although all organ systems can be affected.[5,11] Local tissue destruction and hematologic toxicity are the 2 classic manifestations of crotalid envenomation, although systemic and neurotoxicity are also important.

Tissue toxicity
Crotalid venom injection locally causes vascular endothelial and basement membrane damage, destruction of the extracellular matrix, and an inflammatory cascade leading to swelling, erythema, and pain.[9] Myotoxic components have also been reported and rhabdomyolysis from local and systemic myotoxic venom effects are rare but occur.[9] Only approximately 10% of envenomations (not including dry bites) lack local tissue manifestations.[10] Local effects tend to occur within 30 minutes to 60 minutes; however, they can be delayed for several hours. Ecchymosis, bullae, and necrosis may develop over time (**Figs. 1** and **2**).[5,12] The severity is variable, from mild local pain and swelling to severe pain with rapidly advancing swelling and necrosis with autoamputation, particularly with bites to the fingers.[13] Tissue toxicity from rattlesnake envenomations tends to be more severe than that from cottonmouths or copperheads although there can be considerable overlap.

Hematologic toxicity
Coagulopathy manifesting as hypofibrinogenemia with an elevated prothrombin time (PT) and thrombocytopenia are the major hematologic manifestations of crotalid envenomation.[5,9,11,12] The incidence of such abnormalities has been reported to be 33%, 49%, and 60% (PT >14 seconds), respectively.[12] Although severe bleeding is rare, it can occur.[11,14] Thrombocytopenia and hypofibrinogenemia may be protracted,

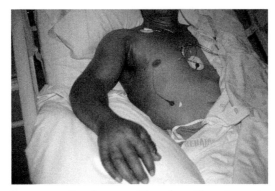

Fig. 1. Dorsal hand envenomation from a rattlesnake with ecchymosis extending into the proximal arm, axilla, and lateral thorax.

recur, or develop late after the envenomation.[5,15] There is some question as to whether late developing hemotoxicity could be due to early antivenom administration, masking initial effects, with subsequent antivenom clearance allowing free venom concentrations to rise and late hemotoxicity to manifest. Delayed hemotoxicity has not been well documented in the absence of antivenom administration. The mechanism of snakebite-induced thrombocytopenia is unclear but is thought to be from platelet membrane damage secondary to venom phospholipases, which results in platelet destruction.[9,12] This theory may conflict with the fact that platelet values often improve significantly after the administration of antivenom.[15] Other evidence points to platelet aggregation as a cause of thrombocytopenia.[10] Rattlesnake venom contains thrombin-like enzymes, which inefficiently cleave fibrinogen, resulting in poorly cross-linked fibers, forming unstable clots while consuming fibrinogen. In addition, venom also contains fibrinolysins, which degrade fibrinogen and fibrin.[9–11] Both mechanisms contribute to coagulopathy and hypofibrinogenemia.

Neurotoxicity

Neurotoxicity is not a major factor in most crotalid envenomations. The Mojave rattlesnake (*Crotalus scutulatus*) is the major exception. It is known to possess a neurotoxic venom component named Mojave toxin that prevents the presynaptic release of

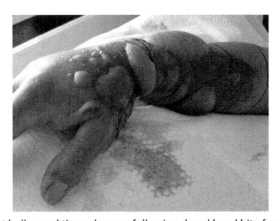

Fig. 2. Significant bullae and tissue damage following dorsal hand bite from *C viridis helleri*.

acetylcholine.[16] Envenomation can produce cranial nerve dysfunction, weakness, and paralysis.[9] Local tissue effects may be nonexistent or mild in such cases.[5] The Southern Pacific rattlesnake (C helleri) has also been shown to possess at least 1 isoform of the Mojave toxin and a neurotoxic presentation has been reported in some cases.[16,17] Timber rattlesnake (C horridus) envenomations are known to cause myokymia, a rippling movement of muscles often noted in the face.[9] Other species of rattlesnakes may also cause myokymia and rarely more significant weakness.[9,10]

Systemic toxicity

Mild systemic symptoms, including nausea, vomiting, and diaphoresis, are most common. More severe manifestations, including hypotension, tachycardia, respiratory distress, angioedema, cardiovascular collapse and confusion, are less frequent.[5,10] Third spacing of fluid secondary to capillary endothelial damage likely contributes to hypotension as does the presence of a protein that depresses myocardial function found in some rattlesnake venoms.[9] This fluid shift does not explain the totality of systemic manifestations (described previously), and severe acute hypersensitivity reactions (anaphylactic and anaphylactoid) are thought to contribute to cases of hypotension, cardiovascular collapse, and angioedema.[10,18] There are many reports of anaphylactic reactions in individuals with previous exposure to rattlesnakes, from prior envenomations, ingestion of rattlesnake meat, or simply handling of the snakes.[18–21] Alternatively, there is at least 1 case report of a similar presentation in an individual with no prior rattlesnake envenomations or exposures, raising the question of an anaphylactoid reaction.[22] Regardless, treatment should include assessment of airway, breathing, and circulation as well as administration of antihistamines, corticosteroids, and epinephrine in addition to antivenom, discussed later. Fortunately, these severe presentations are rare, representing only approximately 1% of envenomations.[18]

Coral Snake Envenomation

Bites by the eastern coral snake are generally more severe than those of the Texas coral snake. Bites by the Arizona coral snake are essentially not medically significant.[8] Envenomation results in little to no local tissue damage. The major manifestation is neuromuscular blockade that can present with ptosis, cranial nerve palsies, dysarthria, and dysphagia and can progress to complete respiratory paralysis and death.[5,23] The mechanism is postsynaptic acetylcholine blockade at the neuromuscular junction.[8] Symptom onset may be delayed for up to 12 hours, but generally patients with significant envenomations develop symptoms within 6 hours.[5,24] No deaths were reported to the American Association of Poison Control Centers from 1983 to 2007 and only 4% of bites were coded as major effects from 2001 to 2005.[6,7] There was not a documented coral snake fatality from 1967 until 2009 (although the envenomation occurred in 2006 in Florida).[8] Interpretation of this data is complicated because incidence of treatment with coral snake antivenom among severity groups is not provided and this could alter the severity of a patient's course. In addition, severity of coral snake bites may be mitigated by more intensive care as represented by a higher rate of admissions to ICUs.[6]

GENERAL TREATMENT CONSIDERATIONS
Crotalid Envenomations

General emergency department care of snakebites begins as usual with attention to airway, breathing, and circulation. Intravenous access should be obtained so that intravenous fluids and parenteral pain control can be administered. Tetanus vaccination should be updated if indicated (this is true of coral snake envenomations as well). Antibiotics are not routinely indicated because the incidence of infections is low, approximately 3%.[5,9,10] Elevation of the affected extremity can help mitigate some of the edema.[10,12] Particular attention to the airway and consideration of early intubation is important in bites to the head, face, or tongue because obstruction from swelling can occur.[9,10]

Initial evaluation should focus on the bite site. One, two, or even multiple puncture marks corresponding to a snake's fangs are often identifiable.[9] Frequent examination of the affected extremity or area of envenomation is important to assess for worsening swelling. Distal pulses and capillary refill should be assessed in extremity envenomations. Many sources advocate circumferential markings on extremities or marking the leading edge of swelling to ensure consistent measurements in the same location.[9,10] Initial laboratory evaluation should include a complete blood count, international normalized ratio (INR), PT, fibrinogen, and fibrinogen degradation products. A creatinine kinase (CK) level can be considered if there is concern for rhabomyolysis. Elevated fibrinogen degradation products can be an early sign of coagulopathy but are not as useful as fibrinogen levels in subsequently assessing coagulopathy or after antivenom response.[10]

Any patients with signs, symptoms, or laboratory evidence of envenomation should be admitted at least for observation even if antivenom is not indicated (discussed later). Although infrequent, local tissue manifestations can be delayed or worsen over time and hematologic toxicity can manifest late.

Coral Snake Envenomations

Given the potentially serious and deadly effects of coral snake envenomation, all patients suffering a bite are recommended to seek medical care immediately. General care in an emergency department includes assessment of airway, breathing, and circulation with preparation to control the patient's airway in cases of respiratory insufficiency. CK levels should be checked in addition to basic laboratory tests because *Micrurus fulvius* venom contains a myotoxic component and CK elevations have been reported in the tens of thousands.[8] Other prehospital interventions are discussed later, as is antivenom treatment.

PHARMACOLOGIC TREATMENT OPTIONS
Crotalid Envenomation

Crotalidae polyvalent immune Fab (CPIF) is 1 of 2 antivenoms currently approved by the Food and Drug Administration (FDA) for the treatment of crotalid envenomation. CPIF is an ovine-derived polyvalent Fab fragment derived from sheep immunized with venom from the eastern diamondback (*C adamanteus*), western diamondback (*C atrox*), Mojave rattlesnake (*C scutulatus*), and the cottonmouth (*Agkistrodon piscivorus*).[5] A Fab fragment is made by digesting a whole antibody with the enzyme papain, cleaving the Fc portion and producing 2 Fab fragments, each of which possesses a single epitope binding site.[5] The Fc portion of whole antibodies is responsible for complement fixation and opsonization. Removal of this portion reduces the risk of anaphylactoid reactions and serum sickness.[9] Allergy to papain is a relative contraindication to CPIF.[25] Although CPIF does not effectively reverse swelling or necrosis, it can halt progression of local tissue damage as well as improve hematologic, neurotoxic, and systemic toxicity.[9,10] Indications for antivenom treatment include progressive local effects, significant hematologic toxicity, and systemic or neurotoxic signs of envenomation.[10] What defines significant hematologic toxicity is not well described in the literature and clinician discretion should be used. For example, significant drops in platelet values despite still in the normal range may warrant antivenom consideration; however, what degree of decline warrants administration is unclear. Limb envenomations with minor isolated local effects can be observed and antivenom administered if swelling progresses or other manifestations of toxicity develop, as described previously.[10]

Crotalidae immune F(ab')$_2$ (CIF) is the other currently FDA-approved crotalid antivenom. It will not be available for purchase in the US until 2018. CIF is raised by the immunization of horses with fer-de-lance (Bothrops asper) and South American rattlesnake (C durissus) venom.[26] Horse allergy is not listed as a contraindication for CIF but caution is advised when administering to allergic individuals.[26] CIF is an F(ab')$_2$ fragment which is produced by digesting whole immunoglobulin with the enzyme pepsin rather than papain. This produces a V-shaped protein with the 2 antigen binding arms of the immunoglobulin still connected rather than being separate as in the Fab fragment. As with the Fab fragment, the Fc portion of the immunoglobulin has been cleaved. The larger mass of the F(ab')$_2$ fragment is thought to confer a longer half-life, with F(ab')$_2$ fragments having been measured in human serum several days longer than Fab fragments.[27] More importantly, 1 comparative trial suggested this longer half-life may correlate with statistically significant higher platelet values during follow-up and a reduced risk of delayed or recurrent coagulopathy compared with Fab fragments.[27,28] In addition to this apparent benefit in preventing delayed or recurrent thrombocytopenia and coagulopathy, there was no difference in ability to achieve initial control of hematologic toxicity between the 2 antivenoms. Also of importance, there was no difference between the antivenoms in incidence of acute or delayed hypersensitivity reactions (discussed later).[27,28] No clinical studies are available comparing CPIF versus CIF with regard to local tissue toxicity. There is a study using a rabbit model comparing the efficacy of CPIF to CIF in preventing local hemorrhagic effects of various North American snakes' venom. In this study, CIF was superior to the Fab fragment in preventing local hemorrhagic effects in 11 of 14 snake venoms, equivalent in 1 instance and inferior in 2 of the 14.[29]

Both antivenoms, discussed previously, are categorized as pregnancy class C.[25,26] CPIF has been used safely in pregnancy and, given the consequential risk to the fetus with envenomation, it should be used when indicated.[30,31] Experience with CIF in pregnancy is lacking and further study is warranted at this time to determine its safety in such a patient population.

With regard to the pediatric population, a review published in 2012 (the most recent to date) looked at CPIF use in 82 pediatric patients. Only 6 had adverse reactions and all of these were mild.[32] This is consistent with other previously published studies of use in children.[33] Given such a safety profile, antivenom should be used in children, consistent with current consensus guidelines.[10] CIF also seems to be safe in the pediatric population. Patients less than 16 years of age made up 24% of all subjects enrolled in CIF phase II and phase III trials. There was no difference in side-effect profile between adults and children in these studies, and, given the overall good safety profile, CIF is reasonable to use in the pediatric population once available commercially.[26]

Antivenom dosing

CIF dosing is not reviewed because it is not commercially available.

Initial CPIF dosing should be 4 vials to 6 vials with further dosing in 4-vial to 6-vial aliquots until local progression of venom effects has halted, there is improvement in hematologic parameters, and neurologic and systemic effects have subsided (**Fig. 3**) (with the exception of myokymia, which can be resistant to antivenom treatment).[10] Each 4-vial to 6-vial dose can be mixed in saline and infused over approximately

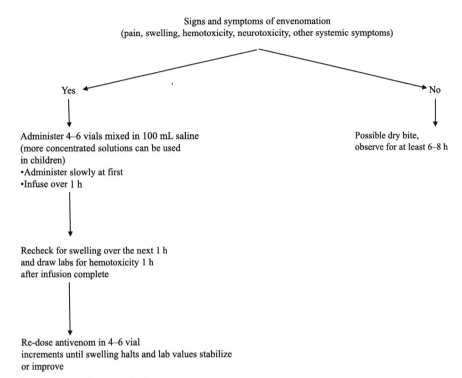

Fig. 3. CPIF antivenom dosing.

1 hour. Hematologic parameters should be repeated approximately 1 hour after each antivenom administration to assess response.[10] The majority of crotalid envenomations can be controlled with 2 doses or less and specifically only 17% of rattlesnake bites and 2% of copperhead and cottonmouth bites require more than 12 vials to achieve control.[10] Although repeat doses may be needed, the response is often muted in comparison to initial doses, particularly pertaining to hematologic effects.[10] Severe life-threatening envenomations presenting with shock or significant bleeding should be treated with an initial dose of 8 vials to 12 vials with subsequent dosing, as described previously.[10] The CPIF package insert recommends 3 maintenance doses, 2 vials each, 6 hours apart, once initial control is achieved.[25] Although initial studies suggested a decreased incidence of recurrence of local tissue effects and hematologic toxicity with maintenance doses, postmarketing experience and recent case reports question the efficacy of empiric maintenance doses. Although the clinical significance of the recurrent effects is unclear, case reports have been published of serious or fatal outcomes.[34] More recent reports suggest recurrence may happen even when maintenance doses are used.[35] Routine use of maintenance dosing varies among institutions and is not uniformly recommended by current consensus guidelines.[10]

Blood products

Blood products should not be considered for coagulopathy and thrombocytopenia resulting from snakebites until treatment with antivenom has occurred (**Fig. 4**). In the absence of antivenom administration, blood products often produce only a transient improvement in hematologic parameters. Patients with life-threatening bleeding warrant blood products, but again they should be given in conjunction with antivenom. As previously stated, thrombocytopenia and coagulopathy are usually well tolerated in crotalid envenomations; however, severe bleeding and death have been reported.[11]

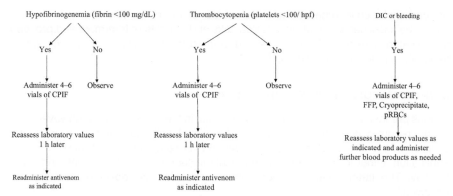

Fig. 4. Treatment of crotalid venom–induced hemotoxicity. DIC, disseminated intravascular coagulation; FFP, fresh frozen plasma; hpf, high power field; pRBC, packed red blood cells.

Coral Snake Envenomation

The current FDA-approved treatment of coral snake envenomation is the Wyeth (now a subsidiary of Pfizer) North American Coral Snake Antivenin (NACSA).[36] It is whole IgG from horses inoculated with *Micrurus fulvius* venom.[24] Patients should be questioned specifically about horse allergy or history of administration of horse-derived products in addition to a history of atopy.[36] In addition, a skin test using horse serum (included with the antivenom) should be injected intradermally prior to antivenom administration to assess for any reaction.[36] Ten percent of individuals can have a false-negative test so vigilance is still required when administering antivenom to nonreactive individuals.[36] Even in an individual with a positive skin test or history of horse allergy, coral snake an-tivenom is not absolutely contraindicated because its use could prevent the need for intubation and a prolonged ICU stay. Given that mechanical ventilation could be an alternative treatment to antivenom, however, a careful assessment of the risks and benefits of antivenom administration is imperative prior to initiation of treatment.

Wyeth no longer manufactures NACSA and there are no other FDA-approved anti-venoms for coral snakes. In an effort to maintain at least some supplies of this anti-venom, there have been multiple extensions of the original expiration date on vials, most recently from April 30, 2016, to April 30, 2017, based on FDA assessment of stability. This extension is specific to lot number 4030024.[37]

Prior to the development of NACSA, mortality from coral snake envenomation was reported to be 10%.[6] As such, empiric antivenom administration was recommended for confirmed or even possible envenomations even in the absence of symptoms.[5,24] Given the finite amount of current antivenom stockpiles and lack of new production, this practice warrants further analysis. A review in 2013 from Florida found no statistically significant difference in the incidence of intubation between those patients empirically administered antivenom after their bite versus those given antivenom only after developing symptoms.[24] Given the risk of acute hypersensitivity reactions as well as delayed serum sickness with NACSA and no significant difference in rates of intubation among groups, it seems reasonable to avoid empiric antivenom administration at this time. There is a question, however, as to how effective the antivenom is in reversing weakness once it develops, so administration should begin at the first sign of neuromuscular toxicity.[24]

NACSA is not currently categorized with respect to use in pregnancy. In addition, there have been no reports of its use in pregnant patients. Given the potential severity of coral snake envenomations and the unclear safety of the antivenom, each case should be assessed individually to weigh risks and benefits of treatment and proceed as indicated. Use of NACSA has been described in the pediatric population and is generally safe for use in children.[24]

NONPHARMACOLOGIC TREATMENT OPTIONS

Various prehospital treatment options are popular in the lay community; however, they are not recommended by experts. Some of the most well-known include tourniquets, excision of the bite site, and venom extraction via some form of negative pressure application. Other less well-known treatments include electroshock, heat, and cryotherapy. The latter have not been shown beneficial, are obscure, and are not reviewed.[9]

True tourniquets that inhibit blood flow are not recommended and can have deleterious effects.[10] Pressure immobilization bandages (PIBs) that allow venous and arterial flow yet prevent lymphatic flow have been hypothesized as potentially helpful in retarding venom distribution through lymphatics.[9] It is useful to divide the discussion between crotalid and elapid envenomations due to the differences in venom effects. Although crotalid venom has systemic activity, the most common manifestation is local tissue damage. In contrast, coral snake envenomation causes little to no local tissue damage but can result in systemic neuromuscular toxicity, leading to weakness and paralysis. This difference has implications in the usefulness of PIB use. Although a small porcine study of crotalid envenomation showed improvement in survivability, the lethal dose (LD) 100 of snake venom was used. Observations in humans have not demonstrated outcome improvement, literature suggests little to no benefit, and most experts do not recommend PIB use in crotalid bites.[38] In contrast, given the risk of respiratory compromise and death in coral snake bites, it seems reasonable to attempt to delay systemic absorption of venom until there is access to definitive medical care. A porcine model of *Micrurus fulvius* envenomation treated with a PIB versus none demonstrated an average delay in toxicity in the treatment arm of 268 minutes compared with controls. Four of five pigs also survived to the study endpoint of 8 hours compared with 0 of 5 in the control arm ($P = .0036$).[23] Although a PIB is not definitive treatment, delaying onset of serious systemic toxicity may allow more time to seek definitive medical care.

Excision of the bite site to remove venom prior to distribution has been advocated in the past. A dog model using radiolabeled venom reported recovery of 79% of venom; however, the article was lacking methodological description.[39] Another rabbit model showed no benefit of early surgical débridement and fasciotomy in conjunction with antivenom versus antivenom alone in long-term outcomes and actually demonstrated worsened functional outcomes.[40] In 1 case series describing outcomes in 54 patients treated with excisional therapy, complication rates were high and efficacy difficult to establish based on limited descriptions.[41] Excisional therapy, therefore, is not recommended.

Use of venom extractors has been described in humans; however, given the nature of case reports, lack of controls, and high incidence of dry bites, no conclusions about their efficacy can be made.[42] A handful of studies have attempted to quantify the amount of venom that can be removed by an extractor. In a case series of 2 individuals, a venom extractor was applied within 1 minute of envenomation by *C atrox* (western diamondback rattlesnake). A maximum concentration of 27.5 μg of venom per milliliter of fluid was removed; however, the total volume of fluid removed was not reported, making determinations of the relative amount of venom removed impossible.[42]

An artificial envenomation rabbit model using radiolabeled venom reported a 34% recovery rate using venom extractors.[43] In contrast, another study using radiolabeled mock venom in a human model retrieved only 0.04% of the total venom load injected into subjects.[44] In addition to the mixed results, extrapolating the benefit of percentage removal of venom to clinical outcomes is problematic. To that end, a porcine model was used to assess leg swelling after artificial rattlesnake envenomation between controls and those treated with a venom extractor. There was no statistically significant difference between the 2 groups. Some pigs in the treatment arm did develop a circular necrotic lesion corresponding with the site of extractor application.[38] In summary, given the lack of proven benefit and question of harm, the use of venom extractors is currently not recommended.

SURGICAL TREATMENT OPTIONS

Compartment syndrome and the role of fasciotomies for treatment of crotalid envenomation has been a contentious topic in some clinical practice settings. Significant swelling, paresthesias, pallor, and pain with passive movement occur in many crotalid bites and are also typical manifestations of compartment syndrome. A true compartment syndrome, however, is rarely encountered with crotalid bites when pressure monitoring is used.[10,12,13] When true elevated compartment pressures occur after a crotalid bite, the clinical presentation is thought to be from myonecrosis due to direct venom effects on the muscular compartment rather than vascular insufficiency secondary to increased compartment pressures. Most bitten patients actually have increased blood flow to affected extremities.[5,9] Despite this, when concern for compartment syndrome is present, compartment pressure measurements can be obtained. When values rise above 30 mm Hg to 50 mm Hg, this may prompt surgical consultation.[9] The utility of fasciotomy in this situation is, however, unclear. In a rabbit model of rattlesnake envenomation, fasciotomy plus antivenom decreased local edema in comparison to antivenom alone; however, functional outcomes were worse in the fasciotomy plus antivenom group and there was no survival benefit.[40] Given that elevated pressures are thought to be from direct venom-induced myonecrosis, prompt administration of antivenom may prevent this effect and the development of elevated pressures. Even when elevated pressures have already developed, antivenom alone has been shown to reduce them and increase perfusion pressure in the compartment.[45] There still may be a role for fasciotomy after a snakebite, when there are persistently elevated pressures despite aggressive antivenom administration. Surgical decompression may include digits.[46]

TREATMENT RESISTANCE/COMPLICATIONS
Recurrence

Clinical improvement usually follows initial antivenom dosing for symptomatic snakebites. Approximately half of patients with crotalid envenomation have recurrence of some clinical aspect. For local tissue effects, recurrence generally occurs 6 hours to 36 hours after initial improvement. Recurrence of hematologic toxicity can be even more delayed and variable with most cases occurring 2 days to 7 days after antivenom administration.[5,10,34,35] In addition to recurrent hematologic toxicity, delayed new-onset hematologic toxicity has been reported in those treated with antivenom.[47] These patients may simply have had masking of initial hematologic toxicity by antivenom, but this is unclear. This recurrent or delayed hematologic toxicity is complicated by the fact that it may not respond well to repeated doses of antivenom administration. The authors' practice is to weigh the risks of bleeding from specific platelet values and fibrinogen values (understanding the dearth of evidence behind some of these decisions) in the context of the individual patient. If the authors are concerned about bleeding, further antivenom is given until a response is no longer seen or the patient's values improve, based on clinical judgment. Thereafter, if bleeding risk is still present due to severe thrombocytopenia or hypofibrinogenemia or bleeding occurs, blood products are considered.

Antivenom Complications

Crotalidae polyvalent immune Fab

Acute hypersensitivity and anaphylactoid reactions, including urticaria, pruritis, and wheezing, have been reported in approximately 6% to 14% of patients treated with CPIF. Reactions are generally mild; however, severe reactions with airway involvement do occur and the initial dose of antivenom should be administered in a setting able to deal with such emergencies.[5,10,48] In cases of such a reaction, antivenom administration should be at least temporarily discontinued and antihistamines and corticosteroids given. Although these therapies are generally adequate treatment, epinephrine may be needed in severe reactions. Once a patient is stabilized, a reassessment of further need for antivenom should take place. Antivenom should be restarted at a lower rate if continued treatment is decided on.

Delayed hypersensitivity reactions, specifically serum sickness, also occur after CPIF. The incidence has been reported to be 5% to 16% and development is usually 7 days to 21 days after antivenom treatment. Manifestations include fever, rash, myalgias, and arthralgias. Serum sickness responds well to oral antihistamines and corticosteroids.[5,10,48]

North American Coral Snake Antivenin

Because it is whole IgG, a higher rate of acute and delayed hypersensitivity reactions is expected with NACSA compared with CPIF. Adverse reactions, however, were reported in only approximately 18% of cases receiving NACSA in 1 series. In addition, a majority of reactions seem to be minor, such as urticaria; however, 2% developed hypotension and 1% developed angioedema, which is exceedingly rare with CPIF use.[24] There was no comment on the development of serum sickness in this article but the manufacturer cautions that it may occur 5 days to 24 days postadministration.[36] As with other acute and delayed hypersensitivity reactions, treatment is with antihistamines, corticosteroids, and epinephrine in severe cases.

EVALUATION OF OUTCOME AND LONG-TERM RECOMMENDATIONS
Crotalid Envenomation

Up to 25% of crotalid bites are considered dry bites, meaning no venom is injected.[5,6,10] In this subset of patients, no effects manifest more than some local pain. These patients should nonetheless have blood work obtained, including a complete blood cell count, fibrinogen, and fibrinogen degradation products, because hematologic effects can at times manifest in the absence of local effects.[9,10] Crotalid bites should be observed for at least 6 hours to 8 hours.[5,10] If no clinical or laboratory manifestations develop, patients may be discharged.[5]

Once initial control of local tissue effects and stabilization of hematologic parameters is obtained, repeat reassessments and laboratory testing are reasonable every 6 hours to 8 hours.[10] Worsening local effects or hematologic parameters should prompt reassessment of the need for further antivenom and more frequent clinical and laboratory assessment. In patients with stable swelling, adequate pain control and stable hematologic parameters after about 24 hours of observation discharge can be considered.[10] Even in the setting of stable swelling, however, ability to maintain adequate pain control and functional status should be considered prior to discharge. Regarding hematologic parameters, "stable values" do not necessarily mean within the normal range because many patients can be safely discharged with abnormal platelet counts or fibrinogen levels that are normalizing.[15] Follow-up at 2 days to 3 days and at 5 days to 7 days after last antivenom dose for repeat testing of hematologic parameters is recommended given the risk of recurrence when CPIF has been administered.[10] No follow-up is needed, per consensus guidelines, for patients with minor envenomations and no evidence of hematologic toxicity who did not require antivenom.[10]

Coral Snake Envenomation

The incidence of dry bites in elapids, including coral snakes, is higher than in crotalids, 40% compared with 25%.[8,24] Given the possibility for more delayed manifestations of coral snake envenomation, all patients suffering a bite should be observed for at least 24 hours. If patients continue to be asymptomatic after this period, then they may be discharged.[8] Patients receiving antivenom who are asymptomatic may be discharged after an asymptomatic period of approximately 24 hours as well. If patients are intubated after a coral snake bite, they may require mechanical ventilation for days to weeks.[8]

SUMMARY

- Native North American venomous snakes fall into 3 categories: crotalids, elapids, and colubrids.
- Crotalids include the rattlesnakes, copperheads, and cottonmouths, and their envenomations are characterized primarily by local tissue destruction and hematologic toxicity.
- All native North American members of the elapid family are coral snakes and their envenomation can be characterized by neuromuscular blockade and subsequent muscular weakness.
- Colubrids are generally considered medically inconsequential.
- Treatment of envenomation of all types of snakes includes good supportive care with antivenom administration when indicated.

REFERENCES

1. Weinstein SA, Keyler DE. Local envenoming by the Western hognose snake (Heterodon nasicus): a case report and review of medically significant Heterodon bites. Toxicon 2009;54:354–60.
2. Uetz P, Freed P, Hosek J, editors. Higher taxa in extant reptiles. Available at: http://www.reptile-database.org/db-info/taxa.html#Ser. Accessed August 8, 2016.
3. Weinstein SA, White J, Keyler DE, et al. Non-front-fanged colubroid snakes: a current evidence-based analysis of medical significance. Toxicon 2013;69:103–13.
4. Cardwell MD. Recognizing dangerous snakes in the United States and Canada: a novel 3-step identification method. Wilderness Environ Med 2011;22(4):304–8.
5. Gold BS, Dart RC, Barish RA. Bites of venomous snakes. N Engl J Med 2002; 347(5):347–56.
6. Seifert SA, Boyer LV, Benson BE, et al. AAPCC database characterization of native US venomous snake exposures, 2001–2005. Clin Toxicol 2009;47(4): 327–35.

7. Walter FG, Stolz U, Shirazi F, et al. Temporal analyses of coral snakebite severity published in the American Association of Poison Control Centers' Annual Reports from 1983 through 2007. Clin Toxicol 2010;48(1):72–8.

8. Norris RL, Pfalzgraf RR, Laing G. Death following coral snake bite in the United States–first documented case (with ELISA confirmation of envenomation) in over 40 years. Toxicon 2009;53(6):693–7.

9. Holstege CP, Miller MB, Wermuth M, et al. Crotalid snake envenomation. Crit Care Clin 1997;13(4):889–921.

10. Lavonas EJ, Ruha AM, Banner W, et al. Unified treatment algorithm for the management of crotaline snakebite in the United States: results of an evidence-informed consensus workshop. BMC Emerg Med 2011;11(1):1.

11. Ruha AM, Curry SC. Recombinant factor VIIa for treatment of gastrointestinal hemorrhage following rattlesnake envenomation. Wilderness Environ Med 2009; 20(2):156–60.

12. Tanen DA, Ruha AM, Graeme KA, et al. Epidemiology and hospital course of rattlesnake envenomations cared for at a tertiary referral center in central Arizona. Acad Emerg Med 2001;8(2):177–82.

13. Hall EL. Role of surgical intervention in the management of crotaline snake envenomation. Ann Emerg Med 2001;37(2):175–80.

14. Lavonas EJ, Khatri V, Daugherty C, et al. Medically significant late bleeding after treated crotaline envenomation: a systematic review. Ann Emerg Med 2014;63(1): 71–8.

15. Bush SP, Wu VH, Corbett SW. Rattlesnake venom-induced thrombocytopenia response to antivenin (crotalidae) polyvalent: a case series. Acad Emerg Med 2000;7(2):181–5.

16. French WJ, Hayes WK, Bush SP, et al. Mojave toxin in venom of Crotalus helleri (Southern Pacific Rattlesnake): molecular and geographic characterization. Toxicon 2004;44(7):781–91.

17. Bush SP, Siedenburg E. Neurotoxicity associated with suspected southern Pacific rattlesnake (Crotalus viridis helleri) envenomation. Wilderness Environ Med 1999;10(4):247–9.

18. Brooks DE, Graeme KA. Airway compromise after first rattlesnake envenomation. Wilderness Environ Med 2004;15(3):188–93.

19. Tanen DA, Ruha AM, Graeme KA, et al. Rattlesnake envenomations: unusual case presentations. Arch Intern Med 2001;161(3):474–9.

20. Hogan DE, Dire DJ. Anaphylactic shock secondary to rattlesnake bite. Ann Emerg Med 1990;19(7):814–6.

21. Kerns W, Tomaszewski C. Airway obstruction following canebrake rattlesnake envenomation. J Emerg Med 2001;20(4):377–80.

22. Nordt SP. Anaphylactoid reaction to rattlesnake envenomation. Vet Hum Toxicol 2000;42(1):12.

23. German BT, Hack JB, Brewer K, et al. Pressure-immobilization bandages delay toxicity in a porcine model of eastern coral snake (Micrurus fulvius fulvius) envenomation. Ann Emerg Med 2005;45(6):603–8.

24. Wood A, Schauben J, Thundiyil J, et al. Review of Eastern coral snake (Micrurus fulvius fulvius) exposures managed by the Florida Poison Information Center Network: 1998–2010. Clin Toxicol 2013;51(8):783–8.

25. Crofab [package insert]. West Conshohocken (PA): BTG International Inc; 2012.

26. Anavip [package insert]. Mexico D.F. (Mexico): Instituto Bioclon S.A. de CV; 2015.

27. Boyer LV, Chase PB, Degan JA, et al. Subacute coagulopathy in a randomized, comparative trial of Fab and F (ab') 2 antivenoms. Toxicon 2013;74: 101–8.

28. Bush SP, Ruha AM, Seifert SA, et al. Comparison of F (ab') 2 versus Fab antivenom for pit viper envenomation: a prospective, blinded, multicenter, randomized clinical trial. Clin Toxicol 2015;53(1):37–45.

29. Sánchez EE, Galán JA, Perez JC, et al. The efficacy of two antivenoms against the venom of North American snakes. Toxicon 2003;41(3):357–65.

30. Dunnihoo DR, Rush BM, Wise RB, et al. Snake bite poisoning in pregnancy. A review of the literature. J Reprod Med 1992;37(7):653–8.

31. LaMonica GE, Seifert SA, Rayburn WF. Rattlesnake bites in pregnant women. J Reprod Med 2009;55(11–12):520–2.

32. Farrar HC, Grayham T, Bolden B, et al. The use and tolerability of crotalidae polyvalent immune FAB (ovine) in pediatric envenomations. Clin Pediatr 2012;51(10): 945–9.

33. Offerman SR, Bush SP, Moynihan JA, et al. Crotaline Fab antivenom for the treatment of children with rattlesnake envenomation. Pediatrics 2002;110(5): 968–71.

34. Miller AD, Young MC, DeMott MC, et al. Recurrent coagulopathy and thrombocytopenia in children treated with crotalidae polyvalent immune fab: a case series. Pediatr Emerg Care 2010;26(8):576–82.

35. Clark RF, O'Connell CW, Villano JH, et al. Severe recurrent coagulopathy following crotaline envenomation refractory to maintenance dosing of antivenom. Am J Emerg Med 2015;33(6):856.e3-e5.

36. North American coral snake Antivenin [package insert]. Marietta (PA): Wyeth Laboratories Inc; 2001.

37. U.S. Food and Drug Administration. Expiration Date Extension for North American Coral Snake Antivenin (Micrurus fulvius) (Equine Origin) Lot 4030024 Through April 30, 2017. Available at: www.fda.gov/biologicsbloodvaccines/ safetyavailability/ucm445083.htm. Accessed August 29, 2016.

38. Bush SP, Green SM, Laack TA, et al. Pressure immobilization delays mortality and increases intracompartmental pressure after artificial intramuscular rattlesnake envenomation in a porcine model. Ann Emerg Med 2004;44(6):599–604.

39. Snyder CC, Pickins JE, Knowles RP, et al. A definitive study of snakebite. J Fla Med Assoc 1968;55:330–7.

40. Stewart RM, Page CP, Schwesinger WH, et al. Antivenin and fasciotomy/debridement in the treatment of the severe rattlesnake bite. Am J Surg 1989;158(6): 543–7.

41. Huang TT, Lynch JB, Larson DL, et al. The use of excisional therapy in the management of snakebite. Ann Surg 1974;179(5):598.

42. Bronstein AC, Russell FE, Sullivan JB. Negative pressure suction in the field treatment of rattlesnake bite victims [abstract]. Vet Hum Toxicol 1986;28:485.

43. Bronstein AC, Russell FE, Sullivan IB, et al. Negative pressure suction in the field treatment of rattlesnake bite [abstract]. Vet Hum Toxicol 1985;28:297.

44. Alberts MB, Shalit M, LoGalbo F. Suction for venomous snakebite: a study of "mock venom" extraction in a human model. Ann Emerg Med 2004;43(2): 181–6.

45. Gold BS, Barish RA, Dart RC, et al. Resolution of compartment syndrome after rattlesnake envenomation utilizing non-invasive measures. J Emerg Med 2003; 24(3):285–8.

46. Watt CH. Treatment of poisonous snakebite with emphasis on digit dermotomy. South Med J 1985;78:694–9.
47. Seifert SA, Cano DN. Late, new-onset thrombocytopenia in a rattlesnake envenomation treated with a Fab antivenom. Clin Toxicol 2013;51(9):911–2.
48. Clark RF, McKinney PE, Chase PB, et al. Immediate and delayed allergic reactions to Crotalidae polyvalent immune Fab (ovine) antivenom. Ann Emerg Med 2002;39(6):671–6.

Arthropod Envenomation in North America

Timothy B. Erickson, MD[a],*, Navneet Cheema, MD[b]

KEYWORDS

- Arthropods • Spiders • Scorpions • Hymenoptera • Bees • Ants • Ticks
- Centipedes

KEY POINTS

- Black widow spider bites cause painful muscle spasms, secondary to neurotoxicity, and are responsive to antivenom therapy.
- Brown recluse spider bites result in hematotoxicity and most commonly manifest locally as skin necrosis.
- Scorpion stings in North America produce severe localized pain with occasional neurotoxic systemic effects.
- Hymenoptera stings from bees and wasps can result in local skin reaction to severe anaphylactic reactions and are responsible for more fatalities than any other venomous arthropod.
- Fire ant stings can cause multiple painful localized skin reaction and pustules.

SPIDERS

There are nearly 40,000 species of spiders worldwide (class Arachnida). Most species cannot inflict serious bites to humans because they do not have fangs long enough to penetrate the human skin.[1,2,3] As a result, most exposures are often unnoticed and do not need treatment. In North America, approximately 50 species of arachnids potentially cause human morbidity. Spiders use their venom to paralyze and liquefy their prey. There are only a few medically relevant spiders that produce toxic venoms that can lead to local reactions, systemic illnesses, hematotoxicity, and neurotoxicity.

[a] Division of Medical Toxicology, Department of Emergency Medicine, Brigham and Women's Hospital, Harvard Humanitarian Initiative & Harvard Medical School, Neville House, 75 Francis Street, Boston, MA 02115, USA; [b] Section of Emergency Medicine, University of Chicago, Chicago, IL, USA
* Corresponding author.
E-mail address: terickson@bwh.harvard.edu

Emerg Med Clin N Am 35 (2017) 355–375
http://dx.doi.org/10.1016/j.emc.2017.01.001
0733-8627/17/© 2017 Elsevier Inc. All rights reserved.

Black Widow Spiders

Introduction

The *Latrodectus* genus of spiders includes 5 primary species found in North America: *Latrodectus mactans*, *Latrodectus bishop*, *Latrodectus geometricus*, *Latrodectus hesperus*, and *Latrodectus variolus*.[3] They live in dimly lit, secluded areas such as woodpiles, stonewalls, cabins, barns, stables, and outhouses. They are present in southern Canada and every US state except Alaska.[4] Black widows are jet black with an iconic red hourglass marking on the ventral aspect of the abdomen (**Fig. 1**). The red hourglass is specific to *L mactans*; other species have distinctive ventral markings, such as triangles and spots. There is a seasonal variation in the number of black widow bites, starting to increase in spring, peaking in September, and reaching a nadir in January to February.[4]

Black widows are docile and nocturnal and bite when their web is disturbed. The female black widow is generally considered poisonous to humans and is more aggressive if guarding her egg sac. The male black widow spider has smaller jaws with minimal venom production and is not significantly poisonous to humans. These spiders use striated muscles to control the amount of venom they inject, and about 15% of bites do not deliver venom.[5] The venom's toxicity is due to the presence of α-latrotoxin. This toxin facilitates exocytosis of synaptic vesicles and the release of the neurotransmitters norepinephrine, γ-aminobutyric acid, and acetylcholine.[6] The toxin also causes degeneration of motor end plates, resulting in denervation. The venom destabilizes nerve cell membranes by opening ion channels, causing a large influx of calcium into the cell and depletion of acetylcholine from presynaptic nerve terminals.

Patient evaluation overview

Latrodectism is the clinical syndrome that follows a black widow bite. The bite produces a pinprick sensation that often goes unnoticed. With careful examination, 2 small fang marks may be noticed. Within the first few hours, local irritation develops, including erythema, urticaria, or a characteristic halo-shaped target lesion. These local symptoms may be followed by generalized symptoms of pain and muscle spasms in the chest, abdomen, and lower back. Typically, the pain is concentrated to the chest with upper extremity bites and abdomen with lower extremity envenomation. Abdominal rigidity can be severe and may be mistaken as an acute abdomen.[7,8] Signs and symptoms in small children are wound erythema, irritability, constant crying, sialorrhea, agitation, and seizures. Victims experience pain on the wound site, muscle

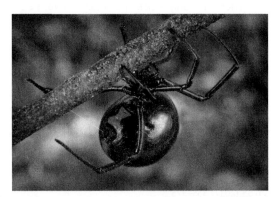

Fig. 1. Black widow spider, *Lactrodectus mactans*. (*Courtesy of* CDC/Paula Smith; and James Gathany.)

spasms, abdominal and thoracic pain, and fine tremors.[9] About one-third of patients will go on to have systemic symptoms.[2] These systemic symptoms include hypertension, sweating, salivation, dyspnea with increased broncho-secretions, and seizures. Less common effects include myocarditis,[10] compartment syndrome of the upper extremity,[11] and priapism.[12,13] Death is rare from black widow envenomation alone, with no recent cases reported in the US literature, and only a few documented worldwide.[14–16]

Pharmacologic treatment options

Tetanus immunization should be updated, but antibiotics are unnecessary unless there is evidence of a wound infection. Oral and parenteral analgesics are administered if pain is severe. Muscle spasms may require large doses of benzodiazepines. With administration of these drugs, attention should be given to the patient's airway status because of the concomitant neurotoxicity of the venom.

Historically, administration of calcium gluconate was considered because of concern for the development of hypocalcemia following black widow envenomation. This practice is currently not advocated, because studies have proven no benefit to the administration of calcium.[7,17] Likewise, dantrolene administration has not been shown to be clinically efficacious for muscle spasms.

Nonpharmacologic treatment options

Pain at the bite site may be relieved with application of an ice pack. The wound can be cleansed with soap and irrigated with water.

Combination therapies

In extreme cases with severe symptoms, *Latrodectus* antivenom is recommended.[18] Currently, in North America, the most widely available product is black widow antivenin (Lyovac, Merck). Black widow antivenin is a horse serum–derived product containing immunoglobulin G antibodies to *L mactans* venom. The dose of antivenom is one vial diluted in 50 mL of normal saline administered intravenously over 15 minutes. A more highly purified equine F(ab)$_2$ antibody black widow spider antivenom is also under investigation.[19] The use of *Latrodectus*-specific antivenom is restricted to patients with severe envenomation (eg, seizures, hypertensive crisis, respiratory compromise, or intractable pain), with no allergic contraindications, in whom opioids and benzodiazepines are ineffective. If available, young children and elderly patients with severe toxicity should receive antivenom early in the clinical course.[20]

Treatment resistance/complications

There has traditionally been reluctance to use antivenom because of concern for anaphylaxis. Two reviews of antivenom use in the United States have demonstrated low rates of adverse reactions.[4,14] There have only been 2 deaths reported after black widow antivenom administration.[7,21] Patients receiving antivenom may experience flu-like symptoms or serum sickness 1 to 3 weeks following treatment. This entity is generally self-limited and responsive to antihistamines and steroids.

Evaluation of outcome and long-term recommendations

In adults, the pain will gradually subside after several hours but may remain for 2 to 3 days. A small child bitten by a black widow spider has a greater chance of morbidity and mortality. As with snake envenomation, the volume of distribution and milligrams per kilograms dose of the venom is relatively larger in children than adults. A dose that may cause painful muscle spasms in an adult may lead to respiratory arrest in a child.[1] Any symptomatic patient who has suffered a bite from a black widow spider should be admitted for observation and pain control. Pregnant patients should undergo fetal monitoring. If there is cardiopulmonary compromise or seizures, the patient should be admitted to the intensive care unit for stabilization and antivenom administration. Symptoms of latrodectism typically last days, but some patients can have intermittent muscle weakness and spasms for weeks.

Brown Recluse Spiders

Introduction

The 6 species of recluse spiders in North America are *Loxosceles arizonica*, *Loxosceles deserta*, *Loxosceles devia*, *Loxosceles laeta*, *Loxosceles rufescens*, and *Loxosceles recluse*. Of these, *L recluse* is the most common. These spiders are reclusive nocturnal hunters and are active from spring to fall.[22,23] Victims typically are bitten on the extremities while rummaging in confined spaces such as a closet or an attic, while putting on a boot, or when using a blanket or sleeping bag that a spider is trapped in.

The brown recluse gets its name because of its reclusive nature and brown- or fawn-colored body. It is approximately 1 to 5 cm in length, with a characteristic violin- or fiddle-shaped marking on the dorsal cephalothorax (**Fig. 2**). They have long, slender legs and 6 eyes rather than eight, which is the norm for other spiders.[24]

The venom of the recluse spider, per volume, is more potent than that of the rattlesnake and can cause extensive skin necrosis. The venom acts directly on cell walls, causing immediate injury and cell death. It contains the calcium-dependent enzyme sphingomyelinase D, which in combination with C-reactive protein has a direct lytic effect on RBCs. The local tissue destructive effects are due to hemolytic enzymes and a levarterenol-like substance that induces vasoconstriction. Following cell wall damage, intravascular coagulation causes a cascade of clotting abnormalities and local polymorphonuclear leukocyte infiltration, culminating in a necrotic ulcer.

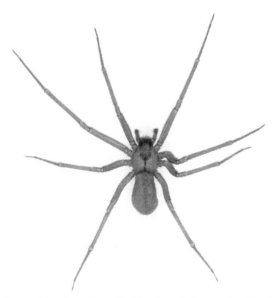

Fig. 2. Brown recluse spider, *L reclusa*. (Public domain image by Alex Wild; "Insects Unlocked" project, University of Texas at Austin.)

Patient evaluation overview

Most brown recluse bites occur in predawn hours and are often painless. The seasonality of brown recluse bites and the geographic area should be considered when making this diagnosis. One study demonstrated that 95% of brown recluse bites occurred between the months of April and October.[22] *L reclusa* is primarily found in the south central United States.[25] The clinical response to loxoscelism ranges from cutaneous irritation (necrotic arachnidism) to a life-threatening systemic reaction. Most signs and symptoms of envenomation are localized to the bite area.[26] Most (90%) result in nothing more than a local reaction and resolve spontaneously.[27] Within a few hours, the patient experiences itching, swelling, erythema, and tenderness over the bite site. Classically, erythema surrounds a dull, blue-gray macule circumscribed by a ring or halo of pallor. Gradually, over 3 to 4 days, the wound forms a necrotic base with a central black eschar. In 7 to 14 days, the wound develops a full necrotic ulceration.[28] Bites that are in fatty areas, such as the thigh or buttocks, tend to cause more extensive necrosis.[29] Several sources call for stricter diagnostic criteria and claim that the diagnosis of necrotic arachnidism secondary to brown recluse spiders is overreported and often mistaken for skin abscesses (eg, MRSA [methicillin-resistant *Staphylococcus aureus*]) and other dermatologic causes.[30–32]

The systemic reaction, which is less common than the cutaneous reaction, is associated with a higher morbidity. The reaction rarely correlates with the severity of the cutaneous lesion. Within 24 to 72 hours following the envenomation, the patient experiences fever, chills, myalgias, and arthralgias. In severe systemic reactions, the patient may suffer coagulopathies, hypotension, jaundice, disseminated intravascular coagulation (DIC), seizures, renal failure, and hemolytic anemia.[33,34] In rare cases, a patient may succumb to the systemic reaction.[27]

Hobo Spider

The Hobo spider (*Eratigena agrestis*, formerly *Tegenaria*), also known as the aggressive house spider, is found in the Pacific Northwest region of the United States and Canada.[35] This spider was traditionally included with *Loxosceles* species when discussing cases of necrotic arachnidism; however, recent studies are calling this into question.[35] Similar symptoms lead many to incorrectly attribute hobo spider bites to that of the brown recluse, which is less indigenous to the northwest United States. This species is more aggressive and bites with minor provocation.[36] Hobo spiders are brown with gray markings and have a herringbone pattern on the abdomen (**Fig. 3**).

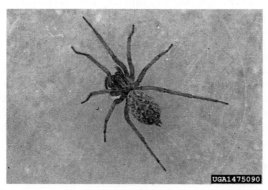

Fig. 3. Hobo spider (*E agrestis*). (*From* Whitney Cranshaw, Colorado State University, Bugwood.org.)

Pharmacologic treatment options

The management of envenomation by the brown recluse or hobo spider depends on whether the reaction is local or systemic. It is difficult to predict which type of wound will eventually progress to a disfiguring necrotic ulcer. Tetanus immunization should be updated, but antibiotics are only indicated if there is a secondary wound infection. Antihistamines and analgesics can be beneficial. Many treatment modalities, including dapsone, triamcinolone, diphenhydramine, colchicine, and trypsin, have been studied, but none have prevented the formation of an ulcerative lesion.[37]

Nonpharmacologic treatment options

Proper care includes wound cleansing, immobilization, and elevation of the affected extremity to reduce pain and swelling. Early application of ice to the bite area will lessen the local wound reaction, whereas heat will exacerbate the symptoms. A suggested method of treating expanding wound necrosis due to brown recluse spider bites is hyperbaric oxygen treatment. However, results with such treatment have been mixed, and little evidence exists to support its use.[27,38]

Combination therapies

Although not proven in clinical trials, glucocorticoids may provide a protective effect on the red blood cell (RBC) membrane, thus slowing hemolysis. The patient should be monitored in a hospital setting for the development of DIC. Transfusion of RBCs and platelets may be necessary. Plasma exchange for refractory hemolysis has been recently described following brown recluse spider envenomation.[33] Urine alkalinization with bicarbonate may lessen renal damage if the patient is experiencing acute hemolysis.

There continues to be ongoing research with brown recluse antivenom.[39] However, there is little evidence to support its efficacy, particularly against local dermatologic effects.[40] Institutions in Mexico and Brazil currently produce antivenom for *Loxosceles* bites, but the product is not commercially available in the United States.

Surgical treatment options

Early excision of ulcers is not recommended because wound healing is slowed and scarring is more severe if excised early in the clinical course. Complications of early surgical intervention include recurrent wound breakdown as well as long-term distal extremity dysfunction. Delayed excision of ulcers after the necrotic process has subsided (usually within 6–8 weeks), followed by secondary closure with skin grafting, is the preferred method of managing necrotic ulcers. In a normal host with appropriate wound care, most bite wounds heal well with only 10% occurrence of major scarring. Immunocompromised patients and those with diabetes mellitus often have a more prolonged and complicated healing process.

Treatment resistance/complications

Historically, the use of the polymorphonuclear leukocyte inhibitor, dapsone, was advocated to diminish scarring and subsequent surgical complications. Its use, however, has not proven effective in any large study with human or animal models.[38] Because of the potential for dapsone to induce methemoglobinemia and hemolytic anemia, particularly in children and those patients with glucose-6-phosphate dehydrogenase deficiency, administration is not advised.

Evaluation of outcome and long-term recommendations

Patients who are asymptotic following a period of observation in the emergency department (ED) and have normal baseline laboratory values may be discharged home with close outpatient follow-up for wound care within 24 to 48 hours. Systemic effects of brown recluse spider bites are rare but can be life threatening, and the patient should be evacuated if in a remote setting.

Tarantulas

Introduction

Tarantulas are feared because they are the largest of all spiders (**Fig. 4**). They inhabit the deserts of the western United States and Mexico, but have been discovered as far east as the Mississippi River Valley. These large, hairy spiders are relatively harmless. They are extremely shy and bite only when vigorously provoked or roughly handled.

Patient evaluation overview

Tarantula bites usually cause minimal pain and surrounding edema with minimal necrosis and no serious systemic effects. Although tarantula bites are usually of little consequence to humans, they can be more severe in domestic animals, especially canines. The growing trade of these arachnids as exotic pets should prompt the clinician to inquire about this as a possible cause an unusual skin lesion.[41]

Pharmacologic treatment options

Tetanus prophylaxis should be updated, and nonsteroidal anti-inflammatory agents can be given to alleviate pain. If needed, the patient is treated with antihistamines and topical glucocorticoids.

Nonpharmacologic treatment options

Treatment of bites consists of local wound care, and involved limbs should be raised and immobilized.

Treatment resistance/complications

Exposure to the hairs on the abdomen of the tarantula is more concerning than the actual bite. These hairs can be flicked off in large numbers as a defense mechanism and are capable of producing urticaria and pruritus that may persist for several weeks. The hairs may also get into the eyes and cause keratoconjuctivitis or ophthalmia nodosa, a nodular, granulomatous lesion in the cornea.[42,43] Patients with these complaints after exposure to a tarantula should be referred to an ophthalmologist. Without appropriate care, these eye lesions may progress to keratitis, uveitis, retinitis, and orbital cellulitis.

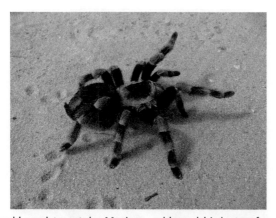

Fig. 4. Mexican red-kneed tarantula, Mexican red-kneed birdeater, female (*Brachypelma smithi*). (Photo by: George Chernilevsky, Vinnytsya, Ukraine.)

SCORPIONS
Introduction

Scorpion stings can cause significant morbidity and mortality.[40] Scorpions are arachnids that resemble crustaceans and are among the oldest terrestrial animals. Worldwide, about 2 billion people are at risk for scorpion envenomation, with over one million stings and thousands of deaths annually.[44] In North America, scorpion deaths only accounted for 0.3% of the venomous and nonvenomous animal deaths reported to the Centers for Disease Control and Prevention in the last decade.[45] Nevertheless, they remain a public health concern throughout the South and southwest United States and among outdoor enthusiasts camping and hiking in desert regions.

The scorpion has a pair of anterior legs with pinchers, a long mobile tail equipped with venom glands and a stinger, known as the telson (**Fig. 5**). Although members of the genera *Hadrurus*, *Vejovis*, and *Uroctonus* are capable of inflicting painful wounds, only the southwestern desert scorpion (*Centruroides exilicauda*, formerly *Centruroides sculpturatus*) poses a serious health threat in the United States. They are called bark scorpions because they cling to the bottom of fallen brush and trees. They are tan-brown in color, vary in length from 1 to 6 cm, and are most active at night. The chitin shell of this scorpion will fluoresce under an ultraviolet or Wood's lamp, aiding in rapid identification (**Fig. 6**). *Centruroides* venoms are neurotoxic, causing repetitive firing of axons by activation of sodium channels. This activation causes spontaneous depolarization of both the sympathetic and the parasympathetic nervous systems.

Patient Evaluation Overview

Unless the scorpion is identified, the diagnosis is based on clinical symptoms. Most victims will have localized tenderness, with an increased sensitivity to touch over the area of the sting, exacerbated by tapping on the area. Patients suffering more serious envenomation manifest the venom effects from overstimulation of the sympathetic, parasympathetic, and central nervous systems. Elevation of blood pressure and heart rate typically occurs within an hour of envenomation, and tachydysrhythmias may develop during this time. Pediatric victims are at a greater risk for severe reactions. Disconjugate, "roving" eye movements are common in children, along with other neurologic findings, including muscle fasciculations, weakness, agitation, and

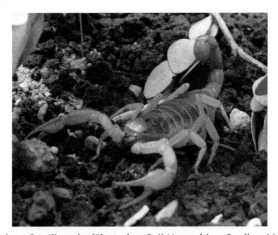

Fig. 5. Bark scorpion, *C exilicauda*. (Photo by: Gail Hampshire, Cradley, Malvern, U.K.)

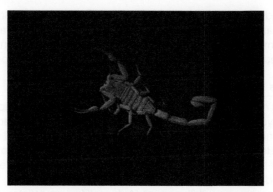

Fig. 6. Arizona bark scorpion glowing under ultraviolet light. (Photo by: Bryce Alexander.)

opisthotonos. Less common sequelae are severe ataxia, respiratory distress, seizures, and posterior reversible encephalopathy syndrome.[46]

Pharmacologic Treatment Options

Analgesics and tetanus prophylaxis should be administered. Benzodiazepines and opioids are indicated for agitation and muscle spasms. Tachydysrhythmias and hypertension may be treated with β-blockers, such as esmolol or labetalol. Advanced life support and airway control may be required for more severe envenomations.

In the United States, *Centruroides*-specific antivenom, an immune F(ab')$_2$ equine injection (Anascorp), was recently approved for severe envonomation by the US Food and Drug Administration.[47] Scorpion antivenom for other species has been produced for clinical use in several other countries. As with all animal-derived antivenoms, both immediate and delayed allergic reactions including serum sickness are possible. In a linked set of prospective trials of an equine F(ab')$_2$ antivenom, more than 1500 patients were treated with antivenom. There were only 1/500 acute adverse reactions and 1/200 delayed reactions, most of which were mild and did not require hospitalization or ED evaluation.[48] Although this study demonstrated antivenom can be administered safely, there remains concern that it may not be cost-effective. For this reason, *Centruroides*-specific antivenom (Anascorp *Centroides* scorpion immune F[ab]$_2$ equine injection) should be reserved for cases of severe systemic toxicity.[49]

Nonpharmacologic Treatment Options

The treatment of *Centruroides* envenomations is supportive. Cool compresses or ice packs and local wound care are used for the local symptoms and pain.

Evaluation of Outcome and Long-Term Recommendations

Clinical score predicting the need for hospitalization in scorpion stings has been described.[50] It is recommended that victims with systemic symptoms be observed for 24 hours, and children be admitted to the hospital for monitoring. Most patients with localized pain at the site of the sting can be safely discharged home with adequate pain medications.

HYMENOPTERA
Introduction

The order Hymenoptera includes bees, vespids (hornets and wasps), and fire ants. Bees and vespids cause more than one-fourth of all reported envenomations in the

United States and an estimated 50 annual deaths.[45] In the United States, 10% of all cases of anaphylaxis are attributed to stinging insects or hymenoptera.[51] Although hymenoptera venoms possess intrinsic toxicity, it is their ability to sensitize the victim and cause subsequent anaphylactic reactions that makes them so potentially lethal.

Bees and Vespids

Honeybees (*Apis mellifera*) are insects with alternating black and yellow body stripes. The female honeybee's stinger is a modified ovipositor that is connected to a venom sac. Because honeybees lose their barbed stinger after stinging and die, they generally only sting in defense when provoked or stepped on. Their venom causes a much greater release of histamine per gram than does other hymenoptera venom and thus is potentially more dangerous.

Africanized honeybees, or "killer bees" (*Apis mellifera scutellata*) (**Fig. 7**), are now found in Texas, Arizona, California, and most of the temperate southern states.[52] In the 1950s, African bees were imported into Brazil for breeding experiments designed to improve honey production and disease resistance. Many escaped and subsequently mated with other imported European honeybees.[53] These hybrids have since migrated northward along the coasts and temperate regions of the continent. Although the toxicity of their venom is equal to that of their native counterpart, they are far more aggressive. A hive can respond to a perceived threat with more than 10 times the number of bees within seconds. When the ovipositor is pulled from the bee's abdomen after stinging a victim, it releases a pheromone, isoamyl acetate. This pheromone attracts other bees to the victim and incites multiple stings. Massive numbers of stings from an attack of Africanized bees can result in multisystem damage and death from severe venom toxicity. Acute tubular necrosis and renal involvement with myoglobinuria are well-known complications of massive envenomation.[54] In swarms, these bees can overwhelm and kill even healthy nonallergic victims.[55] Envenomation from these aggressive arthropods has become a public health issue and is most dangerous to very young or elderly patients and those with concomitant medical conditions.[56]

The most common hornets in the United States are the yellow jackets (*Vespa pennsylvanica*). They are usually seen around garbage cans, beverage containers, and various foods. They are aggressive and sting with little provocation. Wasps (*Polistes annularis*, the paper wasp) have thin, smooth bodies and a formidable sting. They build

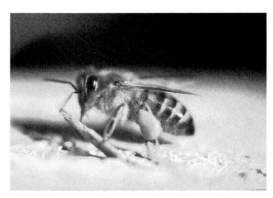

Fig. 7. Adult African killer bee, *A mellifera scutellata*. (*From* Jeffrey W. Lotz, Florida Department of Agriculture and Consumer Services, Bugwood.org.)

their nests in the eaves of buildings. Unlike honeybees, these vespids are carnivorous and able to use their smooth unbarbed stingers multiple times.[57,58]

Hymenoptera venoms contain enzymes (phospholipase A and hyaluronidase) that directly affect vascular tone and permeability. Most of the toxicity of the venom results from bradykinin, acetylcholine, dopamine, histamine, and serotonin. Although their enzymes are similar, there is little immunologic cross-reactivity between bee and vespid venoms. Although a bee sting may not sensitize a person to yellow jacket venom, a yellow jacket sting is more likely to sensitize one to wasp venom.[59]

Patient evaluation overview

Four possible reactions are seen after hymenoptera stings: a local reaction, toxic reaction, systemic anaphylaxis, and a less common delayed-type hypersensitivity reaction.[36,60]

Local reactions

Local reactions are the most common reactions resulting from the vasoactive effects of the venom and are generally mild. The most common response includes pain, erythema, edema, and pruritus at the sting site. Local reactions occurring in the mouth or throat can produce swelling that may compromise and lead to upper airway obstruction.

Toxic reactions

Toxic reactions may occur when a patient suffers from multiple stings. Africanized bees are notorious for such attacks, but an aggressive native hive may elicit a similar response. The essential lethal dose is approximately 20 stings per kilogram in most mammals.[57] Symptoms of a toxic reaction may resemble anaphylaxis, but gastrointestinal manifestations (vomiting and diarrhea) and sensations of light-headedness and syncope may also occur. Headache, fever, drowsiness, involuntary muscle spasms, edema (without urticarial), and seizures may ensue. Although urticaria and bronchospasm are not always present, severe envenomations may lead to respiratory arrest. Hepatic failure, rhabdomyolysis, coagulopathies, and DIC have been reported in victims. In addition, myocardial infarctions, cerebrovascular accidents, and intracranial bleeds have been described.[61] Toxic reactions are thought to occur from a direct multisystem effect of the venom.

Anaphylactic reactions

Anaphylactic reactions are generalized systemic allergic reactions that may occur after envenomation. They are thought to occur from an immunoglobulin E–mediated mechanism, leading to the release of pharmacologically active mediators within mast cells and basophils. Symptoms are initially mild, but severe reactions can lead to death within minutes. Unlike the toxic reaction, there is no correlation between systemic allergic reactions and the number of stings. Most allergic reactions occur within the first 10 to 15 minutes and nearly all occur within 6 hours. Fatalities that occur within the first hour of the sting usually result from airway obstruction or anaphylactic shock. Initial symptoms typically consist of ocular pruritus, facial flushing, and generalized urticaria. Symptoms may intensify rapidly with chest or throat constriction, wheezing, dyspnea, abdominal cramping, diarrhea, vomiting, vertigo, fever, laryngeal stridor, and syncope.

Delayed reactions

Delayed reactions, appearing 1 to 2 weeks after a sting consist of serum sickness–like signs and symptoms of fever, malaise, headache, urticaria, lymphadenopathy, and polyarthritis. This reaction is thought to be immune complex mediated.[60]

Pharmacologic treatment options

With more severe local reactions, there is a more sustained inflammatory response, and the swelling may spread to the entire extremity and persist for several days. A short course of antihistamines and prednisone (1 mg/kg/d for 5 days) may decrease the duration of symptoms. Systemic reactions occur in approximately 1% of hymenoptera stings. No specific antivenom currently exists for Hymenoptera stings. In all but the mildest of systemic reactions, the mainstay of treatment is epinephrine (**Table 1**). Epinephrine counteracts the bronchospastic and vasodilatory effects of histamine. Epinephrine can be given as an intramuscular injection (0.01 mL/kg of 1:1000 solution; not to exceed 0.3 mL). In more severe life-threatening reactions, the intravenous or endotracheal route is preferred (0.1 mL/kg of 1:10,000 solution). The dose may be repeated at 15-minute intervals as needed. Early intubation is indicated if there is evidence of severe laryngeal edema or stridor because airway obstruction is the leading cause of death in anaphylaxis. Antihistamines are given early, but not as a substitute for epinephrine. An H_2-receptor blocker (eg, famotidine or ranitidine), in addition to an H_1-receptor blocker (diphenhydramine), may aid in inhibiting the vasodilatory effects of histamine. Adjunctive therapy for bronchospasm includes inhaled β_2-agonists (eg, albuterol). When hypotension ensues, isotonic fluid resuscitation and pressor agents are instituted.

A biphasic allergic reaction can occur in up to 20% of patients. A general rule is that urticaria plus involvement of any other organ system constitutes anaphylaxis.[62] A delayed serum sickness–like reaction may appear 10 to 14 days following the initial sting. This immune complex disorder may be treated with a short course of prednisone.

Nonpharmacologic treatment options

If present, the embedded stinger should be removed manually. Previous sources recommended cautiously scraping the stinger off with lateral pressure, rather than grasping it, to avoid compression of the venom sac resulting in further venom release. Recent studies have demonstrated that this is erroneous because the venom has likely been completely released within seconds of envenomation.[63] Treatment is symptomatic, with ice or cold compresses.

Combinations therapies

An emergency insect sting kit generally contains a tourniquet, epinephrine in a 1:1000 dilution, and an antihistamine. These kits are widely available, and susceptible patients should carry them whenever they venture into the wilderness or remote settings.

Treatment resistance/complications

Most serious reactions to bee stings occur in the first 30 to 60 minutes. The local effects of a sting may persist for 2 or 3 days, or even weeks if there is a retained stinger. Delayed hypersensitivity may occur 7 to 10 days after the sting.[62]

Table 1
Hymenoptera sting treatment

Medication	Dose
Glucocorticoids	Methylprednisolone 125 mg intravenously (IV)
Antihistamine	Diphenhydramine: 25–50 mg IV or orally (PO)
Epinephrine	0.01 mL/kg of 1:1000 solution, do not exceed 0.3 mL intramuscularly
H2 blocker	Famotidine: 20 mg IV/PO Ranitidine: 50 mg IV/PO
Albuterol	2.5–5 mg every 20 min for 3 doses as needed

Evaluation of outcome and long-term recommendations
Essential to the treatment of any systemic reaction is the prevention of future reactions. Patients who have had a systemic reaction should be instructed to wear protective clothing and avoid hymenoptera-infested habitats. Portable epinephrine kits (Epi-Pen and Epi-Pen Jr) are available. They should be prescribed before the patient leaves the ED. The patient should be urged to carry the kit at all times when in the wilderness setting and to use epinephrine for any systemic symptoms. Even if symptoms are mild, the patient should seek emergency care. The patient should also be instructed to wear a medical alert tag.

Referral to an allergist is indicated for any patient who has experienced life-threatening respiratory symptoms or hypotension. Venom immunotherapy desensitization is very effective in preventing further systemic reactions, with 95% to 100% protection after 3 months of treatment. Victims who have only urticaria or angioedema do not require venom immunotherapy. Only 10% of these patients will have systemic reactions with subsequent stings.[63]

FIRE ANTS
Introduction

Five known species of fire ants belonging to the family Formicidae and genus *Solenopsis* are found in North America. Two of the species were imported into the United States, the red fire ant (*Solenopsis invicta*) and the black fire ant (*Solenopsis richteri*), of which *S invicta* is the predominant species and responsible for 95% of clinical cases (**Fig. 8**). They were imported aboard ships from Brazil in the 1940s and introduced in

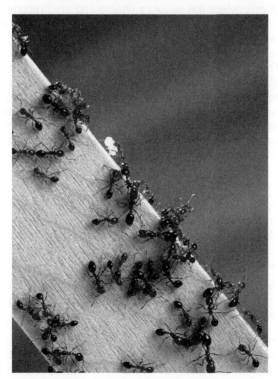

Fig. 8. Fire ants (*S invicta*). (*From* United States Department of Agriculture Agricultural Research Service, Image Number K5388-1. Photo by Scott Bauer.)

Alabama. They subsequently spread throughout the Southeast and are presently found in 13 southern states, from Florida to Texas. Their geographic range is limited by soil, temperature, and moisture.[64]

S invicta are 2 to 5 mm in size and red in color. They live in colonies and build large mounds up to 3 ft in diameter, which are interconnected by underground tunnels up to 100 ft long. These mounds are found most commonly in yards, parks, and open fields.[65] Fire ants are aggressive insects with no natural enemies and tend to attack in swarms, with multiple stings. In endemic areas, nearly 50% of the exposed population is stung each year. Stings occur most frequently on the ankles and feet during the summer months. Fire ants sting in a 2-phase process. The ant first bites the victim with powerful mandibles, then, if undisturbed, will arch the body and swivel around the attached mandibles to sting the victim repeatedly with the stinger or ovipositor. The sting sites produce a characteristic circular pattern of papules around 2 central punctures. Fierce fire ant attacks ensue in response to an alarming pheromone released by an individual or group of ants.

Bee and wasp venoms are made of proteins. Conversely, fire ant venoms are 95% alkaloid,[57] and the remaining 5% is very immunogenic, which can sensitize a victim to the venom. This sensitization creates a risk for future anaphylaxis, and 10% of victims have some degree of hypersensitivity.[66] The venoms have cytotoxic, bactericidal, insecticidal, and hemolytic properties. They also activate the complement pathway and promote histamine release.

Patient Evaluation Overview

Clinical manifestations reflect the venom's effects and are predominantly dermatologic reactions. The initial bites and stings cause a sharp burning pain associated with circular wheals or papules around the central hemorrhagic punctures. The wheal-and-flare reactions resolve within 1 hour, but then develop into sterile pustules within 24 hours. The pustules slough off over 48 to 72 hours, leaving shallow ulcerated lesions. The pustules are pruritic and often become contaminated after the victim scratches the lesions. Secondary infections may ensue but are usually minor. Approximately 25% of victims develop more severe local reactions, characterized by an exaggerated wheal-and-flare response, followed by the development of erythema, edema, and induration greater than 5 cm in diameter. These lesions are intensely pruritic, may resemble cellulitis, and persist for 24 to 72 hours.[65]

Pharmacologic Treatment Options

Topical glucocorticoid ointments, local anesthetic creams, and oral antihistamines are useful for the itching associated with these reactions. No intervention has been shown to prevent or resolve the pustules. Prophylactic antibiotics are generally not indicated.

Nonpharmacologic Treatment Options

Treatment consists of local conservative measures including application of ice or cool compresses for symptomatic relief and gentle, frequent cleansing of the affected areas to prevent secondary infections.

Combination therapies

Immunotherapy may be appropriate for persons with severe hypersensitivity to fire ant venom or those who have had a previous anaphylactic reaction to a fire ant sting. The efficacy of immunotherapy has been variable, but it has been reported to provide protection as high as 98%.[64,67]

Treatment resistance/complications

Anaphylactic reactions have been estimated to occur after as many as 1% of fire ant stings. Anaphylaxis may occur several hours after a sting and is known to occur more frequently in children than in adults. Those victims demonstrating severe allergic reactions should be referred for more comprehensive allergy skin testing.

Ticks

Ticks, which also belong to the class Arachnida, are vectors of human disease. With the recent changes in climate and global warming, they are increasing their North American distribution. Although less feared than spiders, they cause a higher morbidity because of transmission of infectious disease such as Rocky Mountain spotted fever. The bite of a tick is usually painless, but the victim may later have neurologic manifestations, including difficulties walking, weakness, flaccid paralysis, slurred speech, and visual disturbances. The victim usually has a history of recent outdoor activity. Two species responsible in North America are *Dermacentor andersoni* (wood tick) and *Dermacentor variabilis* (dog tick). The blacklegged tick (*Ixodes scapularis*) (**Fig. 9**) transmits *Borrelia burgdrferi* known to cause Lyme disease. Patients with a dermatologic "target lesion" or erythema migrans following a tick bite should be evaluated for Lyme disease (**Fig. 10**). These patients are treated with doxycycline or (other appropriate antibiotics if allergic) to prevent delayed neurologic and cardiotoxic manifestations. Investigations are ongoing with vaccine in development for Lyme disease.[68]

Centipedes, millipedes, and caterpillars

Several species of caterpillars (order Lepidoptera) as well as centipedes and millipedes (class Myriapoda) secrete substances that cause severe burning pain, numbness, pustular dermatitis, edema, vomiting, and headache.[69] Oropharyngeal exposure can cause mucosal edema and irritations. Centipedes are generally considered more venomous than millipedes. A recent case report describes a case of erucism and renal failure following Lonomia caterpillar envenomation.[70]

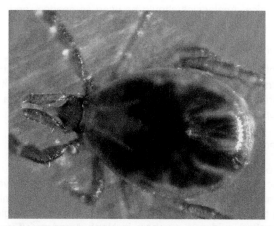

Fig. 9. The blacklegged tick (*I scapularis*), the primary vector for Lyme disease in the central and eastern Unites States. (*From* Gross L. A new view on Lyme disease: rodents hold the key to annual risk. PLoS Biol 2006;4(6):e182.)

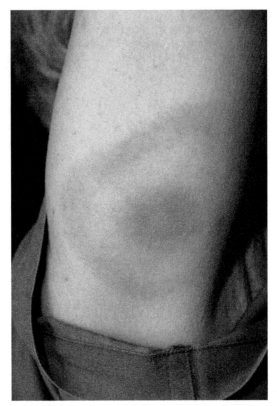

Fig. 10. *Eythema migrans* in Lyme disease depicting the pathognomonic erythematous rash in pattern of a "bull's eye" lesion. (*Courtesy of* CDC/James Gathany; and James Gathany.)

Pharmacologic Treatment Options

Centipedes can inflict bites that cause erythema and edema. Treatment is usually local soaks and analgesics. Analgesics should be used as needed, and more supportive therapy may be needed for severe envenomation.

Nonpharmacologic Treatment Options

Treatment consists of washing the area thoroughly with soap and water and removing any spines or hairs present. Spines of caterpillars can be removed with adhesive tape or by applying white water-soluble glue. Locally applied ice packs, a paste of baking soda paste, or topical lidocaine[71] may be beneficial.

OTHER ARTHROPODS

Many other arthropods such as beetles (order Coleoptera) can cause local skin reactions and allergic reactions, depending on the individual's sensitivity. Patients are treated symptomatically with local steroid creams and antihistamines. Conenose bugs or "kissing bugs" may cause severe local and systemic allergic reactions and have recently reached epidemic numbers in North America[72] (**Fig. 11**). Treatment with antihistamines and local wound care, depending on the degree of reaction, are generally all that is needed.

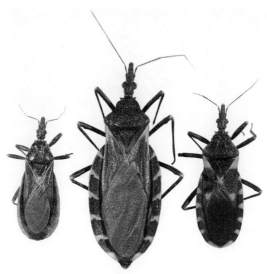

Fig. 11. Three species of kissing bugs: *Triatoma protracta*, the most common species in the western United States; *Triatoma geraeckeri*, the most common in Texas; *Tritoma sanguisuga*, most common in the eastern United States. (*From* Curtis-Robles R, Wozniak EJ, Auckland LD, et al. Combining public health education and disease ecology research: using citizen science to assess Chagas disease entomological risk in Texas. PLoS Negl Trop Dis 2015;9:e0004235.)

Mosquitoes (class Insecta, family Culicidae), although technically not considered venomous arthropods, are abundant and annoying throughout North America. They can be dangerous vectors for diseases such as malaria, dengue fever, Chikungunya, and Zika virus in tropical regions of Africa, Asia, and South and Central America. Recently, Zika virus has been reported in North America in persons traveling from Brazil and the Caribbean.[73,74] Mosquitoes responsible for the transmission of Zika virus include *Aedes albopitus* and *Aedes aegypti* (**Fig. 12**).

Protection and Prevention

Protection from arthropod bites is best achieved by avoiding infested areas, wearing protective clothing, and using insect repellents. Insect repellents containing *N,N*-diethyl-meta-toluamide (DEET) are the most effective products on the market, providing broad-spectrum repellency lasting several hours. DEET's peak duration of action plateaus at a concentration of 50%, with no added benefit from products containing higher concentrations.[75] Topical insect repellents (often combined with sunscreen products) generally do not provide complete protection. However, products containing ethyl butylacetylaminopropionate can provide protection for up to 3 hours and can be safely added to sunscreen lotions without potential side effects.[76] Mosquitoes bite untreated skin and may even bite through clothing. Deerflies, midges, black flies, and ticks prefer to bite around the head and will crawl into the hair to bite unprotected areas. Wearing protective clothing with long sleeves and pants, including a hat, reduces the chance of being bitten. Treating clothes and hats with permethrin in addition to spraying with DEET on the skin offers the greatest protection. Mesh insect tents or bedding provides additional lines of defense. Finally, avoiding hikes or outdoor activities at dawn or dusk can diminish arthropod encounters.

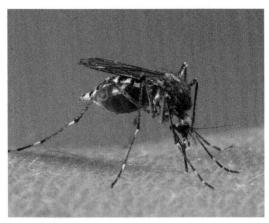

Fig. 12. *A aegypti* mosquito, biting a human. (*From* US Department of Agriculture Agricultural Research Service, Image Number K4705-9.)

Outdoor enthusiasts traveling throughout the wilderness or to a part of the world where insect-borne disease is a potential threat should educate themselves concerning indigenous arthropods as well as the toxicities and diseases they may transmit.

REFERENCES

1. Otten E. Venomous animal injuries. In: Walls RW, Hockberger RS, Gausche-Hill MA, editors. Rosen's emergency medicine: concepts and clinical practice. 9th edition. Philadelphia: Elsevier; 2017. p. 698–714.
2. Isbister GK, Fan HW. Spider bite. Lancet 2011;378(9808):2039–47.
3. Diaz JH, Leblanc KE. Common spider bites. Am Fam Physician 2007;75(6): 869–73.
4. Monte AA, Bucher-Bartelson B, Heard KJ. A US perspective of symptomatic Latrodectus spp. envenomation and treatment: a National Poison data system review. Ann Pharmacother 2011;45(12):1491–8.
5. Peterson ME. Black widow spider envenomation. Clin Tech Small Anim Pract 2006;21(4):187–90.
6. Rash LD, Hodgson WC. Pharmacology and biochemistry of spider venoms. Toxicon 2002;40(3):225–54.
7. Clark RF, Wethern-Kestner S, Vance MV, et al. Clinical presentation and treatment of black widow spider envenomation: a review of 163 cases. Ann Emerg Med 1992;21(7):782–7.
8. Bush SP. Black widow spider envenomation mimicking cholecystitis. Am J Emerg Med 1999;17(3):315.
9. Sotelo-Cruz N, Hurtado-Valenzuela JG, Gomez-Rivera N. Poisoning caused by Latrodectus Mactans (Black Widow) spider bite among children. Clinical features and therapy. Gac Med Mex 2006;142(2):103–8 [in Spanish].
10. Dendane T, Abidi K, Madani N, et al. Reversible myocarditis after black widow spider envenomation. Case Rep Med 2012;2012:794540.
11. Cohen J, Bush S. Case report: compartment syndrome after a suspected black widow spider bite. Ann Emerg Med 2005;45(4):414–6.
12. Hoover NG, Fortenberry JD. Use of antivenin to treat priapism after a black widow spider bite. Pediatrics 2004;114(1):e128–9.

13. Goel SC, Yabrodi M, Fortenberry J. Recognition and successful treatment of priapism and suspected black widow spider bite with antivenin. Pediatr Emerg Care 2014;30(10):723–4.

14. Nordt SP, Clark RF, Lee A, et al. Examination of adverse events following black widow antivenom use in California. Clin Toxicol (Phila) 2012;50(1):70–3.

15. Gonzalez Valverde FM, Gomez Ramos MJ, Menarguez Pina F, et al. Fatal latrodectism in an elderly man. Med Clin (Barc) 2001;117(8):319 [in Spanish].

16. Pneumatikos IA, Galiatsou E, Goe D, et al. Acute fatal toxic myocarditis after black widow spider envenomation. Ann Emerg Med 2003;41(1):158.

17. Prongay R, Kelsberg G, Safranek S. Clinical inquiry: which treatments relieve painful muscle spasms from a black widow spider bite? J Fam Pract 2012; 61(11):694–5.

18. Clark RF. The safety and efficacy of antivenin Latrodectus mactans. J Toxicol Clin Toxicol 2001;39(2):125–7.

19. Dart RC, Bogdan G, Heard K, et al. A randomized, double-blind, placebo-controlled trial of a highly purified equine F(ab)2 antibody black widow spider antivenom. Ann Emerg Med 2013;61(4):458–67.

20. Shackleford R, Veillon D, Maxwell N, et al. The black widow spider bite: differential diagnosis, clinical manifestations, and treatment options. J La State Med Soc 2015;167(2):74–8.

21. Murphy CM, Hong JJ, Beuhler MC. Anaphylaxis with Latrodectus antivenin resulting in cardiac arrest. J Med Toxicol 2011;7(4):317–21.

22. Rader RK, Stoecker WV, Malters JM, et al. Seasonality of brown recluse populations is reflected by numbers of brown recluse envenomations. Toxicon 2012; 60(1):1–3.

23. Vetter RS. Seasonality of brown recluse spiders, Loxosceles reclusa, submitted by the general public: implications for physicians regarding loxoscelism diagnoses. Toxicon 2011;58(8):623–5.

24. Erickson T, Hryhorczuk DO, Lipscomb J, et al. Brown recluse spider bites in an urban wilderness. J Wilderness Med 1990;1:258–64.

25. Saupe EE, Papes M, Selden PA, et al. Tracking a medically important spider: climate change, ecological niche modeling, and the brown recluse (Loxosceles reclusa). PLoS One 2011;6(3):e17731.

26. Dare RK, Conner KB, Tan PC, et al. Brown recluse spider bite to the upper lip. J Ark Med Soc 2012;108(10):208–10.

27. Tutrone WD, Green KM, Norris T, et al. Brown recluse spider envenomation: dermatologic application of hyperbaric oxygen therapy. J Drugs Dermatol 2005;4(4):424–8.

28. Swanson DL, Vetter RS. Bites of brown recluse spiders and suspected necrotic arachnidism. N Engl J Med 2005;352(7):700–7.

29. Tarullo DB, Jacobsen RC, Algren DA. Two successive necrotic lesions secondary to presumed loxosceles envenomation. Wilderness Environ Med 2013;24(2): 132–5.

30. Furbee RB, Kao LW, Ibrahim D. Brown recluse spider envenomation. Clin Lab Med 2006;26(1):211–26, ix-x.

31. Osterhoudt KC. Diagnosis of brown recluse spider bites in absence of spiders. Clin Pediatr (Phila) 2004;43(4):407 [author reply: 407–8].

32. Vetter RS, Swanson DL. Of spiders and zebras: publication of inadequately documented loxoscelism case reports. J Am Acad Dermatol 2007;56(6):1063–4.

33. Abraham M, Tilzer L, Hoehn KS, et al. Therapeutic plasma exchange for refractory hemolysis after brown recluse spider (Loxosceles reclusa) envenomation. J Med Toxicol 2015;11(3):364–7.

34. Elbahlawan LM, Stidham GL, Bugnitz MC, et al. Severe systemic reaction to Loxosceles reclusa spider bites in a pediatric population. Pediatr Emerg Care 2005; 21(3):177–80.

35. McKeown N, Vetter RS, Hendrickson RG. Verified spider bites in Oregon (USA) with the intent to assess hobo spider venom toxicity. Toxicon 2014;84:51–5.

36. Tong TSA, Clark RF. Arthropod bites and stings. In: Erickson TB, editor. Pediatric toxicology: diagnosis and management of the poisoned child. New York: McGraw-Hill, Medical Pub. Division; 2005. p. 624.

37. Cabaniss WW, Bush S, O'Rourke DP, et al. A randomized controlled trial of trypsin to treat brown recluse spider bites in Guinea pigs. J Med Toxicol 2014;10(3):266–8.

38. Phillips S, Kohn M, Baker D, et al. Therapy of brown spider envenomation: a controlled trial of hyperbaric oxygen, dapsone, and cyproheptadine. Ann Emerg Med 1995;25(3):363–8.

39. de Roodt AR, Estevez-Ramirez J, Litwin S, et al. Toxicity of two North American Loxosceles (brown recluse spiders) venoms and their neutralization by antivenoms. Clin Toxicol (Phila) 2007;45(6):678–87.

40. Isbister GK, Graudins A, White J, et al. Antivenom treatment in arachnidism. J Toxicol Clin Toxicol 2003;41(3):291–300.

41. Saucier JR. Arachnid envenomation. Emerg Med Clin North Am 2004;22(2): 405–22, ix.

42. Choi JT, Rauf A. Ophthalmia nodosa secondary to tarantula hairs. Eye (Lond) 2003;17(3):433–4.

43. Yang Y, Christakis T, Mireskandari K. Acute conjunctivitis and corneal foreign bodies secondary to tarantula hairs. CMAJ 2016;188(3):212–4.

44. Chippaux JP, Goyffon M. Epidemiology of scorpionism: a global appraisal. Acta Trop 2008;107(2):71–9.

45. Forrester JA, Holstege CP, Forrester JD. Fatalities from venomous and nonvenomous animals in the United States (1999-2007). Wilderness Environ Med 2012;23(2):146–52.

46. Porcello Marrone LC, Marrone BF, Neto FK, et al. Posterior reversible encephalopathy syndrome following a scorpion sting. J Neuroimaging 2013;23(4):535–6.

47. Quan D. North American poisonous bites and stings. Crit Care Clin 2012;28(4): 633–59.

48. Boyer L, Degan J, Ruha AM, et al. Safety of intravenous equine F(ab')2: insights following clinical trials involving 1534 recipients of scorpion antivenom. Toxicon 2013;76:386–93.

49. Armstrong EP, Bakall M, Skrepnek GH, et al. Is scorpion antivenom cost-effective as marketed in the United States? Toxicon 2013;76:394–8.

50. Quan D, LoVecchio F. A clinical score predicting the need for hospitalization in scorpion envenomation. Am J Emerg Med 2007;25(7):856.

51. Tankersley MS, Ledford DK. Stinging insect allergy: state of the art 2015. J Allergy Clin Immunol Pract 2015;3(3):315–22 [quiz: 323].

52. Ferreira RS Jr, Almeida RA, Barraviera SR, et al. Historical perspective and human consequences of Africanized bee stings in the Americas. J Toxicol Environ Health B Crit Rev 2012;15(2):97–108.

53. Whitfield CW, Behura SK, Berlocher SH, et al. Thrice out of Africa: ancient and recent expansions of the honey bee, Apis mellifera. Science 2006;314(5799):642–5.

54. Bridi RA, Balbi AL, Neves PM, et al. Acute kidney injury after massive attack of Africanised bees. BMJ Case Rep 2014;2014.
55. Bledsoe BE. Unwelcome visitors: is EMS ready for fire ants and killer bees. EMS Mag 2007;36(8):68, 70, 72 passim.
56. Zaluski R, Kadri SM, Souza EA, et al. Africanized honeybees in urban areas: a public health concern. Rev Soc Bras Med Trop 2014;47(5):659–62.
57. Fitzgerald KT, Flood AA. Hymenoptera stings. Clin Tech Small Anim Pract 2006; 21(4):194–204.
58. Vetter RS, Visscher PK, Camazine S. Mass envenomations by honey bees and wasps. West J Med 1999;170(4):223–7.
59. Hamilton RG. Diagnosis of Hymenoptera venom sensitivity. Curr Opin Allergy Clin Immunol 2002;2(4):347–51.
60. Mingomataj EC, Bakiri AH, Ibranji A, et al. Unusual reactions to hymenoptera stings: what should we keep in mind? Clin Rev Allergy Immunol 2014;47(1):91–9.
61. Ciron J, Mathis S, Iljicsov A, et al. Multiple simultaneous intracranial hemorrhages due to hornet stings. Clin Neurol Neurosurg 2015;128:53–5.
62. Lee JK, Vadas P. Anaphylaxis: mechanisms and management. Clin Exp Allergy 2011;41(7):923–38.
63. Erickson T. North American arthropod envenomation and parasitism. In: Auerbach PS, editor. Wilderness medicine. 5th edition. Philadelphia: Mosby Elsevier; 2007. p. 2316.
64. Rhoades R. Stinging ants. Curr Opin Allergy Clin Immunol 2001;1(4):343–8.
65. Kemp SF, deShazo RD, Moffitt JE, et al. Expanding habitat of the imported fire ant (Solenopsis invicta): a public health concern. J Allergy Clin Immunol 2000;105(4): 683–91.
66. Demain JG, Minaei AA, Tracy JM. Anaphylaxis and insect allergy. Curr Opin Allergy Clin Immunol 2010;10(4):318–22.
67. Tankersley MS. The stinging impact of the imported fire ant. Curr Opin Allergy Clin Immunol 2008;8(4):354–9.
68. Contreras M, Villar M, Alberdi P, et al. Vaccinomics approach to tick vaccine development. Methods Mol Biol 2016;1404:275–86.
69. French RN, Brillhart D. Images in clinical medicine. Erucism due to lepidoptera caterpillar envenomation. N Engl J Med 2015;373(18):e21.
70. Schmitberger PA, Fernandes TC, Santos RC, et al. Probable chronic renal failure caused by Lonomia caterpillar envenomation. J Venom Anim Toxins Incl Trop Dis 2013;19(1):14.
71. Haddad V Jr, Lastoria JC. Envenomation by caterpillars (erucism): proposal for simple pain relief treatment. J Venom Anim Toxins Incl Trop Dis 2014;20:21.
72. Klotz SA, Shirazi FM, Boesen K, et al. Kissing Bug (Triatoma spp.) intrusion into homes: troublesome bites and domiciliation. Environ Health Insights 2016;10:45–9.
73. Guerbois M, Fernandez-Salas I, Azar SR, et al. Outbreak of Zika virus infection, Chiapas State, Mexico, 2015, and first confirmed transmission by Aedes aegypti mosquitoes in the Americas. J Infect Dis 2016;214(9):1349–56.
74. Wikan N, Smith DR. Zika virus: history of a newly emerging arbovirus. Lancet Infect Dis 2016;16(7):e119–126.
75. Fradin MS, Day JF. Comparative efficacy of insect repellents against mosquito bites. N Engl J Med 2002;347(1):13–8.
76. Webb CE, Russell RC. Insect repellents and sunscreen: implications for personal protection strategies against mosquito-borne disease. Aust N Z J Public Health 2009;33(5):485–90.

Wilderness Emergency Medical Services Systems

 CrossMark

Michael G. Millin, MD, MPH[a],*, Seth C. Hawkins, MD[b]

KEYWORDS

- Wilderness • Emergency medical services • Medical direction

KEY POINTS

- Wilderness emergency medical services (EMS) programs should be integrated with local emergency response programs.
- Wilderness EMS programs should function with the oversight of a qualified physician medical director.
- Wilderness EMS providers should function with defined scopes of practice as determined by their education, certification of that education, licensure, and local medical director credentialing. These scopes of practice should include provisions to use operationally specific protocols that are approved by the local medical director and the appropriate EMS regulatory authority.

INTRODUCTION

Although one could argue that the history of emergency medical services (EMS) dates back to the Napoleonic Wars or perhaps the US Civil War, when organized systems were developed to move injured soldiers off the battle field, formal wilderness EMS (WEMS) programs in the United States can be traced to 1938 with the work of Charles Minot Dole and the formation of a ski rescue committee with the National Ski Association.[1]

Over the past 75 years, wilderness medicine and EMS have both evolved greatly in their own rights. With the development of the Wilderness Medical Society (WMS), the National Association of EMS Physicians (NAEMSP), and their respective scientific journals, these 2 disciplines have established themselves as bona fide practices of medicine. This is an exciting time as the practice of WEMS is in evolution,

Disclosure: The authors disclose that they are codirectors of the national Wilderness EMS Medical Director's Course mentioned in the body of this article. The authors further report that there are no other financial disclosures relevant to this article.
[a] Department of Emergency Medicine, Johns Hopkins University School of Medicine, Maryland Search and Rescue, 5801 Smith Avenue, Davis Building, Suite 3220, Baltimore, MD 21209, USA;
[b] Department of Emergency Medicine, Wake Forest University School of Medicine, Burke County EMS Special Operations Team, 200 Avery Avenue, Morganton, NC 28655, USA
* Corresponding author.
E-mail address: MichaelGMillin@gmail.com

Emerg Med Clin N Am 35 (2017) 377–389
http://dx.doi.org/10.1016/j.emc.2016.12.001

emed.theclinics.com

combining the creativity of wilderness medicine with the structure of formal EMS systems.

Definition of Emergency Medical Services

The National Association of State EMS Officials (NASEMSO) defines EMS as an "Integrated system of medical response... that includes the full spectrum of response from recognition of the emergency to access of the healthcare system, dispatch of appropriate response, pre-arrival instructions, direct patient care by trained personnel, and appropriate transport or disposition."[2]

Further, in their statement defining EMS, the NASEMSO medical directors council states that anyone participating in any of the activities of EMS, regardless of the environment, is by definition engaging in the practice of EMS medicine, which requires the oversight of a qualified physician.[2]

To those who are not directly involved in their operations, EMS systems may look very different throughout the United States and even the world. These differences become quite pronounced when comparing traditional frontcountry EMS programs to backcountry WEMS programs. Yet, despite these differences, the fundamental elements of EMS systems remain the same.

With the 1964 publication of *Accidental Death and Disability: The Neglected Disease of Modern Society*, the public and Congress began to take notice of the importance of improving the system of emergency care in the United States.[3] This publication identified a fractured emergency care system, beginning with poor quality care provided to patients in the out-of-hospital milieu and a disorganized system of getting patients to acute care hospitals.

In 1973, Congress passed the EMS Act, appropriating federal resources to the development of regional EMS systems.[4] The EMS Act of 1973 identified 15 essential components to an EMS system: personnel, training, communications, transportation, facilities, critical care units, public safety agencies, consumer participation, access to care, patient transfer, coordinated patient record-keeping, public information and education, review and evaluation, disaster planning, and mutual aid. Interestingly, the original development of EMS systems did not stipulate physician involvement, an oversight that would be corrected in future years.

Given the essential components of an EMS system as identified by the 1973 EMS Act and the more recently published definition of EMS by NASEMSO, perhaps the following scenario will clarify the general structure and purpose of an EMS system:

It's a bright sunny day and Mr Jones is out for a bike ride with a bunch of friends. Without notice or a precipitating event, Mr Jones falls off his bike and lies on the ground unresponsive. One of Mr Jones' fellow bike riders recently completed a bystander hands-only cardiopulmonary resuscitation (CPR) course offered by the local fire department and recognized that Mr Jones was having agonal respirations. He quickly began chest compressions and another friend called 9-1-1. The dispatcher mobilized appropriate resources and continued to assist the friends on the telephone. Within minutes the fire department arrived with an automated external defibrillator. Mr Jones was shocked out of ventricular fibrillation, transferred to a hospital where he had emergent percutaneous coronary intervention showing a 100% left anterior descending artery lesion. He was discharged from the hospital 2 days later, neurologically intact, to follow-up with cardiac rehab.

This scenario highlights many important components to an EMS system. Through community engagement, the EMS system was able to educate Mr Jones' friends in the technique of hands-only CPR and how to access the emergency care system. The firefighters that arrived acted on protocols that were developed by an EMS medical director who ultimately provides oversight and responsibility for the care of Mr Jones. Mr Jones was then safely transferred to an acute care hospital that initiated definitive care and follow-up.

Without the essential components of an EMS system previously outlined, Mr Jones would likely have died for lack of community engagement and appropriately trained resources arriving to his side. Analogous medical and traumatic emergencies are seen in wilderness areas as those seen in areas covered by more traditional EMS agencies. It is the challenge and priority of WEMS system medical directors and administrators to develop programs that provide, with reasonable consideration to logistical and environmental factors, similarly high quality of care to patients in the wilderness as is delivered in urban areas.

Definition of Wilderness Emergency Medical Services

The NASEMSO definition of EMS states that anyone engaging in the activities of EMS is practicing EMS medicine, regardless of the environmental constraints. Further, the 1973 EMS Act does not describe specific environments for the development of an EMS system, thereby implying that the requirements to create an EMS system apply for all environments. It follows that the care of patients in a wilderness environment should be supported by a similar organizational structure as care of patients in traditional frontcountry environments.

Considering the scenario with Mr Jones, this patient's greatest chance for neurologically intact survival lies in a system that is able to initiate early CPR, mobilize trained resources, and transport him to an acute care hospital capable of performing cardiac intervention. EMS is this system and in the wilderness such a system is called WEMS.

Defining wilderness, and those circumstances in which WEMS providers are operational and protocols are activated, is critical. In some systems, the same provider might be operating within a specific scope of practice in a traditional system but another when he or she is in a wilderness setting. Many authors have proposed criteria to define wilderness in the sense of a different type of medical care needed. These definitions include distance to definitive care (variably defined but usually somewhere between 1 to 2 hours), the presence of environmental considerations, or austerity (lack of traditional resources). Yet all these definitions have significant barriers to being applied universally and so it must be understood that definitions in WEMS must be contextual. A more compelling definition encompassing multiple situational factors is "medical management in situations where care and prevention are limited by environmental considerations, prolonged extrication, and/or resource availability."[5] A more recent definition, higher in complexity but more specific to EMS care, is the systematic and preplanned delivery of medical care in those areas where fixed or transient geographic challenges reduce availability or alter requirements for medical or patient movement resources.[6]

Clearly, the constraints of the wilderness environment necessitate a different structure compared with traditional frontcountry EMS. Most obviously, EMS providers responding to WEMS events need to be trained and prepared to operate in the extremes of environmental conditions and carry into those environments the equipment needed for their own self-preservation and the care of their patients.

Noting that WEMS systems evolved from volunteers in the skiing and climbing community desiring to help their fellow outdoor enthusiasts, a prevailing attitude has been that something is better than nothing, regardless of the quality of the intervention. This has led to the development of a system of wilderness response agencies that often were not integrated into the emergency care system, that often functioned without physician oversight, and that lacked the essential components to an EMS system.

In an effort to address the lack of integration of wilderness medical response with the rest of the emergency care system, NAEMSP and NASEMSO published a position statement on medical oversight of operational EMS programs, which includes ski patrols, wilderness search and rescue (SAR) teams, urban SAR teams, fast or open water rescue teams, and wildland fire crews.[7] This statement points out that these programs should function within and not outside the health care system and have a qualified medical director that ensures established patient care standards are met.

There is no doubt that it can be logistically and even financially constraining for a volunteer wilderness SAR team or ski patrol to meet all the requirements of an EMS system. However, assuming the ultimate purpose is provision of quality patient care, this goal is quite appropriate. Regardless of the environment, the pathophysiology of acute coronary syndrome, major trauma, or the myriad of emergent conditions is generally the same. Further, the environmental factors of temperature extremes and prolonged extrication that are specific to WEMS response may exacerbate or even accelerate underlying pathophysiology, making patient care management more complex. From a patient care perspective, it makes sense that the health care system designed to manage emergent conditions in the wilderness should also be designed to provide quality and expeditious patient care, physician oversight, and processes for review and continuous improvement.

WILDERNESS EMERGENCY MEDICAL SERVICES SYSTEM STRUCTURE
Review of the Components of an Emergency Medical Services System

When Congress passed the EMS Act in 1973, the primary purpose was to address growing concerns for poor quality care that was being delivered to the public in frontcountry situations. WEMS system development was not a priority in the development of the 15 essential components to an EMS system. Although many of the original essential components fit WEMS, some are less relevant.

The strength of a WEMS program is in its personnel (see later discussion). Many WEMS programs are largely composed of volunteer EMS providers. Although it can at times be difficult to find individuals to volunteer, those that step up are typically very committed to the mission. In addition, these team members tend to come from a variety of personal and professional backgrounds, which help to create robust systems with depth of skills and resources.

A challenge for a volunteer EMS program is training. Team members will have to commit to training time because the case volume is typically low and skills not used in health care tend to dissolve fairly quickly. Thus, a good amount of time in WEMS is spent in training, which is logistically difficult for team members and instructors.

Another logistical challenge is communication. Most frontcountry traditional EMS programs are supported by robust radio systems and cellular telephone communication technologies. In WEMS communication can be difficult and sparse. Thus, programs need to invest in mobile communication platforms and would benefit from coordination with state repeater systems. Communication between field EMS providers and base station physicians at acute care hospitals is typically very difficult to achieve, necessitating allowance for the EMS providers to make more decisions on their own or provide care with operationally specific protocols, supported by after-action patient care review procedures.

The starkest difference between traditional EMS and WEMS is the forms of transportation. Although traditional EMS programs typically transport patients in vehicular ambulances and use rotor-wing air medical transport, WEMS programs usually do not have access to vehicular ambulances. WEMS programs may use rotor wing at times but sometimes the units used for extrication are not designated for patient care and, even when medical helicopters are used, improvised heliports may by necessity be far from the patient. A common misunderstanding of WEMS is that vehicle access is always more limited than traditional EMS. In some wilderness areas, such as the summit of Denali (the highest point in North America), Linville Gorge (the deepest gorge in the Eastern United States), or the base camp of Everest (whose summit is the highest point on the globe), specialized helicopter assets are used that would not be available to the standard frontcountry EMS system or even hospital system. When a vehicle is eventually accessible, it is typical to carry patients out on litters or even make use of techniques for assisted walkouts from remote locations to that vehicle. Other alternate vehicles and transport tools may be used in WEMS, including pack animals, all-terrain vehicles, boats, and litter wheels. Also, importantly, vehicular deployment in the field, especially helicopters is the exception rather than the rule in American WEMS systems (although helicopters are much more widely used in Europe). In the United States, 90% of all rescues are performed on foot.[8]

The destination facility used for the care of sick patients is the same for traditional and WEMS programs: local acute care hospitals and regional specialty centers. However, WEMS programs may also use backcountry first aid tents as an intermediary location for patient evaluation and treatment. When staffed with physicians, or with physician support, these first aid tents may also function as the end location for less sick patients that are treated and released to follow up with primary care physicians.

WEMS programs typically do not make use of their own critical care transport units, identifying a crucial opportunity for system integration between WEMS programs and traditional EMS. WEMS programs may also want to partner with traditional EMS by developing mutual aid agreements with transfer of care plans, support local and regional disaster plans, and engage consumer participation and public information in activities of the agency.

Because a WEMS program is by definition a public safety agency, it is also important that the program have a method for recordkeeping, and for review and evaluation of care provided, and the program itself. Finally, the purpose of a WEMS program is to provide access to health care to the public in an environment that is by definition austere. It is this access to care that is the foundation to the importance for developing a structured program.

Wilderness Emergency Medical Services Providers

Within the context of the National EMS Scope of Practice document, traditional EMS providers derive their scope of practice, or their permission to care for the public, from 4 pillars: education, certification, licensure, and credentialing.[9] Once an EMS provider has graduated from an EMS training program, the provider will take a certification examination verifying their skills that may be based on state or national requirements. Although some states do offer licensure for EMS providers, many do not, leading the provider to acquire licensure through the supervision of a medical director. Regardless of the method of licensure, all EMS providers require local credentialing, which comes from the oversight and supervision of the physician medical director. Nationally, there are 4 levels of EMS providers: emergency medical responder, emergency medical technician, advanced emergency medical technician, and paramedic.

Anticipating that the National EMS Scopes of Practice would not fulfill the needs of all environments, the authors specifically wrote that in "some cases, specialty certifications may be used to respond to local needs" to address the challenges of a specific practice environment.[9] This stipulation opened up the door for future development of specialized training for EMS providers functioning in wilderness environments.

However, to date, most state EMS regulatory authorities do not recognize the specialized training of EMS providers working in wilderness areas, creating a challenge for programs that aim to integrate WEMS with traditional EMS venues.

In an effort to address this gap, the WEMS Committee of the NAEMSP is currently leading an effort to develop WEMS scopes of practice that will meet the unique needs of providers working in the wilderness and the requirements of oversight regulatory bodies.[10] If successful, this project will be an important step forward in advancing WEMS as a recognized and defined component of the emergency care system.

Medical Oversight

WEMS medical directors accomplish the task of medical oversight of the activities of the WEMS providers through 2 primary activities: indirect oversight and direct oversight. Although indirect oversight includes all of the support activities that occur before and after an event, direct oversight includes real-time participation in the care of the patient.

With regard to indirect oversight, the physician tasks are divided into 3 categories: protocol development, education, and quality improvement (QI).

Protocols are written documents that provide direction on how the providers should address specific situations. These protocols should, as much as possible, be evidence-based and grounded in science. Yet, because the science of WEMS is still quite new, many WEMS protocols will require the protocol development team to draw on literature from other practice environments, typically traditional EMS or emergency medicine. In many cases, a committee, chaired by the medical director and including the involvement of team providers and other important stakeholders, such as local trauma surgeons, cardiologists, and other public health officials, should write the protocols for the WEMS team. Written EMS protocols typically follow a standard format, addressing critical issues such as resuscitation, trauma, and medical emergencies. WEMS protocols should also focus on environmental emergencies relevant to the operational environment. Historically, WEMS protocols have permitted medical operators to pursue activities beyond those of traditional providers, such as antibiotic administration or dislocation reduction. In some cases such protocols, like termination of resuscitation or ruling out the need for spinal motion restriction, preceded the introduction of similar protocols in traditional systems by many years.[11,12] WEMS protocols are a living document, subject to periodic changes based on evolving literature and lessons learned from team deployments.

Perhaps the easiest way for physicians to get involved with a WEMS program is to participate in the education of the providers. WEMS providers, like all members of the health care team, require initial and continuing education to achieve and maintain clinical competence within their defined scope of practice. Whereas many WEMS agencies outsource initial education to a recognized wilderness medical training school, most provide opportunities for continuing education in-house or a combination of outsourced and in-house training. Physicians are well placed to participate, and in some cases lead, continuing education programs for the providers because they are able to bridge the gap between textbook learning and real patient care experiences. As with protocol development, continuing education should focus on standard skills for all EMS providers as outlined in the National EMS Scope of Practice Document, and also include skills specific to the wilderness.

In an effort to maintain a culture focused on continuous improvement in the delivery of patient care, a robust QI program should be integrated into the overall structure of the program. All patient care encounters should be documented in an electronic, searchable format, which will provide a foundation for case-by-case and aggregate analysis of the care provided by the team. Because the case volume for WEMS responses tends to be fairly low, it should be possible to perform 100% case review by the medical director and QI team. Cases should be reviewed for completeness of charting; care delivered; and areas for growth, improvement, or celebration. Ideally, the medical director and team educators should meet with the entire team on a regular basis to integrate the QI activities into normal educational activities. Other QI activities include integration of the WEMS program with the local traditional EMS programs, community CPR training, and other community outreach programs.

Direct medical oversight, the process of real-time physician participation in the care of the patient, is perhaps the most interesting role for the medical director. This type of medical oversight may be achieved via cellular telephone communication when the medical director is off-site, radio communication when the medical director is in the field stationed at a base camp location, or in-person when the medical director has responded with the team to the patient's side. Within the context of WEMS, compared with traditional EMS, direct medical oversight via cellular telephone communication may be difficult because there is often poor cellular telephone reception deep in wilderness tracts.

As identified by the NAEMSP/NASEMSO position on operational EMS, WEMS medical directors who deploy into the field should become fully trained and integrated members of the response team.[7] This represents a significant time commitment for the physician medical director, yet also ensures that the medical director stays in touch with the capabilities of the team and the challenges of the work environment.

Understanding that many physicians who have a desire to work with a response team as a WEMS medical director may not have experience or expertise in WEMS system design and oversight, the NAEMSP in partnership with the WMS have cosponsored a course designed to bridge this gap. The WEMS Medical Director Course is designed as a 16-hour course providing an overview of WEMS system structure and the complexities of both indirect and direct medical oversight.[13,14] The course also covers matters of regulatory compliance and avoidance of legal pitfalls.

Equipment

Equipment needed to safely and effectively complete the mission of WEMS response includes operational equipment for personnel and group response, as well as medical equipment for patient care. Although a medical director may have an opinion on operational equipment, it is ultimately the decision of administrative team leaders to determine what equipment not related to patient care will be carried in a response pack. However, the medical director should have ultimate decision-making authority for the equipment needed to care for potential patients, assuming that medical supplies and equipment are within the expected needs based on preapproved protocols and that appropriate considerations are made toward financial and logistical constraints.

With regard to the supplies and equipment needed to manage anticipated patient encounters, it is important to reflect on the expected environment of the response and the scope of practice of the providers. Understanding that it can be quite difficult to establish and maintain intravenous lines in a wilderness environment, medications are often administered by oral or intranasal routes. When parenteral medications are necessary, the preferred choice of medication route (ie, intramuscular, intraosseous routes, or intravenous) should be up to the program medical director given local needs and within the environmental and operational context.

Beyond medication administration, the medical director should consider the appropriate equipment for the environment to manage airway emergencies, traumatic emergencies, and environmental emergencies. Further, especially with an aging population that is increasingly using the outdoors for recreation, medical directors should prepare the team to manage a myriad of medical emergencies. The medical director should also ensure that responders are prepared to mitigate the effects of environmental extremes on their patients by carrying electrolytes for hydration, protein bars for nutrition, and disposable blankets or insulation for warmth.

Every wilderness environment will have unique operational needs and anticipated patient encounters. Understanding that it is beyond the scope of this article to list appropriate equipment for every potential wilderness event, **Table 1** provides some insight toward important operational equipment based on pack recommendations made by the National Association for Search and Rescue,[15] and **Table 2** lists suggested medical equipment for a typical SAR response pack. With regard to the medical equipment listed in **Table 2**, it should be understood that every medical director has individual preferred methods for managing injuries and illness. Thus, this list is meant to provide the reader ideas for building a WEMS medical kit (**Figs. 1** and **2**) and not meant to be all-inclusive or a definitive list of best practice.

SPECIAL PROGRAMS

Briefly previously described, the National Ski Patrol (NSP) is perhaps the largest WEMS system operating at a basic life support (BLS) level. With more than 25,000 patrollers in the system, the NSP provides education and certification programs in outdoor emergency care, mountain rescue, avalanche control, and leadership.[16] Because patrollers work for local ski areas, the NSP does not provide medical oversight, licensure, or credentialing. Patrollers should look locally for physician medical oversight, protocol development, and QI activities.

Created in the mid-1970s, the National Park Service Parkmedic program provides an advanced life support (ALS) level of care, training skills in wilderness medicine, emergency medicine, and SAR techniques. Students spend time in the classroom, emergency department, and field to gain a comprehensive understanding of the principles of emergency medicine as applied to the wilderness environment.[17] Most importantly, in contrast to the NSP programs, the Parkmedic program uses physician leadership on national and local levels to ensure quality of care. In this manner, the Parkmedic program has similar oversight structure as a traditional EMS program.

Table 1 Operational equipment	
Rain Shell	
Insulation	Hat, warm layer
Hydration	Electrolyte solution
Nutrition	Protein bars
Shelter	Tarp, reusable space blanket
Navigation	Compass, Universal Transverse Mercator grid marker, electronic Global Positioning System
Fire starter	Waterproof matches, magnesium fire starter
Signaling	Whistle, mirror, flagging tape
Light	Headlamp, hand-held flashlight, red light
Tools	Knife, pliers
Communications	Cellular telephone, radio
Personal first aid kit	Personal medications, bandages, mole skin, gauze, tape, scissors, tweezers

Table 2 Medical equipment	
Equipment	**Medications**
Basic Life Support Medical Gear	
Bandages	Aspirin
Gauze 4 × 4 in	Epinephrine
Roller gauze 4 in	Acetaminophen
Pelvic binder	Ibuprofen
Kendrick traction splint	Albuterol
Cervical collar	
Structural aluminum malleable splints	
Automated external defibrillator	
Bag-valve-mask with nasal and oral pharyngeal airways	
Duct tape	
Scissors	
Tweezers	
Advanced Life Support Medical Gear	
Advanced airway	Oral steroids
	Antibiotics
	Topical ophthalmic proparacaine
	Ondansetron
	Fentanyl
	Midazolam
	Ketamine

EMERGENCY MEDICAL SERVICES SYSTEM INTERFACE

Although WEMS systems exist to provide emergency care to sick and injured patients in an environment that is quite different from that of patients managed by traditional EMS systems, the goal of care are essentially the same: to provide the highest possible care. Ultimately, WEMS systems do not exist in an isolated bubble. Rather, a WEMS program is the entry point into a complex system and, hence, is actually part of the continuum of care. It is, therefore, essential that a WEMS program be integrated with local traditional EMS programs.

It is important to recognize that many state EMS medical directors and officials from traditional EMS programs may not fully understand the operational constraints and protocol needs of a WEMS program. Therefore, it is incumbent on the WEMS medical

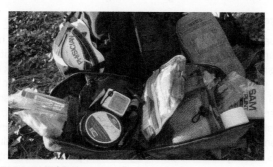

Fig. 1. Maryland SAR WEMS kit contents.

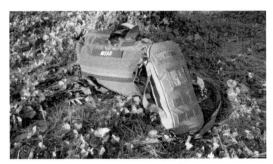

Fig. 2. Maryland SAR WEMS kit contents with medical bag.

director and other leadership to invest time and resource toward educating the rest of the emergency care community so that the team is able to operate unencumbered for the benefit of the wilderness community.

LEGAL ISSUES

There are several legal issues to consider when a physician decides to engage with a WEMS program. Importantly, the medical director should ensure that the program is in compliance with local and state regulations with regard to EMS system design. Providers should have established scopes of practice and the medical director and system leadership should ensure that the providers do not exceed these scopes of practice. Within the context of scope of practice, there is value in the program medical director developing and obtaining regulatory approval for the use of operationally specific protocols that address the needs of the wilderness environment, while maintaining a predetermined standard of care and defined scope of practice.

Medical directors for WEMS programs should have professional liability coverage for their duties as a WEMS program manager. This coverage should include malpractice for direct patient care, as well as oversight of the care of the providers. Medical directors' liability coverage should also include sexual harassment coverage, wrongful termination coverage, and other administrative duties. Programs that provide ALS care must have tight procedures for securing controlled dangerous substances.

CHALLENGES

WEMS systems are growing more numerous and more sophisticated. However, they also face several significant challenges to their growth and improvement.

Provider Shortages

Like many BLS-based services in the United States, WEMS depends heavily on volunteerism. However, national volunteer hours in general have been steadily declining following a brief spike following the 9/11 terrorist attacks in New York City.[18] In particular, fire rescue numbers have declined and these are services often involved in providing WEMS personnel.[6] Coupled with a decline in volunteerism is a declining number of rangers and an increasing ratio of visitors to rangers in parks (both state and national), a shortage of paramedics, a shortage of lifeguards, and a shortage of board-certified emergency physicians, as well as a shortage of training opportunities to provide WEMS training for those providers who are present. Currently, all these provider and training shortages represent a challenge to WEMS operations.

Insufficient Funding

As with EMS as a whole, the WEMS industry and volunteer provider base is under-funded relative to the activities they are tasked with completing. This ubiquitous challenge is addressed differently in each region, depending on resources available and characteristics of the team and providers involved but it is rare that it is not an issue for WEMS systems.

Appropriateness of Rescue

There is an ongoing debate in the United States as to whether rescue is even appropriate for certain categories. These include egregious or reckless behavior, and expensive rescues in known remote or extremely dangerous locations ventured into willingly by participants. The degree to which such individuals should be required to prepurchase insurance or be responsible for the cost of their rescue is also a challenge. In general, most SAR teams and rescue agencies would prefer WEMS operations not be fee-based (for the rescue portion), to avoid increased morbidity and mortality from individuals calling for help late or not at all due to concern about cost. This also reflects the heavily volunteer nature of this work in the United States. On the other hand, many stakeholders and community members believe billing for rescues, or not mounting rescues at all, would be more financially appropriate and would deter behavior they see as reckless. Indeed, no-rescue areas where rescue cannot reasonably be expected have been cited in the medical literature. Defining that threshold and the appropriate financial obligations for all WEMS patients remains a challenge for the industry as a whole and a contested intellectual topic.

SUMMARY

Over nearly a century, WEMS has evolved from basic first aid care provided by laypersons that were not part of the organized health care system to a system that is integrated and designed to provide high-quality complex patient care given environmental constraints. WEMS is now much more than a group of volunteers wanting to provide help to outdoor enthusiasts with common interests. WEMS is now an organized process designed to provide care to sick and injured patients in a wilderness environment, transport the patients out of the environment, and expedite transfer to definitive care. In short, WEMS is now specialized health care in which teams work to bring high-quality care, under physician oversight and integrated into the overall health care system, to the patient rather than expect that somehow the patients will get themselves to definitive care.

Yet, although WEMS should be organized with system integration and physician oversight, the landscape is still very much in evolution. Some programs achieve, and even exceed, the goal of system integration and quality care review, whereas other programs continue to argue that care in the wilderness need not be integrated into the mainstream health care system or require physician oversight.

To ensure quality patient care, integration, and continuous improvement, WEMS providers should have defined scopes of practice that are established by local medical directors and approved by state or regional regulatory authorities. These programs should have active involvement of physicians who are trained to operate in the specific environment of the team and are integrated into the team structure. WEMS program medical directors should ultimately be responsible for the indirect oversight programs of protocol development, education, and QI activities. Further, the medical director should ideally be accessible to provide on-call coverage for direct oversight needs of the program. To account for the reality that a single medical director may not able to provide continuous coverage, it is advisable to have a system of redundancy with associate medical directors or a fail-safe in which a local emergency department is available to provide direct oversight coverage when absolutely necessary.

Sorting through local politics and resistance to change, when the focus is on the patient, it is clear that there is no other choice than to evolve WEMS into a system that mirrors traditional EMS in its commitment to provide the highest quality patient care possible.

REFERENCES

1. National Ski Patrol. NSP background and evolution. Available at: http://www.Nsp. Org/about/background.Aspx. Accessed February 28, 2014.
2. National Association of State EMS Officials — Medical Director's Council. The definition of EMS. Available at: https://http://www.Nasemso.Org/councils/medical directors/documents/definition-of-ems-2012.Pdf. Accessed September 8, 2016.
3. Accidental death and disability: The neglected disease of modern society. Washington (DC): National Academy of Sciences; 1966.
4. Shah MN. The formation of the emergency medical services system. Am J Public Health 2006;96:414–23.
5. Hawkins SC. Wilderness EMS. St. Louis (MO): Mosby-JEMS; 2010.
6. Hawkins SC, Millin MG, Smith WR. Wilderness EMS systems. Philadelphia: Elsevier; 2016.
7. National Association of EMS Physicians and the National Association of State EMS Officials. Medical direction for operational emergency medical services programs. Prehosp Emerg Care 2010;14:544.
8. Russell MF. Wilderness emergency medical services systems. Emerg Med Clin North Am 2004;22:561–73, x–xi.
9. National Highway Transportation Administration. National EMS scope of practice model. 2006.
10. Wilderness Emergency Medicial Services Committee. Scopes of practice of wilderness EMS providers Delphi project. National Association of Emergency Medical Services Physicians Annual Meeting. New Orleans, Louisiana. January 22, 2015.
11. Goth P, Garnett G. Clinical guidelines for delayed or prolonged transport: IV wounds. Rural Affairs Committee, National Association of Emergency Medical Services Physicians. Prehospital Disaster Med 1993;8:253–5.
12. Goth P, Garnett G. Clinical guidelines for delayed or prolonged transport: II. Dislocations. Rural Affairs Committee, National Association of Emergency Medical Services Physicians. Prehospital Disaster Med 1993;8:77–80.
13. Wilderness EMS medical director course. Available at: http://wemsmdcourse. Com. Accessed May 18, 2016.
14. Bennett BL. A time has come for wilderness emergency medical service: a new direction. Wilderness Environ Med 2012;23:5–6.
15. National Association for Search and Rescue. Colsolidated pack guide. Available at: https://d3n8a8pro7vhmx.Cloudfront.Net/nasar/pages/53/attachments/original/1467900943/consolidatedpackguide_v1.Pdf?1467900943. Accessed October 2, 2016.
16. The National Ski Patrol. Available at: http://www.Nsp.Org. Accessed September 8, 2016.

17. Kaufman TI, Knopp R, Webster T. The Parkmedic program: prehospital care in the national parks. Ann Emerg Med 1981;10:156–60.
18. Bureau of Labor statistics, United State Department of Labor: Economic news release: volunteering in the United States, 2015. Available at: http://www.Bls.Gov/news.Release/volun.Nr0.Htm. Accessed September 27, 2016.

Tactical Combat Casualty Care and Wilderness Medicine

Advancing Trauma Care in Austere Environments

Frank K. Butler, MD[a],*, Brad Bennett, PhD[b],
Colonel Ian Wedmore, MD[c]

KEYWORDS

- Tactical combat casualty care • TCCC • Wilderness medicine
- Battlefield trauma care • Tourniquets • Hemostatic dressings

KEY POINTS

- The Joint Trauma System helped the US military achieve unprecedented success in casualty survival during the wars in Afghanistan and Iraq.
- Tactical Combat Casualty Care (TCCC) is the prehospital component of the Joint Trauma System.
- Since most combat fatalities occur before the casualty reaches the care of a surgeon, TCCC plays a key role in ensuring that casualties have a maximal chance of survival.
- The realization that extremity hemorrhage, a leading cause of preventable death on the battlefield, could be effectively and safely addressed with limb tourniquets was the primary driving factor for the Special Operations medical research effort that gave rise to TCCC.
- Organizations advocating for the translation of TCCC concepts to the civilian sector include the Wilderness Medical Society, the National Association of Emergency Medical Technicians, the American College of Surgeons' Hartford Consensus working group, the White House Stop the Bleed campaign, and the Committee on Tactical Emergency Casualty Care.

Disclaimers: The opinions or assertions contained herein are the private views of the authors and are not to be construed as official or as reflecting the views of the Department of the Army or the Department of Defense.
Release: This document was reviewed by the Public Affairs Office and the Operational Security Office at the US Army Institute of Surgical Research. It is approved for unlimited public release.
Disclosures: The authors have no disclosures.
[a] Committee on Tactical Combat Casualty Care, Joint Trauma System, US Army Institute of Surgical Research, 3698 Chambers Pass, JBSA Fort Sam Houston, TX 78234-6315, USA; [b] Uniformed Services University of the Health Sciences, 4301 Jones Bridge Rd, Bethesda, MD 20814, USA; [c] Madigan Army Medical Center, 9040 Jackson Ave., Tacoma, WA 98431, USA
* Corresponding author.
E-mail address: fkb064@yahoo.com

Emerg Med Clin N Am 35 (2017) 391–407
http://dx.doi.org/10.1016/j.emc.2016.12.005
0733-8627/17/Published by Elsevier Inc.

INTRODUCTION

In 1992, the Naval Special Warfare Biomedical Research and Development program undertook a review of battlefield trauma care. The primary driver for this research effort was the realization that, although extremity hemorrhage was a leading cause of preventable death in combat casualties[1,2] and tourniquets could be applied safely for short periods, tourniquet use was universally disparaged in both civilian and military prehospital trauma care.[3–5] A thorough review of battlefield trauma care recommendations at the time resulted in the development of the first set of Tactical Combat Casualty Care (TCCC) Guidelines, a set of evidence-based, best-practice trauma care guidelines designed specifically for use on the battlefield, which were published in *Military Medicine* in 1996.[3] The Wilderness Medical Society (WMS) assisted in reviewing the TCCC recommendations, reevaluating the interpretation of the available evidence that supported these recommendations, and discussing their implications for the battlefield and other austere environments.[6]

After 2001, the lessons learned from the battlefields of Iraq and Afghanistan allowed continuous refinement of the TCCC Guidelines through the efforts of the Committee on Tactical Combat Casualty Care (CoTCCC). Importantly, combat medics, corpsmen, and pararescuemen (PJs) have consistently been a strong presence in the CoTCCC.

Now, in 2016, TCCC has been well-documented to have played a major role in achieving the highest casualty survival rate in the history of modern warfare in military units that train all of their members in TCCC.[4,7–11]

TCCC is presently the standard for battlefield trauma care in the US Military and for many allied nations. CoTCCC members work closely with civilian trauma colleagues in the Hartford Consensus effort and the White House Stop the Bleed campaign to translate trauma care lessons learned on the battlefield to lives saved at home. In cooperation with the National Association of Emergency Medical Technicians (NAEMT), the CoTCCC has helped to develop TCCC-based trauma courses to assist in training civilian emergency medical services systems, fire and rescue, and law enforcement organizations in trauma care.

TACTICAL COMBAT CASUALTY CARE AND WILDERNESS MEDICINE

The wilderness environment presents some of the challenges experienced by medics on the battlefield: both patient and provider are typically in remote locations where evacuation is neither quick nor easy; there may be ongoing hazards to contend with; equipment is limited; the environment may be cold, hot, or aquatic; and the providers are often not trauma care specialists.[6,12] The extreme diversity of nature that makes the wilderness so alluring complicates the care of patients with trauma in a myriad of ways, from whitewater rescue to high-angle rescue to avalanche rescue. Although many of these challenges are distinct from those encountered on the battlefield, there is a good deal of overlap in the approach to patients in these two settings. A selected subset of the trauma care recommendations in TCCC and their applicability to the wilderness environment are reviewed and discussed later. The current TCCC Guidelines may be found on the Joint Trauma System (JTS) and NAEMT Web sites and in the Prehospital Trauma Life Support (PHTLS) textbook that is published every 3 to 4 years by NAEMT.[13]

APPROACH TO PATIENTS

TCCC recognizes that battlefield trauma care must combine good medicine with good small unit tactics and divides its recommendations into 3 phases: Care under Fire (while the unit is actively taking hostile fire), Tactical Field Care (the unit and the casualty are still in a prehospital combat environment but not actively engaging the enemy), and Tactical Evacuation Care (during which time the casualty is being transported to definitive care).[3,13] In the wilderness, the terrain, environment, the location, and the nature of the activity in which the group is engaged provide variation and complexity to prehospital trauma care. An open fracture sustained during a multi-day caving expedition must be approached differently than one that occurs in an urban setting.

In both environments, the well-known ABC (airway, breathing, circulation) sequence of initial steps should be replaced with the acronym MARCH (massive bleeding, airway, respirations, circulation, and head/hypothermia.)

In patients with trauma, control of massive external hemorrhage is the most important initial step. Injury to a major vessel may result in death within as little as 5 to 10 minutes. When the hemorrhage is external, first responders have the ability to effectively intervene to stop the bleeding and should do so.

EXTERNAL HEMORRHAGE CONTROL: TOURNIQUETS

The renewed focus on prehospital tourniquet use is one example of the lifesaving potential of the TCCC Guidelines. Until recently, military medics were taught that tourniquets should be used as a last resort, if at all, to control extremity hemorrhage. During the Vietnam conflict and at the start of the war in Afghanistan, tourniquet use was strongly discouraged. As a result, preventable death from extremity hemorrhage was common. Maughon's[1] study of 2600 combat fatalities in the Vietnam conflict found that 7.4% of the deaths examined resulted from extremity hemorrhage. Kelly and colleagues'[14] 2008 study of 982 combat fatalities sustained during the early years in Afghanistan and Iraq found that the incidence of death from extremity hemorrhage as a percentage of the total was essentially unchanged from the Maughon[1] study at 7.8%. Holcomb and colleagues'[15] 2007 study of Special Operations fatalities noted that 3 of the 12 potentially preventable deaths were from extremity hemorrhage. These findings prompted the US Special Operations Command TCCC Transition Initiative in 2005, which expedited the fielding of tourniquets and hemostatic dressings to deploying Special Operations units.[16] As a result, tourniquet and hemostatic dressing use increased in Afghanistan and Iraq and extremity hemorrhage deaths decreased.[4] Eastridge and colleagues'[9] 2012 study of 4596 US combat fatalities from 2001 to 2011 noted that only 2.6% of total combat fatalities resulted from extremity hemorrhage; a 67% decrease.[4,9,17] Kragh and colleagues'[18,19] landmark studies in 2008 and 2009 documented that extremity tourniquets saved lives and did not result in loss of limbs caused by tourniquet ischemia.

Tourniquets have proved to be lifesaving in the civilian and wilderness sectors as well.[20–22] If a person attacked by an animal or a climber with an open fracture sustains a vascular injury with massive external hemorrhage, immediate application of an extremity tourniquet is required. The first responder then has time to convert the tourniquet to other methods of hemostasis when feasible.[23]

EXTERNAL HEMORRHAGE CONTROL: HEMOSTATIC DRESSINGS

When external hemorrhage occurs at sites that are not amenable to tourniquet use, another modality for achieving control of bleeding is the use of hemostatic dressings. The current TCCC Guidelines recommend Combat Gauze as the hemostatic dressing of choice and Celox Gauze and ChitoGauze as alternative choices. All of these hemostatic dressings should be applied with at least 3 minutes of firm, direct pressure.[13,24–29]

Combat medics on the CoTCCC have consistently expressed a strong preference for gauze-type dressings rather than powdered or granular hemostatic agents, especially for wounds in which the bleeding vessel is at the bottom of a narrow wound tract. Gauze-based hemostatic dressings are more easily packed into the depths of such wounds where they can make direct contact with the bleeding vessel. Further, powdered or granular agents may present an ocular hazard if used in a windy environment or in the presence of rotor wash from helicopters. The Israeli Defense Force has reported excellent success in treating external hemorrhage in their combat wounded with Combat Gauze.[30]

Zietlow and colleagues[20] described the Mayo Clinic experience with Combat Gauze in civilian trauma, reporting a 95% success rate after the failure of standard dressings. Both TCCC-recommended tourniquets and hemostatic dressings should be included in all wilderness first aid kits.

THE PREHOSPITAL TRAUMA AIRWAY

In trauma, managing the airway entails different considerations than those encountered in medical patients. Most airway fatalities in combat are related to direct maxillofacial trauma.[31] Endotracheal intubation in the traumatized airway is challenging, even for experienced intubationists, and most military medics have little experience in intubating patients with airway trauma. Airway trauma on the battlefield is often best managed by allowing the casualty to maintain the sit-up-and-lean-forward position if the patient is conscious and able to do so. This position allows gravity and the patient's protective reflexes to maintain a patent airway.[13] The use of supraglottic airways in the prehospital setting is increasing, but these devices have not been well studied in trauma.

When the measures discussed above do not provide an adequate airway in a casualty with direct trauma to the maxillofacial region, a surgical airway is the intervention of choice.[13,32,33] Combat medics have been shown to be able to perform this procedure with 100% success in a cadaver model when they are well trained and use a CricKey device, which is the recommended device in TCCC.[32,34]

Should the need to secure the airway arise from unconsciousness secondary to traumatic brain injury (TBI) or hemorrhagic shock, nasopharyngeal airways (NPAs) have proved to be a good option.[13] The NPA is an easily trained intervention and no airway fatalities were identified in the 2010 Mabry and colleagues[31] review of this topic as being caused by NPA failure in nontraumatized airways.

In the wilderness setting, a lower incidence of direct maxillofacial trauma and a higher incidence of unconsciousness caused by TBI would be expected. Thus the use of an NPA is a good option in wilderness settings in which a skilled and equipped intubationist is not typically present. A surgical airway remains the emergent airway of last resort for patients with trauma in the wilderness.[35,36]

RESPIRATIONS/BREATHING
Tension Pneumothorax

In the Vietnam conflict, tension pneumothorax was reported to be the second leading cause of preventable battlefield death.[2] The incidence of death has decreased with the use of body armor that provides significant (but not complete) protection to the chest and back. In addition, combat medical personnel are now taught to use needle decompression (NDC) aggressively to treat suspected tension pneumothorax. The Eastridge and colleagues[9] study noted that tension pneumothorax comprised only

0.2% of deaths among US combat fatalities, which represents a decrease of more than 90% in preventable deaths from this cause.[13]

Current TCCC Guidelines call for casualties who have progressive respiratory distress following torso trauma to be suspected of having a tension pneumothorax and considered for NDC on the side of the injury with a 14-gauge, 8-cm (3.25-inch) needle/catheter unit. NDC is performed at the second intercostal space at the midclavicular line or the fourth or fifth intercostal space at the anterior axillary line. Needle entry into the chest should not be medial to the nipple line and the needle should not be directed toward the heart.[13]

Use of an 8-cm (3.25-inch) needle rather than the previously used 5-cm (2-inch) needle was introduced after the Harcke and colleagues[37] article in 2008. Those investigators noted that several of the cases in their autopsy series had failed attempts at NDC because the needle/catheter units used for the procedure were too short and did not reach the pleural space. This observation was followed by a virtual autopsy computed tomography (CT) study of chest wall thickness that found a mean chest wall thickness of 5.36 cm in the 100 military fatalities studied. Harcke and colleagues[37] recommended that an 8-cm (3.25-inch) needle/catheter unit be used for NDC in order to achieve a 99% assurance of reaching the pleural space.[37] Other investigators have presented similar findings and concerns.[38,39] Harcke and colleagues'[37] findings led to the TCCC recommendation to use an 8-cm (3.25-inch), 14-gauge needle/catheter unit inserted to the hub.[13] The authors are unaware of any reports of death from tension pneumothorax in US combat casualties caused by failed NDC since this change was made almost a decade ago.[13] Bilateral NDC should be performed before resuscitation efforts are abandoned when a casualty with torso trauma or polytrauma has a prehospital cardiopulmonary arrest.[13]

In the wilderness setting, death from tension pneumothorax is expected to be less common, although penetrating chest trauma may occur from hunting accidents and blunt chest trauma may result from falls, avalanche, or mountain bike accidents. Inclusion of an 8-cm (3.25-inch), 14-gauge needle in wilderness medical kits is a reasonable measure in order to be able to perform NDC in the unlikely event that this uncommon but life-threatening disorder is encountered in the wilderness. Improved success using an 8-cm (3.25-inch) needle (83%) compared with a 5-cm (2-inch) needle (41%) was reported by the Mayo Clinic.[40] No complications were reported with either length needle.

Open Pneumothorax

An open pneumothorax (also sometimes referred to as a sucking chest wound) may result from a penetrating injury to the chest wall. When the defect in the chest wall is sufficiently large (usually two-thirds or more of the diameter of the trachea), air preferentially flows into the chest cavity via the defect in the chest wall, instead of into the lung via the trachea, as the casualty inhales. Air entering through the defect in the chest wall allows the lung on the affected side to collapse and impairs oxygen exchange.[13]

Although there is little evidence that an open pneumothorax by itself (ie, without injury to underlying lung tissue and major vascular structures), is a potentially lethal injury,[9,41] the impaired pulmonary gas exchange could potentially result in pulmonary compromise in a polytrauma casualty and contribute to secondary hypoxic brain injury in casualties with TBI.[13]

Treatment of an open pneumothorax consists of applying a vented occlusive chest seal over the defect in the chest wall, thus preventing air from entering the pleural space through the defect in the chest wall.[41] The vent in the chest seal prevents the development of a tension pneumothorax in the presence of an underlying lung injury and air leak. Commercially available vented and nonvented chest seals have been evaluated in animal studies.[42,43] In the Kheirabadi study, chest seals were applied and then 200-mL increments of air were injected into the pleural cavity of thoracotomized swine every 5 minutes until either tension pneumothorax developed or the volume of air injected equaled 100% of the animal's estimated total lung capacity.[42] Tension pneumothorax did not develop in animals treated with vented chest seals (incorporating a 1-way valve that allowed air to leave but not to enter the pleural space). However, tension pneumothorax did occur in the animals with chest seals without valves. Vented chest seals, then, are preferred for the prehospital management of open pneumothorax, to be followed by tube thoracostomy when time, skills, and circumstances allow.[13,41]

For wilderness medicine providers, open pneumothorax and the need for a vented chest seal is an injury pattern that might result from gunshot wounds sustained in hunting accidents. This injury, in the setting of delays to evacuation, is one that should be treated with prophylactic antibiotics, as described later.

INTRAVENOUS AND INTRAOSSEOUS ACCESS

It has been a long-standing prehospital trauma care practice to establish intravenous (IV) access for individuals with significant trauma. TCCC has reconsidered this intervention. Starting IV lines inflicts significant cost in both time and logistics and may delay a combat unit's ability to maneuver when needed. TCCC recommends that IV lines be started only for individuals who require fluid resuscitation as a result of hemorrhagic shock or who need IV medications, especially tranexamic acid (TXA) or analgesics. IV lines are easily dislodged, especially during combat operations. The TCCC curriculum describes a technique developed by medics in the 75th Ranger Regiment that helps to ensure that IV lines are not dislodged during casualty movement.[13,44]

INTRAOSSEOUS ACCESS

Establishing IV access is a fairly easy procedure unless the patient is obese, a small child, or in shock, or the person attempting to start the IV does not perform this procedure routinely. However, the last 2 caveats often apply to the battlefield setting. Another way to achieve vascular access is to use an intraosseous (IO) device.[45,46]

This technique is easily trained[47] and can be performed by prehospital providers with a high rate of success.[48] Because the technique is performed based on bony landmarks rather than by visualizing peripheral veins, it is more easily performed under low light and night vision device conditions.[13] The IO approach was proposed by TCCC as an alternative to IV lines on the battlefield in 2002 and quickly became widely used by combat medical personnel because the procedure is quickly and easily performed. IO access is now a widely used technique in the civilian sector as well.[49] The Pyng FAST-1 and the EZ-IO devices have been the most widely used by the US Military in the recent conflicts.[13] Although the risk of osteomyelitis is very low and the authors are unaware of any reports of this complication from the conflicts in Iraq and Afghanistan, both the potential for infection and the patient discomfort experienced with an IO procedure make using peripheral IV access the option of first choice when circumstances allow.

For practitioners of wilderness medicine, the indications for IV and IO access are basically the same as for the battlefield, except that it may be less common for medical providers in the wilderness setting to be prepared to perform fluid resuscitation from hemorrhagic shock.

TRANEXAMIC ACID

Noncompressible hemorrhage is the leading cause of preventable death in combat casualties.[9] The large, prospective, randomized Clinical Randomization of an Antifibrinolytic in Significant Hemorrhage (CRASH-2) study examined the effect of TXA administration in trauma patients at risk of bleeding and documented a small but statistically significant survival benefit. Although deep venous thrombosis is a known complication of trauma, there was no increase in the rate of vascular occlusive events in the TXA group.[50] The subsequent subgroup analysis of the CRASH-2 data focused on deaths caused by bleeding rather than all-cause mortality and examined the effect of the timing of TXA administration on outcomes. The greatest benefit of TXA administration was obtained when the medication was given within 1 hour of the time of injury. TXA administered between 1 and 3 hours after the time of injury also reduced the risk of death caused by bleeding. However, TXA administered later than 3 hours after injury was observed to increase the risk of death from exsanguination.[51]

The Military Application of Tranexamic Acid in Trauma Emergency Resuscitation Study (MATTERS) was performed at a role 3 facility in Afghanistan.[52] The MATTERS investigators found a decreased mortality among combat casualties who received TXA, despite their being more seriously injured. In the subgroup of casualties who received massive transfusions (more than 10 units of red cells within the first 24 hours), mortality in the TXA group was markedly lower (14.4%) compared with the control group (28.1%). The CRASH-2 and MATTERS findings both supported the use of TXA in combat casualties who are either in hemorrhagic shock or at significant risk of that condition. As a result of these two studies, TXA was added to the TCCC Guidelines in 2011.[53]

A subsequent report found a benefit from administering TXA in the prehospital setting.[54] Studies examining the effect of giving TXA before elective surgical procedures associated with significant blood loss have consistently found that TXA reduces blood loss in these procedures and does not increase the risk of deep venous thrombosis.[55] TXA is recommended in the TCCC Guidelines for casualties who are anticipated to need significant blood transfusion (eg, casualties with hemorrhagic shock, 1 or more major amputations, penetrating torso trauma, or evidence of severe bleeding.)[44] The recommended dose is 1 g of TXA in 100 mL of normal saline or Lactated Ringers solution. TXA should be infused over 10 minutes to avoid the risk of hypotension and should be given as soon as possible after injury but not later than 3 hours after injury. In the event that evacuation to a medical treatment facility is delayed, a second infusion of 1 g of TXA should be administered after fluid resuscitation has been performed.[13]

In the wilderness environment, TXA administration should be considered for trauma patients in shock, as well as those with penetrating torso trauma, severe external hemorrhage, or blunt trauma with suspicion of non-compressible hemorrhage. Falls and TBI are common in the wilderness and the value of TXA in reducing intracranial hemorrhage is currently an area of active investigation.

FLUID RESUSCITATION FROM HEMORRHAGIC SHOCK

Hemorrhagic shock is the most common cause of potentially preventable death on the battlefield.[9] In the hospital setting, hemorrhagic shock is treated by resuscitation with blood or blood components until adequate tissue perfusion is restored. A large, prospective, randomized study at Ben Taub Hospital in Houston examined the benefit of early, aggressive fluid resuscitation in patients with penetrating torso trauma and shock.[56] This study found that early fluid resuscitation group had decreased survival as compared to the group of patients in whom fluid resuscitation was delayed until after surgical hemostasis had been achieved.[56] TCCC originally recommended that fluid resuscitation for casualties with shock from noncompressible bleeding sites be delayed until after surgical control of the bleeding and that 1000 mL of Hespan be used to resuscitate casualties in shock from external bleeding sites after hemorrhage control.[3]

However, in 1999, subject matter experts reviewing battlefield trauma care issues from the Battle of Mogadishu recommended that casualties who were experiencing unconsciousness or mental status changes caused by hemorrhagic shock should be fluid resuscitated to an end point of improved mentation, even in the presence of ongoing noncompressible (internal) hemorrhage.[57] Further recommendations from subsequent Department of Defense (DoD) fluid resuscitation workshops on fluid resuscitation led to a single hypotensive fluid resuscitation strategy for combat casualties in shock, whether their hemorrhage was controlled or uncontrolled. The synthetic hetastarch solution Hextend replaced the previously used Hespan because of the former solution's lesser impact on coagulation status.[58,59]

Both of the strategies mentioned earlier made the implicit assumption that blood products would not be available in the tactical field care phase of combat casualty care. In the ensuing years, a number of events have occurred: (1) the value of whole blood as the preferred fluid for fluid resuscitation has been documented[60–63]; (2) transfusing red blood cells in a 1:1 or 1:1:1 ratio with plasma and platelets has been shown to be superior to a transfusion strategy using a predominance of RBCs[64,65]; (3) large volumes of crystalloid have been shown to worsen outcomes in patients with trauma,[66,67]; (4) questions have been raised about the safety of using hetastarch solutions in critically ill patients[68,69]; (5) both military units and civilian trauma systems have shown that blood products can be used in the prehospital setting[61,70–77] and that this practice improves casualty outcomes[74]; and (6) a preponderance of the literature has found that plasma resuscitation is a better choice for resuscitation than either crystalloids or colloids.[78,79] Accordingly, a recent review of fluid resuscitation options in TCCC has recommended a preference list of options for fluid resuscitation, going from the most desirable (whole blood) to the least desirable (crystalloids).

In the wilderness setting, as with ground-based combat medical personnel, blood components are unlikely to be readily available. In this circumstance, the best strategy for treating hemorrhagic shock is hypotensive resuscitation using a reconstituted dried plasma product. Although dried plasma products (French FyLP or German LyoPlas) have been used widely by coalition forces in Afghanistan and Iraq, they are not currently approved by the US Food and Drug Administration for use in the United States (Butler FK: Fluid resuscitation in tactical combat casualty care – yesterday and today. Submitted for publication to *Wilderness and Environmental Medicine*).[78] As long as dried plasma remains unavailable in the United States, if a prolonged evacuation is anticipated, Hextend will provide a more sustained intravascular volume expansion than crystalloids.[80]

HYPOTHERMIA AND COAGULOPATHY ON THE BATTLEFIELD

As noted previously, hemorrhage is the leading cause of preventable death in combat casualties. Hypothermia may contribute to the coagulopathy of trauma by decreasing platelet function, decreasing the activity of enzymes in the coagulation cascade, and causing alterations of the fibrinolytic system.[81,82] Hypothermia (defined as a core temperature $<36^\circ C$) was present in 18% of 2848 combat casualties and was an independent predictor of mortality.[83] Hypothermia may occur even in warm environments and may be exacerbated by long evacuation times, helicopter transport, and wet clothing. Hemorrhagic shock also contributes to hypothermia by reducing the body's ability to produce metabolic heat.[13]

The body temperature in combat casualties should be maintained as close to 37°C as possible.[84] Hypothermia prevention should be started early in the management of combat casualties, after external hemorrhage has been controlled and TXA adminis-tered, if indicated. The casualty should be protected against the environment to the greatest extent possible. Clothing should be retained where that is consistent with treating injuries. Conductive heat loss should be prevented by not having the casu-alty lying directly on the ground or on the floor of an evacuation helicopter. Personal protective equipment should be kept on or with the casualty as feasible. After massive hemorrhage has been controlled, the airway opened, and breathing diffi-culties addressed, wet clothing should be removed and replaced with dry clothes, if feasible.

TCCC recommends the Hypothermia Prevention and Management Kit (HPMK) to minimize heat loss in combat casualties. The HPMK combines an active heating de-vice (the Ready-Heat blanket) with a passive device (the Heat Reflective Shell) to pro-duce a synergistic heat-conserving effect for the casualty. The HPMK has been shown in United States Army Institute of Surgical Research testing to effectively prevent heat loss.[85] Care should be taken to place the Ready-Heat blanket over the uniform shirt, not directly on the skin, because the device may cause burns if placed on bare skin.

If purposed hypothermia prevention devices are not available, then blankets, pon-chos, sleeping bags, or other items at hand should be used to keep the casualty as warm and dry as possible. Controlling hemorrhage and providing adequate fluid resuscitation, with blood components if possible, will restore tissue perfusion and help to maintain the casualty's ability to generate metabolic heat.

The HPMK or similar devices may be very useful in the wilderness, but often are not available. Extra clothing, sleeping bags, insulating blankets, and other items may be more readily available and should be applied in layers to achieve effective hypothermia prevention for patients with trauma in the wilderness.

The WMS Practice Guidelines for the prevention and treatment of hypothermia offer additional treatment options and perspectives.[86]

EYE TRAUMA

Penetrating eye injuries are frequently encountered on the battlefield, especially when exposed to improvised explosive devices (IEDs) with small rock or metallic items embedded in the device to increase the incidence of fragment injuries from the blast. Providers should have a heightened index of suspicion in the presence of multiple punctate facial wounds (peppering). When injury to the globe is sus-pected, first-responder management of these injuries includes a rapid field evaluation and documentation of vision, covering the injured eyes with a rigid eye shield, and prompt administration of TCCC-recommended antibiotics. Eye shields are essential in this setting but have been reported to be underused in the management of eye in-juries during the recent conflicts.[87] If no rigid eye shield is available, a set of protec-tive eyewear will serve this purpose well. A point of emphasis is that pressure patches and other dressings that may come into direct contact with an injured eye should be avoided.[13] Also, avoid manipulating the eye during evaluation and treat-ment in any way that might increase intraocular pressure and result in the expulsion of intraocular contents through the corneal or scleral defect.[13,88] Moxifloxacin 400 mg once a day, given immediately after injury, is the antibiotic of choice in the prehospital environment. This medication has good coverage of the typical causative organisms for intraocular infections and penetrates well into the vitreous cavity. No topical antibiotics (ointments or eye drops) should be used on an unrepaired penetrating injury of the eye.[13,88]

Wilderness medicine practitioners are unlikely to encounter any IEDs, but may have to treat patients with fishhook or impaling thorn injuries to the eye. In both cases, the most important additional point of management is not to try to remove the fishhook or thorn.[88] Wilderness patients with known or suspected penetrating eye injuries should be evacuated as soon as feasible. A more complete discussion of the management of eye injuries and medical disorders in a wilderness setting may be found in the new seventh edition of Auerbach's[88] *Wilderness Medicine* as well as the WMS practice guidelines for eye injuries.[89]

ANALGESIA

At the onset of the Afghanistan conflict, the state of the art for battlefield analgesia in most of the US Military was the same as it had been at the Battle of Bull Run in the US Civil War.[13,90] Intramuscular (IM) morphine was the primary medication used to relieve the pain of combat wounds despite that fact that it is very slow-acting and prolongs the casualty's pain.[3] This, in turn, increases the likelihood of repeated dosing and eventual overdose.[91] Early adopters of TCCC in 2001 were using morphine administered intravenously for rapidity of analgesia and improved ability to titrate the dosage administered.[3]

After demonstration that oral transmucosal fentanyl (OTFC) could safely provide rapid and powerful analgesia in combat casualties without the need to establish an IV, this medication was added to the TCCC Guidelines.[92,93] Wedmore and colleagues[94] subsequently provided additional documentation of the safety of OTFC on the battlefield. OTFC had been recommended for use in wilderness settings as early as 1999.[95]

Ketamine is an excellent analgesic alternative for casualties either in, or at risk of, hemorrhagic shock because this medication does not cause hemodynamic or respiratory depression. Ketamine was added as an analgesic option in TCCC in 2012.[90]

In 2014, the TCCC triple-option analgesia approach to battlefield analgesia was developed. This concept originated at the direct request from combat medical personnel that the CoTCCC provide them with an inclusive but simplified approach on how best to use the available options for analgesia.[17] Thus, oral medications (acetaminophen and meloxicam, a platelet-sparing nonsteroidal analgesic) are recommended for analgesia when pain is not severe and the casualty can continue to function effectively as a combatant for his or her unit. When there is more severe pain, but the casualty is not in, or at significant risk for, shock, OTFC is the analgesic of choice. If there is moderate to severe pain, and the casualty is in shock, or at risk of shock or pulmonary compromise, ketamine is the agent of choice.[92] Ondansetron is recommended for the nausea and vomiting that may result either from opioid administration or from the combat wounds.[96]

The TCCC triple-option analgesia approach lends itself well to the wilderness environment. A practice guideline that mirrors the TCCC triple-option approach was recently approved by the American College of Emergency Physicians.[97] The WMS practice guidelines for pain management also include a discussion of the analgesic options noted earlier.[98]

ANTIBIOTICS

Open combat wounds are prone to infection and are a late cause of morbidity and mortality in combat casualties.[99] Antibiotics are indicated for combat trauma and should be started as soon as feasible. Fourth-generation oral fluoroquinolones are the prehospital antibiotic of choice when the casualty is able to take oral medications.[99] The current recommendation is 400 mg of moxifloxacin when oral medications are feasible and IM or IV ertapenem when the casualty is not able to take oral medications.[13,44,100] Both antibiotics were selected because of their excellent spectrum of activity and their minimal serious adverse effects. In addition, moxifloxacin has excellent bioavailability when taken orally and both medications penetrate well into the vitreous cavity, which is important in treating casualties with penetrating eye injuries.

For injuries that occur in the wilderness environment, as in combat, evacuation is likely to be delayed and oral or parenteral antibiotics are indicated for any trauma that includes infection-prone injuries such as open fractures or animal bites.

TRAUMATIC CARDIOPULMONARY ARREST

Although cardiopulmonary resuscitation (CPR) has been lifesaving in patients with nontraumatic cardiac arrest, CPR is much less likely to be successful in victims of traumatic cardiac arrest.[101–103] On the battlefield, performing CPR on casualties in cardiac arrest may result in additional lives lost as combat medical personnel are exposed to hostile fire while performing CPR and care is withheld from casualties with potentially survivable wounds. In addition, delays in unit movement in order to perform CPR may result in mission compromise.[3,13] CPR should be considered in the tactical prehospital setting only if the arrest is associated with hypothermia, near drowning, or electrocution, or when the casualty is in the tactical evacuation phase of care and arrival at a medical treatment facility is imminent.[13,104] Unrecognized tension pneumothorax is a potentially reversible cause of traumatic cardiac arrest in combat casualties. Any combat casualty who sustains torso trauma or polytrauma and is found to have no pulse or respirations should have bilateral needle decompression performed to ensure they do not have a tension pneumothorax before discontinuation of care.[13,104]

DOCUMENTATION OF CARE

The lack of adequate documentation of prehospital care rendered to US casualties in Iraq and Afghanistan is problematic in ensuring optimal care for casualties and has been a clear obstacle to CoTCCC and Joint Trauma System efforts to improve TCCC.[105] The TCCC Card was developed by the 75th Ranger Regiment to document prehospital care and was adopted by TCCC in 2008. This card is simple, cost-effective, and easily fielded. It has been used widely throughout the wars in Iraq and Afghanistan and is now approved for use throughout the DoD. The recently updated TCCC card allows for a casualty Battle Roster Number (to link the casualty to the DoD Trauma Registry), provides better definition of the mechanism of injury, improves the documentation of tourniquet and hemostatic dressing use, and contains a space for types and doses of analgesics used as well as for several other commonly used elements of combat casualty care.

The TCCC card is commercially available on ruggedized paper stock that enables it to be used with reduced incidence of becoming damaged or unreadable in the harsh combat environment. Documentation of care is an important aspect of caring for casualties in the wilderness as well and either a TCCC card or some other durable record of care should be maintained throughout the time that the patient is receiving prehospital care and subsequently should be transported with the patient to the treating hospital.

ACKNOWLEDGMENTS

The authors gratefully acknowledge ongoing efforts of the CoTCCC, the TCCC Working Group, and the Joint Trauma System to improve the care provided to US casualties on the battlefield and to patients with trauma in the United States.

REFERENCES

1. Maughon JS. An inquiry into the nature of wounds resulting in killed in action in Vietnam. Mil Med 1970;135:8–13.
2. Bellamy RF. The causes of death in conventional land warfare: implications for combat casualty care research. Mil Med 1984;149:55–62.
3. Butler FK, Hagmann J, Butler EG. Tactical Combat Casualty Care in Special Operations. Mil Med 1996;161(Suppl):3–16.
4. Butler FK. The US military experience with tourniquets and hemostatic dressings in the Afghanistan and Iraq conflicts. Bull Am Coll Surg 2015;100(Hartford Consensus Supplement):60–5.
5. Kragh J, Walters T, Westmoreland T, et al. Tragedy into drama: an American history of tourniquet use in the current war. J Spec Oper Med 2013;13:5–25.
6. Butler FK, Zafren K. Tactical management of wilderness casualties in Special Operations. Wilderness Environ Med 1998;9:62–117.
7. Butler FK. Two decades of saving lives on the battlefield: Tactical Combat Casualty Care turns 20. Mil Med, in press.
8. Butler FK, Blackbourne LH. Battlefield trauma care then and now: a decade of tactical combat casualty care. J Trauma 2012;73:S395–402.
9. Eastridge BJ, Mabry RL, Seguin P, et al. Death on the battlefield (2001-2011): implications for the future of combat casualty care. J Trauma 2012;73(6 Suppl 5):S431–7.
10. Kotwal RS, Montgomery HR, Kotwal BM, et al. Eliminating preventable death on the battlefield. Arch Surg 2011;146:1350–8.
11. Savage E, Forestier C, Withers N, et al. Tactical Combat Casualty Care in the Canadian Forces: lessons learned from the Afghan War. Can J Surg 2011;59: S118–23.
12. Sward D, Bennett BL. Wilderness medicine. World J Emerg Med 2014;5:5–15.
13. Butler FK, Giebner SD, McSwain N, et al, editors. Prehospital trauma life support manual. 8th edition (Military). Burlington (MA): Jones and Bartlett Learning; 2014.
14. Kelly JF, Ritenour AE, McLaughlin DF, et al. Injury severity and causes of death from Operation Iraqi Freedom and Operation Enduring Freedom: 2003-2004 versus 2006. J Trauma 2008;64(Suppl):S21–6.
15. Holcomb JB, McMullen NR, Pearse L, et al. Causes of death in Special Operations Forces in the Global War on Terror. Ann Surg 2007;245:986–91.
16. Butler F, Holcomb J. The tactical combat casualty care transition initiative. Army Med Department J 2005;April-June:33–8.
17. Kotwal RS, Butler FK, Edgar EP, et al. Saving lives on the battlefield: a Joint Trauma System review of pre-hospital trauma care in combined joint operating area – Afghanistan. J Spec Oper Med 2013;13:77–80.
18. Kragh JF, Walters TJ, Baer DG, et al. Practical use of emergency tourniquets to stop bleeding in major limb trauma. J Trauma 2008;64(Suppl):S38–50.
19. Kragh JF, Walters TJ, Baer DG, et al. Survival with emergency tourniquet use to stop bleeding in major limb trauma. Ann Surg 2009;249:1–7.

20. Zietlow J, Zietlow S, Morris D, et al. Prehospital use of hemostatic bandages and tourniquets: translation from military experience to implementation in a civilian trauma center. J Spec Oper Med 2015;15:48–53.

21. Scerbo MH, Mumm JP, Gates K, et al. Safety and Appropriateness of Tourniquets in 105 Civilians. Prehosp Emerg Care 2016;20:712–22.

22. Pons O, Jerome J, McMullen J, et al. The Hartford Consensus on active shooters: implementing the continuum of prehospital trauma response. J Emerg Med 2015; 49:878–85.

23. Shackelford S, Butler F, Kragh J, et al. Optimizing the use of limb tourniquets in Tactical Combat Casualty Care: TCCC guidelines change 14-02. J Spec Oper Med 2015;15:17–31.

24. Bennett BL, Littlejohn LF, Kheirabadi BS, et al. Management of external hemorrhage in Tactical Combat Casualty Care: chitosan-based hemostatic gauze dressings. J Spec Oper Med 2014;14:12–29.

25. Bennett BL, Littlejohn L. Review of new topical hemostatic dressings for combat casualty care. Mil Med 2014;179:497–514.

26. Littlejohn L, Bennett B, Drew B. Application of current hemorrhage control techniques for backcountry care: part 2: hemostatic dressings and other adjuncts. Wilderness Environ Med 2015;26:246–54.

27. Drew B, Bennett B, Littlejohn L. Application of current hemorrhage control techniques for backcountry care: part 1: tourniquets and hemorrhage control adjuncts. Wilderness Environ Med 2015;26:236–45.

28. Kheirabadi BS, Edens JW, Terrazas IB, et al. Comparison of new hemostatic granules/powders with currently deployed hemostatic products in a lethal model of extremity arterial hemorrhage in swine. J Trauma 2009;66:316–26.

29. Kheirabadi B, Mace J, Terrazas I, et al. Safety evaluation of new hemostatic agents, smectite granules, and kaolin-coated gauze in a vascular injury wound model in swine. J Trauma 2010;68:269–78.

30. Shina A, Lipsky A, Nadler R, et al. Prehospital use of hemostatic dressings by the Israel Defense Forces Medical Corps: a case series of 122 patients. J Trauma 2015;79:S204–9.

31. Mabry RL, Edens JW, Pearse L, et al. Fatal airway injuries during Operation Enduring Freedom and Operation Iraqi Freedom. Prehosp Emerg Care 2010; 14:272–7.

32. Mabry R, Frankfurt A, Kharod C, et al. Emergency cricothyroidotomy in Tactical Combat Casualty Care. J Spec Oper Med 2015;15:11–9.

33. Hessert MJ, Bennett BL. Optimizing emergent surgical cricothyrotomy for use in austere environments. Wilderness Environ Med 2013;24:53–66.

34. Mabry R, Nichols M, Shiner D, et al. A comparison of two open surgical cricothyroidotomy techniques by military medics using a cadaver model. Ann Emerg Med 2014;63:1–5.

35. Wharton D, Bennett B. Surgical cricothyrotomy in the wilderness: a case report. Wilderness Environ Med 2013;24:12–4.

36. Johnson CA, Goodwine DS, Passier I. Improvised cricothyrotomy on a mountain using hiking gear. Wilderness Environ Med 2016;27(4):500–3.

37. Harcke HT, Pearse LA, Levy AD, et al. Chest wall thickness in military personnel: implications for needle thoracentesis in tension pneumothorax. Mil Med 2008; 172:1260–3.

38. Zengerink I, Brink PR, Laupland KB, et al. Needle thoracostomy in the treatment of tension pneumothorax in trauma patients: what size needle? J Trauma 2008; 64:111–4.

39. Givens ML, Ayotte K, Manifold C. Needle thoracostomy: implications of computed tomography chest wall thickness. Acad Emerg Med 2004;11:211–3.

40. Aho J, Thiels C, El Khatin M, et al. Needle thoracostomy: clinical effectiveness is improved using a longer angiocatheter. J Trauma 2016;80:272–7.

41. Butler F, Dubose J, Otten E, et al. Management of open pneumothorax in Tactical Combat Casualty Care: TCCC guidelines change 13-02. J Spec Oper Med 2013;13:81–6.

42. Kheirabadi BS, Terrazas IB, Koller A, et al. Vented versus unvented chest seals for treatment of pneumothorax and prevention of tension pneumothorax in a swine model. J Trauma 2013;75:150–6.

43. Kotora JG Jr, Henao J, Littlejohn LF, et al. Vented chest seals for prevention of tension pneumothorax in a communicating pneumothorax. J Emerg Med 2013;45:686–94.

44. National Association of Emergency Medical Technicians Web site: TCCC guidelines. Available at: http://www.naemt.org/education/TCCC/guidelines_curriculum; Accessed September 27, 2016.

45. Dubick MA, Holcomb JB. A review of intraosseous vascular access: current status and military application. Mil Med 2000;165:552–9.

46. Calkins MD, Fitzgerald G, Bentley TB, et al. Intraosseous infusion devices: a comparison for potential use in special operations. J Trauma 2000;48:1068–74.

47. Benson G. Intraosseous access to the circulatory system: an under-appreciated option for rapid access. J Perioper Pract 2015;25:140–3.

48. Byars DV, Tsuchitani SN, Erwin E, et al. Evaluation of success rate and access time for an adult sternal intraosseous device deployed in the prehospital setting. Prehospital Disaster Med 2011;26:127–9.

49. Lewis P, Wright C. Saving the critically injured trauma patient: a retrospective analysis of 1000 uses of intraosseous access. Emerg Med J 2015;32:463–7.

50. CRASH-2 Collaborators. Effects of tranexamic acid on death, vascular occlusive events, and blood transfusion in trauma patients with significant hemorrhage. (CRASH-2); a randomized, placebo-controlled trial. Lancet 2010;376:23–32.

51. CRASH-2 Collaborators. The importance of early treatment with tranexamic acid in bleeding trauma patients: an exploratory analysis of the CRASH-2 randomized controlled trial. Lancet 2011;377:1096–101.

52. Morrison JJ, Dubose JJ, Rasmussen TE, et al. Military Application of Tranexamic Acid in Trauma Emergency Resuscitation Study (MATTERS). Arch Surg 2012; 147:113–9.

53. Dickey NW, Jenkins D. Defense Health Board recommendation for the addition of tranexamic acid to the Tactical Combat Casualty Care guidelines. Defense Health Board Memorandum 2011:1–12. Available at: http://www.naemt.org/docs/default-source/education-documents/tccc/10-9-15-updates/dhb-memo-110923-txa.pdf?sfvrsn=2. Accessed January 19, 2017.

54. Wafaisade A, Lefering R, Bouillon B, et al. Prehospital administration of tranexamic acid in trauma patients. Crit Care 2016;20:1–9.

55. Huang F, Wu D, Ma G, et al. The use of tranexamic acid to reduce blood loss and transfusion in major orthopedic surgery: a meta-analysis. J Surg Res 2014;186:318–27.

56. Bickell WH, Wall MJ, Pepe PE, et al. Immediate versus delayed fluid resuscitation for hypotensive patients with penetrating torso injuries. N Engl J Med 1994; 331:1105–9.

57. Butler FK, Hagmann J. Tactical management of urban warfare casualties in special operations. Mil Med 2000;165:1–48.

58. Champion HR. Combat fluid resuscitation: introduction and overview of conferences. J Trauma 2003;54(Suppl):S7–12.
59. Holcomb JB. Fluid resuscitation in modern combat casualty care: lessons learned from Somalia. J Trauma 2003;54(Suppl):S46–51.
60. Spinella P, Pidcoke H, Strandenes G, et al. Whole blood transfusion for hemostatic resuscitation of major bleeding. Transfusion 2016;56:S190–202.
61. Cap A, Pidcoke H, DePasquale M, et al. Blood far forward: time to get moving! J Trauma 2015;78:S2–6.
62. Stubbs J, Zielinski M, Jenkins D. The state of the science of whole blood: lessons learned at Mayo Clinic. Transfusion 2016;56:S173–81.
63. Spinella PC, Perkins JG, Grathwohl KW, et al. Warm fresh whole blood is independently associated with improved survival for patients with combat-related traumatic injuries. J Trauma 2009;66:S69–76.
64. Holcomb J, Spinella P. Optimal use of blood in trauma patients. Biologicals 2010;38:72–7.
65. Borgman MA, Spinella PC, Perkins JG, et al. The ratio of blood products transfused in patients receiving massive transfusions at a combat support hospital. J Trauma 2007;63:805–13.
66. Ley E, Clond M, Srour M, et al. Emergency department crystalloid resuscitation of 1.5 L or more is associated with increased mortality in elderly and non-elderly trauma patients. J Trauma 2011;70:398–400.
67. Duke MD, Guidry C, Guice J, et al. Restrictive fluid resuscitation in combination with damage control resuscitation: time for adaptation. J Trauma 2012;73:674–8.
68. Lissauer ME, Chi A, Kramer ME, et al. Association of 6% hetastarch resuscitation with adverse outcomes in critically ill trauma patients. Am J Surg 2011; 202:501–8.
69. Zarychanski R, Abou-Setta A, Turgeon A, et al. Association of hydroxyethyl starch administration with mortality and acute kidney injury in critically ill patients requiring volume resuscitation. JAMA 2013;309:678–88.
70. Morrison JJ, Oh J, Dubose JJ, et al. En-Route Care Capability From Point of Injury Impacts Mortality After Severe Wartime Injury. Ann Surg 2013;257:330–4.
71. Spinell P, Cap A. Whole blood – back to the future. Curr Opin Hematol 2016; 23(6):536–42.
72. Strandenes G, Cap A, Cacic D, et al. Blood far forward - a whole blood research and training program for austere environments. Transfusion 2013;53:S124–30.
73. Holcomb J, Donathan D, Cotton B, et al. Prehospital transfusion of plasma and red blood cells in trauma patients. Prehosp Emerg Care 2015;19:1–9.
74. Powell E, Hinckley W, Gottula A, et al. Shorter times to packed red blood cells transfusion are associated with decreased risk of death in traumatically injured patients. J Trauma Acute Care Surg 2016;81(3):458–62.
75. Fisher A, Miles E, Cap A, et al. Tactical damage control resuscitation. Mil Med 2015;180:869–75.
76. Wild G, Anderson D, Lund P. Round Afghanistan with a fridge. J R Army Med Corps 2013;159:24–9.
77. Kim B, Zielinski M, Jenkins D, et al. The effects of prehospital plasma on patients with injury: a prehospital plasma resuscitation. J Trauma Acute Care Surg 2012; 73:S49–53.
78. Butler FK, Blackbourne LH, Gross KR. The combat medic aid bag – 2025: CoTCCC top ten recommended battlefield trauma care research, development, and evaluation priorities for 2015. J Spec Oper Med 2015;15:7–19.

79. Butler FK, Holcomb JB, Kotwal RS, et al. Fluid resuscitation for hemorrhagic shock in Tactical Combat Casualty Care: TCCC guidelines change 14-01. J Spec Oper Med 2014;14:13–38.

80. Mortelmans Y, Merckx E, van Nerom C, et al. Effect of an equal volume replacement with 500cc 6% hydroxyethyl starch on the blood and plasma volume of healthy volunteers. Eur J Anesthesiol 1995;12:259–64.

81. Wolberg AS, Meng ZH, Monroe DM, et al. A systematic evaluation of the effect of temperature on coagulation enzyme activity and platelet function. J Trauma 2004;56:1221–8.

82. Watts DD, Trask A, Soeken K, et al. Hypothermic coagulopathy in trauma: effect of varying levels of hypothermia on enzyme speed, platelet function, and fibrinolytic activity. J Trauma 1998;44:846–54.

83. Arthurs Z, Cuadrado D, Beekley A, et al. The impact of hypothermia on trauma care at the 31st combat support hospital. Am J Surg 2006;191:610–4.

84. Winkenwerder W. Defense-wide policy on combat trauma casualty hypothermia prevention and treatment. Assistant Secretary of Defense for Health Affairs Memorandum dated February 16, 2006. Available at: http://www.health.mil/libraries/HA_Policies_and_Guidelines/06-005.pdf. Accessed 14 August 2013.

85. Allen PB, Salyer SW, Dubick MA, et al. Preventing hypothermia: comparison of current devices used by the U.S. Army with an in vitro warmed fluid model. J Trauma 2010;69(Suppl):S154–61.

86. Zafren K, Giesbrecht GG, Danzl DF, et al. Wilderness Medical Society practice guidelines for the out-of-hospital evaluation and treatment of accidental hypothermia: 2014 update. Wilderness Environ Med 2014;25(Suppl):S66–85.

87. Mazzoli RA, Gross KR, Butler FK. The use of rigid eye shields (fox shields) at the point of injury for ocular trauma in Afghanistan. J Trauma 2014;77:S156–62.

88. Butler FK, Chalfin S. The eye in the wilderness. In: Auerbach PS, editor. Wilderness medicine. 7th edition. St Louis (MO): Mosby; 2016. p. 1109–27.

89. Paterson R, Drake B, Tabin G, et al. Wilderness Medical Society practice guidelines for treatment of eye injuries and illnesses in the wilderness: 2014 update. Wilderness Environ Med 2014;25(Suppl):S19–29.

90. Dickey N, Jenkins D, Butler F. Prehospital use of ketamine in battlefield analgesia. Defense Health Board Memorandum 2012:1–11. Available at: http://www.naemt.org/docs/default-source/education-documents/tccc/10-9-15-updates/dhb-memo-120308-ketamine.pdf?sfvrsn=2. Accessed January 19, 2017.

91. Beecher H. Delayed morphine poisoning in battle casualties. JAMA 1944;124:1193–4.

92. Butler FK, Kotwal RS, Buckenmaier CC III, et al. A triple-option analgesia plan for Tactical Combat Casualty Care. J Spec Oper Med 2014;14:13–25.

93. Kotwal R, O'Connor K, Johnson T, et al. A novel pain management strategy for combat casualty care. Ann Emerg Med 2004;44:121–7.

94. Wedmore I, Kotwal R, McManus J, et al. Safety and efficacy of oral transmucosal fentanyl citrate for prehospital pain control on the battlefield. J Trauma 2012;73:S490–5.

95. Weiss E. Medical considerations for wilderness and adventure travelers. Med Clin North Am 1999;83:885–902.

96. Onifer DJ, Butler FK, Gross KR, et al. Replacement of Phenergan (promethazine) with Zofran (ondansetron) for treatment of opioid and trauma-related nausea and vomiting in Tactical Combat Casualty Care: TCCC guidelines change 14-03. J Spec Oper Med 2015;15:17–24.

97. American College of Emergency Physicians Policy Statement. Out of hospital use of analgesia and sedation. Ann Emerg Med 2016;67:305–6.
98. Russell KW, Scaife CL, Weber DC, et al. Wilderness Medical Society practice guidelines for the treatment of acute pain in remote environments: 2014 update. Wilderness Environ Med 2014;25(Suppl):S96–104.
99. O'Connor K, Butler F. Antibiotics in tactical combat casualty care 2002. Mil Med 2003;168:911–4.
100. Hospenthal DR, Murray CK, Anderson RC, et al. Guidelines for prevention of infection after combat-related injuries. J Trauma 2008;64(Suppl):S211–20.
101. Battistella FD, Nugent W, Owings JT, et al. Field triage of the pulseless trauma patient. Arch Surg 1999;134:742–5.
102. Branney SW, Moore EE, Feldhaus KM, et al. Critical analysis of two decades of experience with post-injury emergency department thoracotomy in a regional trauma center. J Trauma 1988;45:87–94.
103. Rosemurgy AS, Norris PA, Olson SM, et al. Prehospital traumatic cardiac arrest: the cost of futility. J Trauma 1993;35:468–73.
104. Dickey N, Jenkins D. Needle decompression of tension pneumothorax and cardio-pulmonary resuscitation in Tactical Combat Casualty Care. Defense Health Board Memorandum 2011:1–11. Available at: http://www.naemt.org/docs/default-source/education-documents/tccc/10-9-15-updates/dhb-memo-120706-needle-decompression.pdf?sfvrsn=2. Accessed January 19, 2017.
105. Kotwal RS, Butler FK, Montgomery HR, et al. The Tactical Combat Casualty Care Casualty Card. J Spec Oper Med 2013;13:82–6.

Point-of-Care Ultrasound in Austere Environments

A Complete Review of Its Utilization, Pitfalls, and Technique for Common Applications in Austere Settings

Laleh Gharahbaghian, MD[a],*, Kenton L. Anderson, MD[b], Viveta Lobo, MD[a], Rwo-Wen Huang, MD[a], Cori McClure Poffenberger, MD[a], Phi D. Nguyen, MD[c]

KEYWORDS

- Point of care • Ultrasound • Austere • High altitude • Resource limited • Disaster
- Battlefield • Military

KEY POINTS

- Ultrasound systems must be handheld, battery operated, durable, and able to withstand extremes of temperature and altitude, while additional equipment may be necessary to help prevent battery degradation and equipment damage.
- Point-of-care ultrasound is portable and lightweight, and can be used to screen for a wide variety of pathology and injury common to austere environments, disaster situations, and resource-limited settings.
- Common point-of-care ultrasound applications used in austere environments include the Extended Focused Assessment with Sonography in Trauma, musculoskeletal and soft tissue injury, high-altitude pulmonary edema, high-altitude cerebral edema, pneumonia, volume status, and various procedural guidance applications.
- The various point-of-care applications used in austere environments for procedural guidance include peripheral vascular access, nerve blocks for pain control, foreign body removal, and abscess drainage.
- Point-of-care ultrasound is a reliable tool to assist in triage, resource allocation decisions, and screening for conditions common in austere environments.

Disclosures/Conflicts of Interests: The authors have nothing to disclose. None have any commercial or financial conflicts of interest.
[a] Emergency Ultrasound Program, Department of Emergency Medicine, Stanford University School of Medicine, 300 Pasteur Drive, Alway Building M121, Stanford, CA 94304, USA;
[b] Emergency Ultrasound Research and Scholarly Activity, Department of Emergency Medicine, Stanford University School of Medicine, 300 Pasteur Drive, Alway Building M121, Stanford, CA 94304, USA; [c] Stanford/Kaiser Emergency Medicine Residency Program, 300 Pasteur Drive, Alway Building M121, Stanford, CA 94304, USA
* Corresponding author.
E-mail address: Lalehg@stanford.edu

Emerg Med Clin N Am 35 (2017) 409–441
http://dx.doi.org/10.1016/j.emc.2016.12.007
0733-8627/17/© 2017 Elsevier Inc. All rights reserved.

emed.theclinics.com

Video content accompanies this article at http://www.emed.theclinics.com.

INTRODUCTION: POINT-OF-CARE ULTRASOUND AND HANDHELD SYSTEMS

Ultrasound technology continues to advance and has come a long way from large wall-mounted systems with poor image quality to small handheld devices with good image quality. Ultrasound systems were optimized for medical military use in the 1980s. Due to its successful utilization at the point-of-care, its lack of ionizing radiation, and the expansion of computer technology, point-of-care ultrasound (POCUS) rapidly spread to trauma, emergency department, and "out-of-hospital" settings, including in austere environments where other imaging modalities cannot be carried.[1,2]

There are various handheld systems that can fit into a large coat pocket, and the power supply and case can fit into any backpack. Their power timing and image quality is less than that of laptop-based systems, but their portability and ability to transfer images wirelessly to electronic mailing or via text messaging make these systems unique. The GE (Chicago, IL) VScan was one of the first handheld devices to come to market with a "flip-open" and touch-sensor style, now with a dual probe for both high-frequency and low-frequency imaging. The SonoSite (Bothell, WA) iViz is one of the newest devices on the market with a larger screen, good image quality, and touch-screen capability. The Philips (Andover, MA) Lumify is another new system that currently requires a subscription. Other devices, including handheld devices by Clarius (Burnaby, Canada) and Signostics (Bothell, WA) provide a probe and require a smart phone for scanning.

POINT-OF-CARE ULTRASOUND IN AUSTERE ENVIRONMENTS: UTILITY AND PITFALLS

The first portable ultrasound machine weighed just over 5 pounds, was the first battery-operated ultrasound machine, and was durable enough to withstand unpredictable battlefield environments.[3] Austere environments continue to pose special challenges to ultrasound equipment, including battery degradation, hard-drive failure, and physical abuse. Advances in equipment design and environment-specific care have allowed successful use of ultrasound in these extreme situations.

MILITARY AND COMBAT ENVIRONMENTS
Ultrasound on the Battlefield

The battlefield is an unforgiving environment for ultrasound machines. In Iraq and Afghanistan, ambient temperatures fluctuate greatly, resulting in battery degradation.[4,5] The environment is also sandy and dusty, contributing to overheating. Ultrasound machines are often treated roughly out of necessity. There are space limitations in medical treatment facilities, so equipment may inadvertently be jostled or knocked to the ground during a mass casualty incident (MCI). Medics may carry small portable ultrasound machines in their packs to the point of injury. Therefore, machines must be handheld, use cooling fans, and have extra batteries available.

Because most battlefield deaths are caused by hemorrhage, the most common role for ultrasound in this environment is the focused assessment with sonography in trauma (FAST) examination, which parallels the civilian MCI experience in which triage of casualties is the priority.[6] Computed tomography (CT) may not be available, and physicians in war zones found ultrasound to be invaluable during triage.[7] The FAST examination can identify occult blood loss in young, highly conditioned patients whose physiologic reserve undermines the reliability of vital signs until late stages of shock.[8]

Pneumothorax assessment of the extended FAST (eFAST) is also useful, especially when planning medical evacuations, because even small pneumothoraces, which might otherwise be considered insignificant, can benefit from thoracostomy to prevent in-flight decompensation.

A variety of other emergency-related ultrasound applications, including fracture assessment and its reduction, inferior vena cava (IVC) collapsibility for resuscitative decision in nontraumatic shock states, optic nerve sheath diameter (ONSD) for intracranial pressure assessment when CT or neurosurgical consultation is unavailable, and procedural guidance for venous access, regional anesthesia, pericardiocentesis, cricothyrotomy, and foreign body detection and removal, have all been found useful.[2,9–13]

Ultrasound in Flight

Because of noise and space limitations in the field with limited physical examination performance ability, POCUS in flight is highly valuable to care for patients in transit to higher levels of care, as they may deteriorate due to their tenuous physiology and stressors of flight (hypoxia, hypobaria, constant movement, noise, and hypothermia or hyperthermia). Ultrasound equipment in flight must be lightweight, take up little space, and be able to tolerate vibrations and large fluctuations in temperature and elevation. Ultrasound has not been found interfere with aircraft avionics and can be used on multiple rotary and fixed-wing airframes.[9,14–16]

Helicopters are often used to transport trauma patients from the field or from a smaller hospital to a larger trauma center. Both small and large fixed-wing aircraft have been used to transport medical patients over longer distances or to areas outside disaster zones. These aircraft are often staffed by medical personnel who can use ultrasound to determine the etiology of undifferentiated hypotension or hypoxia (eFAST, cardiac echo, IVC) and perform ultrasound-guided procedures.[16–20]

DISASTER AND MASS CASUALTY INCIDENTS

During MCIs the volume and severity of casualties overwhelms the capabilities and resources of the response effort. POCUS is ideally suited for MCI conditions when other imaging is often not available due to the remoteness of the mission, destruction of previously available equipment, or interruption of the region's ability to produce electricity. Early in disaster missions, ultrasound is often used as a triage tool. Later, it is more frequently used to diagnose common conditions like pneumothoraces, long bone fractures, and dehydration. Portability becomes an even greater priority when the disaster-relief team has to hand-carry their equipment over a long distance.

Natural Disasters

Several reports from various earthquakes, including the 1988 magnitude 6.9 earthquake in Armenia (one of the first studies to quantify POCUS use during a natural disaster), concluded that POCUS is invaluable since medical care often takes place outdoors for safety reasons, CT scanners may be reserved for head trauma cases, ultrasound provides procedural guidance, and ultrasound has been used to decipher which patients needed dialysis and their likelihood of recovery from crush-related acute renal failure. Furthermore, there were low false-negative rates of the FAST examination for traumatic injuries requiring surgical intervention, with most being due to retroperitoneal or solid organ injuries, a known limitation of the FAST scan.[21–26]

After several more studies from mudslides, cyclones, and earthquakes, a wider range of ultrasound applications was found to be useful, including pelvic, right upper quadrant, renal, orthopedic, cardiac, deep venous thrombosis, and lung scans.[27,28] Decisions regarding patient management and transport were made, and clinical management was changed in a large percentage of patients following POCUS.[9,28]

Man-Made Disasters

The utility of the FAST examination after the bombings in Madrid, London, Lebanon, and Boston have been reported.[29–34] The report from the Boston Marathon bombing describes how the volume of critically wounded and unregistered patients overwhelmed standard radiography processes, causing an emergency physician to go "bed to bed," performing eFAST exams on each patient and leaving the hand-written results taped to the gurneys; 24% of these ultrasound-triaged patients received immediate operative intervention. This report also noted that an older ultrasound machine was limited in utility due to a lack of battery backup and long boot time. This report concluded there should be a battery-operated ultrasound machine in each clinical area, and alternative image documentation protocols should be used during MCIs.

Tropical Environments

Portable ultrasound has been carried on multiple humanitarian missions to remote tropical locations (**Fig. 1**). Portability and battery power are needed, and solar electrical chargers are ideal while attempting to prevent battery degradation. Tropical environments pose the added challenge of prolonged humidity and/or frank wetting, which can destroy batteries and other electrical equipment. A report from the Amazon jungle noted that 7 of the 25 examinations performed (1 FAST, 6 hepatobiliary, 5 transabdominal, and 7 endovaginal pelvic, 3 renal, 3 aorta) changed management; 4 patients avoided a potentially dangerous 2-day evacuation, and 3 were referred for rapid surgical intervention.[27]

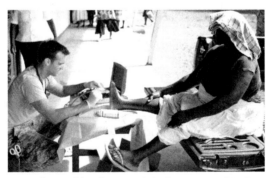

Fig. 1. A battery-operated portable ultrasound device was used to locate and remove the foreign body from a nonambulatory patient in a facility without electricity in the Suriname jungle. (*Courtesy of* K.L. Anderson, MD.)

THE INTERNATIONAL SPACE STATION AND REMOTE TELEMONITORED ULTRASOUND

Ultrasound has been used in some remote areas where it is not feasible to have a clinician or even a technician with specialized training present. The International Space Station (ISS) is probably the epitome of remote locations, and the National Aeronautics and Space Administration pioneered remote telemonitored ultrasound (RTUS), which uses live video streaming of ultrasound examinations performed by nonmedical personnel and reviewed by clinicians in real-time on Earth.[35] This technology has subsequently proven feasible in other remote locations, including high-elevation mountains and inside flying aircraft.[36–39] The number of ultrasound applications possible is limited only by the expert's ability to verbally instruct the operator.

HIGH ALTITUDE

Ultrasound has been most commonly used as a research tool in 2 environments at high altitude (above 1500 m): ski resort health clinics, and base camp clinics for climbers. At ski resort clinics, other radiologic options such as radiograph, CT, or

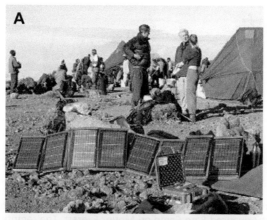

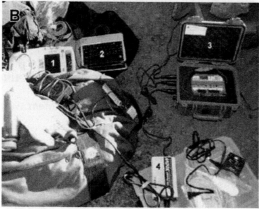

Fig. 2. Electronic devices used on a solar-powered, high-altitude ultrasound research expedition to Mt Kilimanjaro. (*A*) These rigid solar arrays weigh less than 5 kg and provide more than 50 W of power under equatorial sun on Mt Kilimanjaro. This power is controlled by an electronic voltage regulator using a lead-acid battery storage system, housed in the waterproof case in the foreground. (*B*) From left to right: (1) the ultrasound unit (Sonosite 180-plus; Sonosite, Bothell, WA), (2) laptop data storage (Dell Inspiron 910; Dell, Round Rock, TX), (3) 300 W DC-to-AC converter (box in foreground, Go Power!; Carmanah, Victoria, British Columbia, Canada), and (4) electronic voltage regulator with lead-acid battery storage (CT Solar LLC, Palm City, FL). Total weight of all electronic and power storage equipment is less than 18 kg. (*Reprinted from* Fagenholz PJ, Murray AF, Noble VE, et al. Ultrasound for high altitude research. Ultrasound Med Biol 2012;38:5; with permission from Elsevier.)

MRI also may be available. However, at very high altitude (3500 m to 5500 m) or extreme altitude (above 5500 m) the clinics are usually remote, with the only imaging modality being ultrasound that was carried there by foot. Spinning hard drives may cause machine failure, likely due to the cold and decreased barometric pressures; solid state memory devices are recommended, as they do not have any moving parts. Sleeping with cold batteries or soaking transducers in warm water to keep them functioning reliably have been described. Light, portable solar arrays can be used to recharge batteries[40] **(Fig. 2)**. Ultrasound applications can be performed within minutes, limiting patient exposure to the cold environment. Additionally, RTUS techniques can be used, demonstrating that an experienced sonographer does not need to be physically present **(Fig. 3)**.

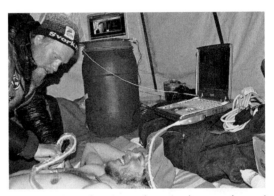

Fig. 3. A nonexpert operator is performing a thoracic ultrasound examination on a fellow climber in a tent at Advanced Base Camp on Mount Everest. The remote expert is seen on the computer screen in the background directing the examination. (*From* Otto C, Hamilton DR, Levine BD, et al. Into thin air: extreme ultrasound at Mt Everest. Wilderness Environmental Med 2009;20:285; with permission from Elsevier.)

COMMON CLINICAL APPLICATIONS OF POINT-OF-CARE ULTRASOUND IN AUSTERE ENVIRONMENTS: TECHNIQUE AND PATHOLOGY
Trauma and Injury Assessment: Extended Focused Assessment with Sonography in Trauma Scan and Musculoskeletal Ultrasound

Extended focused assessment with sonography in trauma
The eFAST examination is a screening tool for intraperitoneal, intrathoracic, and pericardial fluid plus an assessment for pneumothorax. It includes 6 views and does not evaluate the retroperitoneal space. Supine patient positioning is required.[41,42]

- Right upper quadrant (RUQ) **(Figs. 4** and **5**, Videos 1 and 2)
  - Pathology: This is the most sensitive view for free fluid (FF) detection, best seen in the paracolic gutter and Morison pouch. FF is black (anechoic), but can be gray (echogenic) if there are clots **(Fig. 6**, Video 3). Pleural fluid is seen as an anechoic area above the diaphragm causing the spine to be visible, as opposed to normal mirror image of the liver seen above the diaphragm **(Fig. 7)**.
- Left upper quadrant (LUQ) **(Fig. 8**, Videos 4 and 5)
  - Pathology: Fluid is best seen in the subdiaphragmatic region. A left pleural effusion can be seen as described previously **(Figs. 9** and **10**, Video 6).
- Suprapubic (SP) **(Figs. 11** and **12**, Videos 7–9)

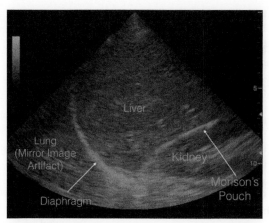

Fig. 4. Normal RUQ view showing above and below the diaphragm, and Morison's pouch.

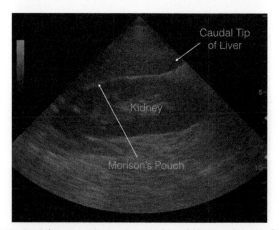

Fig. 5. Normal RUQ view showing Morison's pouch and the caudal tip of the liver.

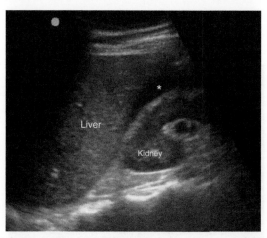

Fig. 6. Positive RUQ view showing black (anechoic) free fluid (*asterisk*) in Morison pouch and around caudal tip of liver.

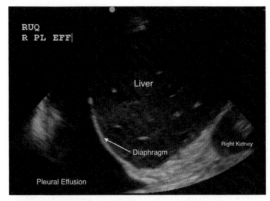

Fig. 7. Positive right thoracic view showing pleural effusion.

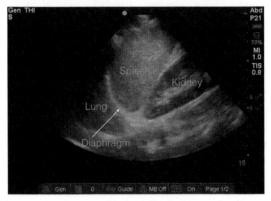

Fig. 8. Normal LUQ anatomy above and below diaphragm and splenorenal space.

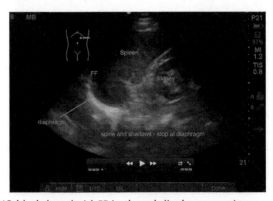

Fig. 9. Positive LUQ black (anechoic) FF in the subdiaphragm region.

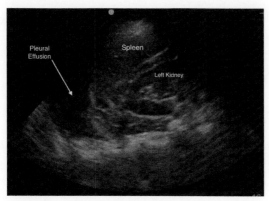

Fig. 10. Positive left thoracic view showing pleural effusion.

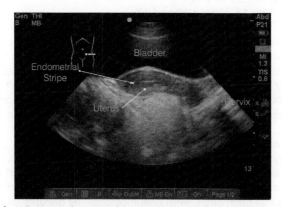

Fig. 11. Normal female sagittal suprapubic anatomy with full bladder.

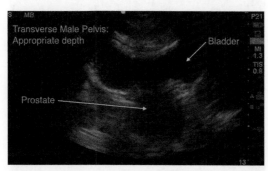

Fig. 12. Normal male suprapubic transverse anatomy showing appropriate depth and prostate.

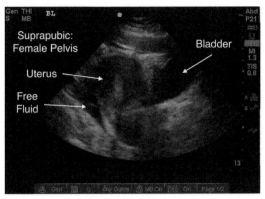

Fig. 13. Positive suprapubic sagittal view of female pelvis.

- ○ Pathology: FF is most likely to be present posterior to the bladder (male individuals) and in the cul-de-sac (Pouch of Douglas in female individuals) (**Figs. 13** and **14**; Videos 10 and 11).
- Subxiphoid (**Fig. 15**, Videos 12 and 13):
  - ○ Pathology: Pericardial effusion (PCE) appears as an anechoic band inferior to the right ventricle (RV, **Fig. 16**). If a suboptimal view, a parasternal long view is used in which PCE is visualized posterior to the heart above the hyperechoic pericardium, which can help differentiate PCE from epicardial fat that will be seen only anteriorly (**Fig. 17**; Video 14). An assessment of left ventricular (LV) contractility and RV strain can be added if the eFAST is used for patients with unexplained shock. Normal is 40% to 50% contraction and an RV:LV ratio of 0.7:1.0.
- Thoracic view for pneumothorax (**Fig. 18**, Videos 15 and 16):
  - ○ Pathology: With 2 ribs in view, each a hyperechoic curve with posterior shadowing, the pleural line is a bright horizontal line between and below the ribs. With normal lung sliding, it "shimmers" as the parietal and visceral pleura move against each other. With pneumothorax, air disrupts ultrasound waves: no movement is seen at the pleural line (Video 17). In motion (M)-mode, lung sliding shows up as a "seashore sign" (**Fig. 19**), whereas pneumothorax has a "barcode sign": only straight horizontal lines demonstrating the lack of

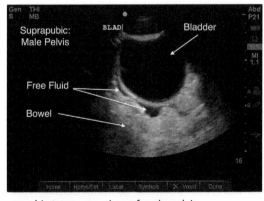

Fig. 14. Positive suprapubic transverse view of male pelvis.

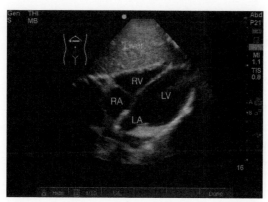

Fig. 15. Normal subxiphoid anatomy showing the 4-chamber heart with liver as an acoustic window.

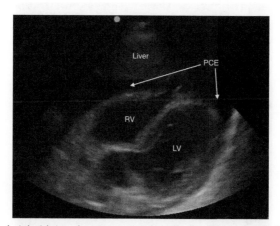

Fig. 16. Positive subxiphoid view showing pericardial effusion inferior to the right ventricle (RV).

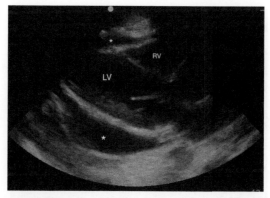

Fig. 17. Positive parasternal long view showing pericardial fluid (*asterisks*) anterior and posterior to the left ventricle (LV).

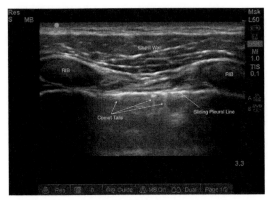

Fig. 18. Normal chest showing comet tail artifact of pleural line from lung sliding between 2 rib shadows.

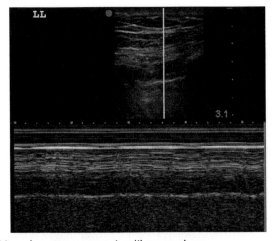

Fig. 19. Normal M-mode pattern appearing like a seashore.

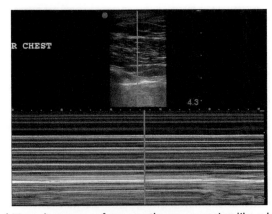

Fig. 20. Abnormal M-mode pattern of pneumothorax appearing like a barcode.

movement (**Fig. 20**). The "lung point" is the junction in which the pneumothorax ends and sliding is again seen, pathognomonic for pneumothorax (Video 18).

The eFAST scan can change differential diagnoses and patient management in a significant number of patients in remote settings.[43] Deciding on evacuations, patients saved from thoracostomy, and identification of emergent conditions masked by normal vital signs have all proved eFAST to be invaluable.[43–45]

Musculoskeletal injury

Austere environments can have treacherous terrain, placing people at risk for musculoskeletal injury. The high-frequency linear probe is often used because most injuries do not require increased depth.

- Subcutaneous or deep tissue hematoma
  - Pathology: Normal skin is echogenic with varying levels of brightness with linear arrays separating various fascial planes (Video 19). Hematomas tend to be initially hypoechoic with mixed echogenicity as the clotting process progresses[46,47] (Video 20). Use color Doppler to differentiate it from a solid mass, as hematomas will lack vascularity. Compression cause the internal echoes of a hematoma to move.
- Fractures/Effusions: POCUS is useful for occult fractures and more sensitive than radiograph for scaphoid, hip, long bone, and sternal fractures, as well as joint effusions.[48–52]
  - Pathology: Fractures are seen as a cortical discontinuity. Another suggestive sign is an adjacent hematoma (**Fig. 21**). The nearby joint space can be assessed for associated joint effusions, seen as a larger anechoic joint space fluid compared with the contralateral side[7] (Video 21).
  - Fracture reduction and hematoma blocks: Ultrasound can be used to identify the location for hematoma blocks for pain control, as well as assess alignment of the bone after reduction attempts.[53]
- Dislocation: POCUS has been studied in shoulder and hip dislocations with high sensitivities.[54,55]
  - Technique and pathology: By placing the probe in longitudinal orientation to the humerus or femur at the joint space, a dislocation can be seen as a

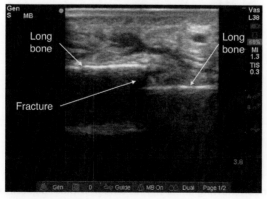

Fig. 21. Fracture seen as a cortical disruption.

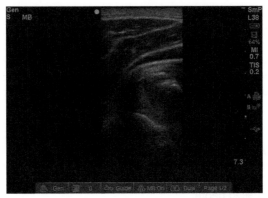

Fig. 22. Anterior shoulder dislocation showing humeral head lateral and inferior to glenoid.

separation of bones. Ultrasound can provide confirmation after dislocation reduction (**Fig. 22**).

- Tendon tear: Tendon tears, especially those of large muscle groups, such as the triceps, quadriceps/patella, and biceps, is accurately diagnosed with POCUS.[56] Tendons appear differently depending on the angle and tilt of the ultrasound transducer relative to the tendon. When oblique against tendon fibers, a hypoechoic artifact is observed, leading to a false-positive interpretation.[56]
  - Pathology: Normal tendon has a linear striped fibrillar appearance and is more echogenic than muscle. Findings suggestive of a tendon tear include local swelling around the tendon fibers, fiber discontinuation, irregularity of the tendon, and hypoechogenicities within the tendon bed itself[56] (**Fig. 23**). Accurate diagnosis is reached by comparing to the contralateral side.[57] Ranging the patient's joints throughout the examination will show the 2 severed ends in a tendon tear separating from one another[58] (**Fig. 24**).

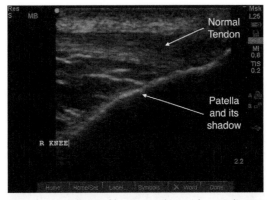

Fig. 23. Normal tendon showing linear fibrous tendon without adjacent fluid of soft tissue edema.

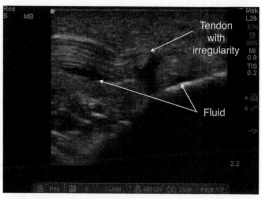

Fig. 24. Partial patella tendon tear seen as disruption of normal tendon linearity with adjacent fluid.

High-Altitude Pulmonary Edema

Lung and cardiac ultrasound can identify individuals with high-altitude pulmonary edema (HAPE) susceptibility and distinguish HAPE from other causes of dyspnea. Cardiac ultrasound has replaced pulmonary artery catheterization for assessing the increased pulmonary artery pressures, allows detection of a patent foramen ovale, and allows assessment of LV and RV myocardial performance to hypoxia because they may contribute to or are associated with HAPE.[59–62] Sonographic B-lines, diagnostic of interstitial fluid, are linear vertical rays arising from the pleural line and extending to the end of the screen, with the number of B-lines correlating with degree of hypoxia and symptom severity in patients with known HAPE.[63] The number increases with each ascend and improves with either the descend or treatment for HAPE.[64] Also, B-lines can appear in all lung zones within minutes of arrival at high altitude, suggesting hypobaria alone could lead to interstitial fluid accumulation before symptoms (subclinical HAPE).[65] Additionally, findings on ultrasound that suggest etiologies of dyspnea, such as pneumothorax, pneumonia, heart failure, pulmonary embolus, or

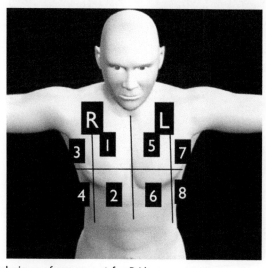

Fig. 25. 8-zone technique of assessment for B-Lines.

myocardial infarction, require immediate evacuation, whereas patients with HAPE may descend until symptoms resolve.

- An 8-zone technique is used, avoiding the need for patients to undress in the cold (**Fig. 25**). The anterior chest wall is delineated from the sternum to the anterior axillary line and subdivided into upper and lower halves (the clavicle to the third intercostal space, and from the third intercostal space to the diaphragm). The lateral zone is delineated from the anterior to the posterior axillary line and subdivided into upper and lower halves. One scan is obtained from each area.
- Pathology: Normal lung will show linear horizontal reverberation artifact, called A-lines (**Fig. 26**). B-lines are defined as discrete laser-like vertical hyperechoic reverberation artifacts that arise from the pleural line, extend to the bottom of the screen without fading, and move synchronously with lung sliding (**Fig. 27**). They

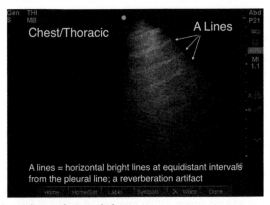

Fig. 26. Sonographic A-lines of normal chest.

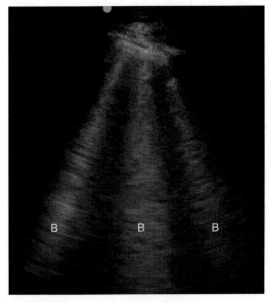

Fig. 27. Sonographic B-lines showing pulmonary edema.

arise from the pleural line, move with lung sliding, spread to the edge of the screen without fading, and erase A-lines. Interstitial syndrome (including pulmonary edema) has been defined as more than 2 B-lines in more than 2 zones, bilaterally. Also, the total sum of all B-lines yields a B-line score which is another indicator of the extent of extravascular lung water.[40,66–68] It is currently unclear if the number of B-lines is able to predict or assess the extent of pulmonary edema at altitude.

Acute Mountain Sickness and High-Altitude Cerebral Edema

Increasing ONSD measurements have been associated with severity of acute mountain sickness (AMS).[69,70] This finding supports the theory that AMS is due to increased intracranial pressure (ICP); however, significant individual variations, at baseline and at altitude, as well as interobserver variation exists with this technique.[71,72] ONSD increases with altitude alone in subjects both with and without AMS, but to a higher degree in the former.[69,70,73] In those who do have AMS, ONSD has a positive correlation with the severity of symptoms, including the Lake Louise score, oxygen saturation, and resting heart rate.[70] However, more recent research failed to demonstrate any association between ONSD and headache, which is often considered the most significant AMS symptom.[74] Other pathologies can be seen with ocular ultrasound, including retinal detachment, vitreous hemorrhage, retrobulbar hematoma, and orbital rupture. The high-frequency linear probe is used (Video 22).

- Pathology: The optic nerve will be visualized in the axial plane as a linear hypoechoic structure extending posteriorly from the anechoic circular globe, surrounded by echogenic retrobulbar fat. ONSD measurement is taken 3 mm behind the papilla, the location with the highest distensibility with increased ICP (**Fig. 28**). Each eye is scanned both sagittally and transversely, and the ONSD is compared with the unaffected eye. The normal cutoff for adults is 5 mm, whereas younger children can be higher.[75,76]

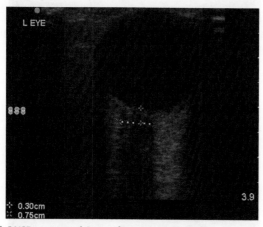

Fig. 28. Abnormal ONSD measured 3 mm from posterior orbit.

Pneumonia

Lung ultrasound is shown to be superior to radiography, and comparable to CT for the diagnosis of pneumonia.[77–79] Compared with traditional imaging used to identify pneumonia, sonography is the preferred method in children.[80–82] Researchers regard POCUS as the reference standard for lung consolidation and concluded that the World Health Organization case management algorithm is inferior in comparison.[81] Considering that pulmonary infection is quite common in patients infected with the human immunodeficiency virus (HIV), ultrasound is especially valuable in countries with high HIV prevalence.[82] The low-frequency phased array or curvilinear probe is used.

- Pathology: Consolidation is seen as a hypoechoic area with tissuelike heterogeneous texture, oftentimes described as "hepatization." It usually has irregular or blurred borders and hyperechoic dendritic or punctate structures representing air bronchograms (**Figs. 29** and **30**). B-lines also can be seen extending from the consolidation (**Fig. 31**). If the consolidation reaches the pleura, the pleural line will have decreased or absent lung sliding. There also may be a parapneumonic pleural effusion in the dependent thorax. It can appear anechoic, or echogenic in the case of empyema, hemorrhage, or clots[77–83] (**Fig. 32**).

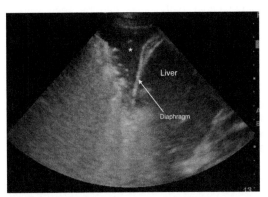

Fig. 29. Right lower lobe pneumonia seen as a hypoechoic triangular region (*asterisk*) with hepatization and hyperechoic borders.

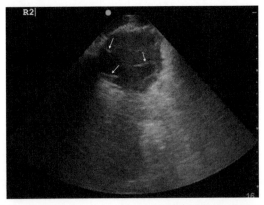

Fig. 30. Air bronchograms (*arrows*) seen within consolidation consistent with pneumonia.

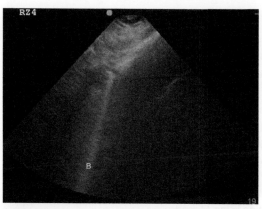

Fig. 31. Small area of pneumonia with resultant B-line extending from the consolidation.

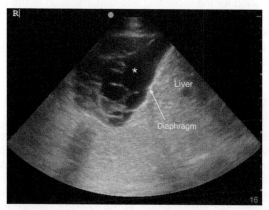

Fig. 32. Loculated parapneumonic pleural effusion (*asterisk*) adjacent to consolidation.

Volume/Hydration Status

Intravascular volume and fluid tolerance is assessed by ultrasound by an evaluation of either the internal jugular (IJ) vein or IVC. Extremes of volume status are correlated to IVC respiratory variation.[28,84–86] Patients with undifferentiated hypotension will benefit from POCUS to assess hydration status, as intravenous fluids may not be widely available.[28] The aorta-to-IVC ratio is associated with volume status in children, even though reports diverge on whether ultrasound alone accurately identifies dehydration in resource-limited settings.[84,85]

- IJ assessment
  - Probe and technique: a high-frequency linear probe is placed on the mid to lower anterior neck, perpendicular to the skin in transverse plane of the vein with the patient supine or semi-upright to 30°. Only gentle pressure should be applied. Under M-mode, the maximum (Dmax) and minimum (Dmin) diameter of the vein can be measured to obtain the collapsibility index (CI)[87–89]: CI = [(Dmax − Dmin)/Dmax] × 100%.
- IVC assessment
  - The IVC will be seen entering the right atrium, with measurements of respiratory variation taken 2 cm caudal to the right atrial inlet. Similar to the IJ,

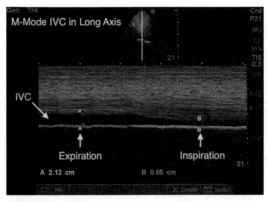

Fig. 33. IVC evaluation using M-mode.

M-mode is used for the recording and determination of the CI (**Fig. 33**). If the maximum diameter of the IVC is less than 2 cm with greater than 50% respiratory variation, the patient may be hypovolemic; if the maximum diameter of the IVC is greater than 2 cm with less than 50% respiratory variation, the patient may be hypervolemic[90,91] (Videos 23 and 24).

COMMON PROCEDURAL ULTRASOUND IN AUSTERE ENVIRONMENTS
Nerve Blocks/Regional Anesthesia

In the wilderness, traumatic injuries to the upper or lower extremities account for approximately 65% of all musculoskeletal/soft tissue injuries, with most of these being lacerations, traumatic pain, sprains or strains, abrasions, fractures, or dislocations. Pain medications are frequently unavailable and can pose medical problems, making nerve blocks an excellent choice for pain control.[92,93] These blocks have demonstrated effectiveness in the combat setting, because patients with significant injuries can be treated in the field while awaiting evacuation.[94] Complications from inadequate pain control include impaired sleep, impaired immune function, increased risk of developing chronic pain, and increased time to recovery.[94,95] The primary challenges include an inability to clearly identify the nerve, intraneural penetration, and intravascular injection. In the wilderness environment, additional challenges include nonsterility and inability to monitor for signs of local anesthetics systemic toxicity, a rare condition causing neurologic and/or cardiovascular excitation (agitation, seizure, tachycardia, and hypertension) then depression (respiratory depression, coma, bradycardia, asystole).[93,96]

- Probe: High-frequency linear probe for superficial nerves; low-frequency curvilinear probe for deeper nerves.
- Technique: Nerves have a "honeycomb" appearance on ultrasound due to hypoechoic (dark) areas embedded within the hyperechoic (bright) nerve sections (**Fig. 34**). Place the probe in transverse orientation to the nerve, at a safe distance from the vascular bundle to avoid inadvertent vascular injection. Using a longitudinal approach in relation to the needle, penetrate the skin, visualizing the needle on the screen at all times as it gets closer to the nerve, being careful to never penetrate the nerve (**Fig. 35**). Draw back on the syringe to avoid injecting within a vascular structure, then slowly inject the anesthetic, creating a "halo" appearance of fluid surrounding nerve (**Fig. 36**).

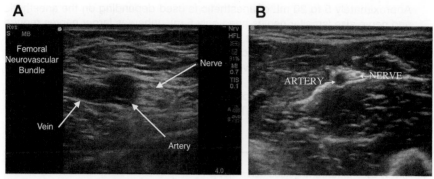

Fig. 34. (*A*) Femoral nerve with its "honeycomb" appearance next to the femoral vessels. (*B*) Ulnar nerve with its characteristic honeycomb appearance next to the ulnar artery.

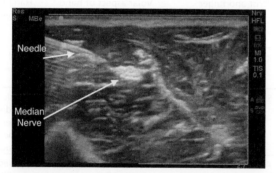

Fig. 35. The length of the needle is seen due to the probe oriented in-plane to the needle. Its tip is seen approaching the median nerve.

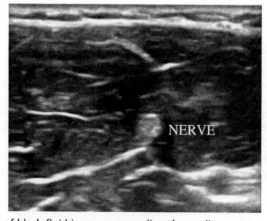

Fig. 36. A "halo" of black fluid is seen surrounding the median nerve.

Approximately 5 to 20 mL of anesthetic is used depending on the anesthetic and nerve size (smaller nerves need only 5 mL, whereas larger nerves require up to 20 mL). Retract if patient notes significant pain with injection, as intraneural penetration may have occurred. Intralipids can be used if toxicity occurs. Contraindications to nerve blocks include coagulopathy or allergy to anesthetic.

- Nerve function: The nerve's motor and sensory functions must be assessed before and after the procedure (**Table 1**).

Table 1
Commonly used ultrasound-guided nerve blocks

Nerve	Motor	Sensory	Injuries Treated
Radial	Wrist extension	Dorsal aspect of hand from thumb to radial half of ring finger	Hand injuries to affected area
Median	Wrist and finger flexion	Volar aspect of hand from thumb to radial half of ring finger	Hand injuries to affected area
Ulnar	Intrinsic muscles of hand	Sensation to 5th digit, and ulnar half of ring finger	Hand injuries to affected area
Interscalene brachial plexus	Superior and middle trunks of the brachial plexus (C5–C7), shoulder and upper arm	Superior and middle trunks of the brachial plexus (C5–C7), shoulder and upper arm	Shoulder, humerus, and elbow injuries; does not reliably block forearm or hand injuries
Sciatic (popliteal)	All movements of foot and toes (via tibial and peroneal nerves)	Foot and most of leg, excludes most medial aspect (innervated by saphenous)	Injuries to lower leg, ankle, and foot
Femoral	Flexion at hip and extension at knee	Medial aspect of distal thigh and leg	Hip fractures, proximal femur, and knee injuries

Peripheral Vascular Access

Vascular access in the hypovolemic patient can be difficult to achieve. Using ultrasound to guide peripheral vascular access has provided success rates from 91% to 97% after prior failed attempts, and initially perceived difficult peripheral access cases are often deemed easier when ultrasound is used.[97–100] In the austere environment, when transfer to the nearest medical facility may be delayed, beginning resuscitative efforts in the field is important. Ultrasound-guided vascular access is easy to learn, with novice users trained to proficiency after minimal training.[101] Complications are the same as those associated with traditional methods: local infiltration, cellulitis, thrombophlebitis, and hematoma formation.[102]

- Technique: The most common area for ultrasound-guided vascular access is the antecubital fossa, although any visible vein can be used. A tourniquet is placed proximally. A longer 1.5-inch catheter may be needed for deeper veins. After cleaning the skin with an alcohol swab, the nondominant hand holds the probe with its indicator toward the sonographer's left in transverse orientation to the vein, a short-axis technique.[101] Then, centering the vein on the screen by sliding the probe and adjusting the screen depth, compressing it with the probe to distinguish it from an artery, and noting the vein's depth from the skin, all will optimize successful cannulation. The dominant hand holds the catheter and places it at the center of the probe and penetrates the skin (**Fig. 37**, Video 25). The needle tip must be seen as it advances toward the vein. This requires the probe to also slide in the direction of needle advancement. You may notice a tenting of the anterior wall of the vein. Once the needle punctures the vessel wall, blood return will be seen, and you can place the probe down, advance the catheter over the needle, and secure the line using standard methods (**Fig. 38**).

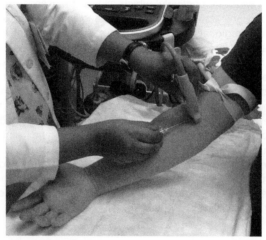

Fig. 37. Short-axis single-operator technique. The nondominant hand holds the probe while the dominant hand holds the catheter.

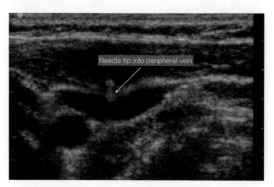

Fig. 38. Needle tip seen tenting the anterior wall of the vein.

Foreign Body (Identification and Removal)

In the wilderness, foreign objects are estimated to account for 2% of all soft tissue injuries.[92] Delay in identification or removal of foreign bodies has been shown to increase associated pain, infection, and inflammation. Ultrasonography is a reliable diagnostic mode for foreign bodies assessment, as well as for guiding their removal.[103,104] It has proven to be superior to plain film radiography, detecting both radiopaque and radiolucent objects with sensitivities of 94% to 98%.[105,106] Unsuspecting fragments and adjacent musculoskeletal and neurovascular structures also can be seen, and once detected, ultrasound can be used to guide the removal of the foreign body with reliability and less complication.[106] During foreign body removal, you are able to accurately identify the location and its measurements, as it may not be in the area of the puncture site, so you are able to make your incision length more precise.[107]

- Technique: The probe is placed over the injury, or the assumed entrance site if visible, and a wide margin is evaluated. Once the hyperechoic foreign body is identified, evaluate it in both its longitudinal and transverse axis, and measure its length and width respectively, which allows the assessment of its position, orientation, and any potential fragments alongside it (**Figs. 39** and **40**). After appreciating the regional structures, identify the closest distance of the object in longitudinal axis from the skin's surface and mark the skin; this will be your entry point for removal. After wiping the area with an alcohol wipe, and injecting local anesthetic if available or performing a nerve block, use a number 11 scalpel and make a small incision as wide as the width of the foreign body. Applying gel and the probe over the skin adjacent to the incision site allows for direct visualization while blunt dissection is done by forceps through the incision and advancing toward the foreign body for its capture and removal. Irrigate the wound again, and allow it to heal by secondary intention.
- Water bath technique: If a foreign body is suspected in the hand or foot, placing the region in a bucket of water and inserting the probe in the water without applying pressure on the region can prevent further pain elicitation and improved foreign body removal technique[108] (**Fig. 41**, Video 26).

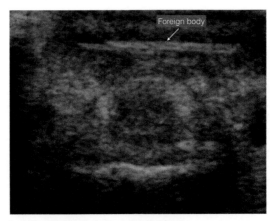

Fig. 39. Ultrasound of foreign body in longitudinal axis.

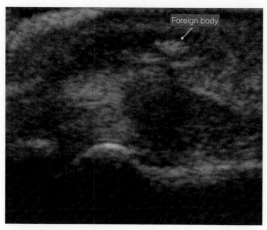

Fig. 40. Ultrasound of foreign body in transverse axis.

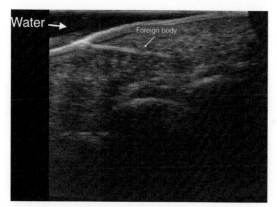

Fig. 41. Ultrasound of foreign body using water bath.

Abscess (Diagnosis)

Differentiating abscess versus cellulitis can be difficult with physical examination alone. Using POCUS will improve accuracy of diagnosis from 86% for physical examination alone to 98% with POCUS.[109] This improvement will save certain patients from unnecessary invasive procedures if cellulitis or an abscess smaller than 1 cm is seen, and reserve an incision and drainage for those who really need it.[110] In addition, abscesses may be deeper than previously anticipated, or may be communicating with deeper infective pockets that require surgical drainage,[111] allowing appropriate management decisions on evacuation need in austere environments.

- Pathology: Normal soft tissue will have well-delineated tissue planes (**Fig. 42**). Cellulitis is seen as anechoic layers of fluid within the soft tissue causing a characteristic "cobblestone" appearance, or in some cases you may only see a loss of well-demarcated tissue planes caused by tissue thickening and inflammation (**Figs. 43** and **44**). Abscesses are seen as anechoic or hypoechoic irregularly bordered structures, often with echogenic purulent material (**Fig. 45**). When the

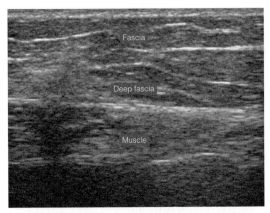

Fig. 42. Normal soft tissue with well-delineated tissue planes.

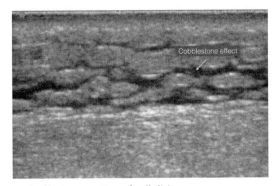

Fig. 43. "Cobblestone" effect suggestive of cellulitis.

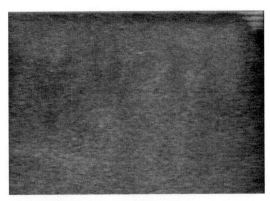

Fig. 44. Cellulitis with loss of well-delineated tissue planes.

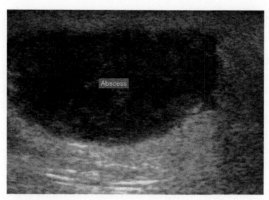

Fig. 45. Hypoechoic fluid-filled structure consistent with an abscess.

probe is directly over the abscess, and gentle pressure is applied, the purulent material will move within the abscess (Video 27). Take note of any adjacent structures, such as nerve bundles, vascular structures, muscle, or tendons, and their relative location to the abscess to assist in incision and drainage.

SUMMARY

Ultrasound systems must be handheld, battery operated, durable, and able to withstand extremes of temperature and altitude, and additional equipment may be necessary to help prevent battery degradation and equipment damage. POCUS is portable and lightweight, and can be used to screen for a wide variety of pathologies common to austere environments, disaster situations, and resource-limited settings. Common POCUS applications used in austere environments include the eFAST scan, musculoskeletal and soft tissue applications, an assessment for HAPE, high-altitude cerebral edema, pneumonia, volume status, and various procedural guidance applications. The various POCUS applications used in austere environments for procedural guidance include peripheral vascular access, nerve blocks for pain control, foreign body identification and removal, and abscess identification and drainage. POCUS is a reliable tool to assist in triage, resource allocation decisions, screening for conditions, and management of patients with pathology common in austere environments.

SUPPLEMENTARY DATA

Supplementary data related to this article can be found at http://dx.doi.org/10.1016/j.emc.2016.12.007.

REFERENCES

1. Newman PG, Rozycki GS. The history of ultrasound. Surg Clin North Am 1998; 78(2):179–95.
2. Nations JA, Browning RF. Battlefield applications for handheld ultrasound. Ultrasound Q 2011;27(3):171–6.
3. Hwang J, Quistgaard J, Souquet J, et al. Portable ultrasound device for battlefield trauma. Proc IEEE Ultrason Symp 1998;240:1663–7.
4. Brooks AJ, Price V, Simms M. FAST on operational military deployment. Emerg Med J 2005;22:263–5.

5. Nelson BP, Melnick ER, Li J. Portable ultrasound for remote environments, part I: feasibility of field deployment. J Emerg Med 2011;40(2):190–7.

6. Bellamy RF. The causes of death in conventional land warfare: implications for combat casualty care research. Mil Med 1984;149:55–62.

7. Berger E. Lessons from Afghanistan and Iraq: the costly benefits from the battle-field for emergency medicine. Ann Emerg Med 2007;49:486–8.

8. Stinger H, Rush R. The Army forward surgical team: update and lessons learned, 1997–2004. Mil Med 2006;171:269–72.

9. Mazur SM, Rippey J. Transport and use of point-of-care ultrasound by a disaster medical assistance team. Prehosp Disaster Med 2009;24:140–4.

10. Harke T, Statler J, Montilla J. Radiology in a hostile environment: experience in Afghanistan. Mil Med 2006;171:194–9.

11. Rozanski TA, Edmonson JM, Jones SB. Ultrasonography in a forward-deployed military hospital. Mil Med 2005;170:99–102.

12. Buckenmaier CC. Interview: 21st century battlefield pain management. Pain Manag 2013;3:269–75.

13. McNeil CR, McManus J, Mehta S. The accuracy of portable ultrasonography to diagnose fractures in an austere environment. Prehosp Emerg Care 2009;13: 50–2.

14. Heegaard W, Plummer D, Dries D, et al. Ultrasound for the air medical clinician. Air Med J 2004;23:20–3.

15. Price DD, Wilson SR, Murphy TG. Trauma ultrasound feasibility during helicopter transport. Air Med J 2000;19:144–6.

16. Melanson SW, McCarthy J, Stromski CJ, et al. Aeromedical trauma sonography by flight crews with a miniature ultrasound unit. Prehosp Emerg Care 2001;5: 399–402.

17. Polk JD, Fallon WF Jr, Kovach B, et al. The "Airmedical F.A.S.T." for trauma pa-tients—the initial report of a novel application for sonography. Aviat Space En-viron Med 2001;72:432–6.

18. Polk JD, Fallon WF Jr. The use of focused assessment with sonography for trauma (FAST) by a prehospital air medical team in the trauma arrest patient. Prehosp Emerg Care 2000;4:82–4.

19. Roline CE, Heegaard WG, Moore JC, et al. Feasibility of bedside thoracic ultra-sound in the helicopter emergency medical services setting. Air Med J 2013;32: 153–7.

20. Ketelaars R, Hoogerwerf N, Scheffer GJ. Prehospital chest ultrasound by a Dutch helicopter emergency medical service. J Emerg Med 2013;44:811–7.

21. Sarkisian AE, Khondkarian RA, Amirbekian NM, et al. Sonographic screening of mass casualties for abdominal and renal injuries following the 1988 Armenian earthquake. J Trauma 1991;31:247–50.

22. Dan D, Mingsong L, Jie T, et al. Ultrasonographic applications after mass casu-alty incident caused by Wenchuan earthquake. J Trauma 2010;68:1417–20.

23. Zhang S, Zhu D, Wan Z, et al. Utility of point-of-care ultrasound in acute man-agement triage of earthquake injury. Am J Emerg Med 2014;32:92–5.

24. Hu H, He Y, Zhang S, et al. Streamlined focused assessment with sonography for mass casualty prehospital triage of blunt torso trauma patients. Am J Emerg Med 2014;32:803–6.

25. Gregan J, Balasingam A, Butler A. Radiology in the Christchurch earthquake of 22 February 2011: Challenges, interim processes and clinical priorities. J Med Imaging Radiat Oncol 2016;60:172–81.

26. Keven K, Ates K, Yagmurlu B, et al. Renal Doppler ultrasonographic findings in earthquake victims with crush injury. J Ultrasound Med 2001;20:675–9.
27. Dean AJ, Ku BS, Zeserson EM. The utility of handheld ultrasound in an austere medical setting in Guatemala after a natural disaster. Am J Disaster Med 2007;2: 249–56.
28. Shorter M, Macias DJ. Portable handheld ultrasound in austere environments: use in the Haiti disaster. Prehosp Disaster Med 2012;27:172–7.
29. Turegano-Fuentes F, Caba-Doussoux P, Jover-Navalon JM, et al. Injury patterns from major urban terrorist bombings in trains: the Madrid experience. World J Surg 2008;32:1168–75.
30. Aylwin CJ, Konig TC, Brennan NW, et al. Reduction in critical mortality in urban mass casualty incidents: analysis of triage, surge, and resource use after the London bombings on July 7, 2005. Lancet 2006;368(9554):2219–25.
31. Beck-Razi N, Fischer D, Michaelson M, et al. The utility of focused assessment with sonography for trauma as a triage tool in multiple-casualty incidents during the second Lebanon war. J Ultrasound Med 2007;26:1149–56.
32. Kimberly HH, Stone MB. Clinician-performed ultrasonography during the Boston marathon mass casualty incident. Ann Emerg Med 2013;62:199–200.
33. Eikermann M, Velmahos G, Abbara S, et al. Case records of the Massachusetts general hospital. Case 11-2014. A man with traumatic injuries after a bomb explosion at the Boston Marathon. N Engl J Med 2014;370(15):1441–51.
34. Brunner J, Singh AK, Rocha T, et al. Terrorist bombings: foreign bodies from the Boston Marathon Bombing. Semin Ultrasound CT MR 2015;36:68–72.
35. Foale CM, Kaleri AY, Sargsyan AE, et al. Diagnostic instrumentation aboard ISS: just-in-time training for non-physician crewmembers. Aviat Space Environ Med 2005;76:594–8.
36. McBeth PB, Hamilton T, Kirkpatrick AW. Cost-effective remote iPhone tethered telementored trauma telesonography. J Trauma 2010;69:1597–9.
37. Crawford I, McBeth PB, Mitchelson M, et al. Telementorable "just-in-time" lung ultrasound on an iPhone. J Emerg Trauma Shock 2011;4(4):526–7.
38. McBeth PB, Crawford I, Blaivas M, et al. Simple, almost anywhere, with almost anyone: remote low-cost telementored resuscitative lung ultrasound. J Trauma 2011;71:1528–35.
39. Biegler N, McBeth PB, Tevez-Molina M, et al. Just-in-time cost-effective off-the-shelf remote telementoring of paramedical personnel in bedside lung sonography—a technical case study. Telemed J E Health 2012;18:807–9.
40. Fagenholz PJ, Murray AF, Noble VE, et al. Ultrasound for high altitude research. Ultrasound Med Biol 2012;38(1):1–12.
41. Wongwaisayawan S, Suwannanon R, Prachanukool T, et al. Trauma ultrasound. Ultrasound Med Biol 2015;41(10):2543–61.
42. American Institute of Ultrasound in Medicine, American College of Emergency Physicians. AIUM practice guideline for the performance of the focused assessment with sonography for trauma (FAST) examination. J Ultrasound Med 2014; 33(11):2047–56.
43. Blaivas M, Kuhn W, Reynolds B, et al. Change in differential diagnosis and patient management with the use of portable ultrasound in a remote setting. Wilderness Environ Med 2005;16(1):38–41.
44. Roberts J, Mcmanus J, Harrison B. Use of ultrasonography to avoid an unnecessary procedure in the prehospital combat environment: a case report. Prehosp Emerg Care 2006;10(4):502–6.

45. Miletić D, Fuckar Z, Mraović B, et al. Ultrasonography in the evaluation of hemo-peritoneum in war casualties. Mil Med 1999;164(8):600–2.

46. Shokoohi H, Boniface K, Taheri MR, et al. Spontaneous rectus sheath hematoma diagnosed by point-of-care ultrasonography. CJEM 2013;15(2):119–22.

47. Ryu JK, Jin W, Kim GY. Sonographic appearances of small organizing hema-tomas and thrombi mimicking superficial soft tissue tumors. J Ultrasound Med 2011;30(10):1431–6.

48. You JS, Chung YE, Kim D, et al. Role of sonography in the emergency room to diagnose sternal fractures. J Clin Ultrasound 2010;38(3):135–7.

49. Yousefifard M, Baikpour M, Ghelichkhani P, et al. Comparison of ultrasonogra-phy and radiography in detection of thoracic bone fractures; a systematic re-view and meta-analysis. Emerg (Tehran) 2016;4(2):55–64.

50. Medero colon R, Chilstrom ML. Diagnosis of an occult hip fracture by point-of-care ultrasound. J Emerg Med 2015;49(6):916–9.

51. Yıldırım A, Unlüer EE, Vandenberk N, et al. The role of bedside ultrasonography for occult scaphoid fractures in the emergency department. Ulus Travma Acil Cerrahi Derg 2013;19(3):241–5.

52. Vieira RL, Levy JA. Bedside ultrasonography to identify hip effusions in pediatric patients. Ann Emerg Med 2010;55(3):284–9.

53. Fathi M, Moezzi M, Abbasi S, et al. Ultrasound-guided hematoma block in distal radial fracture reduction: a randomised clinical trial. Emerg Med J 2015;32(6):474–7.

54. Akyol C, Gungor F, Akyol AJ, et al. Point-of-care ultrasonography for the man-agement of shoulder dislocation in ED. Am J Emerg Med 2016;34(5):866–70.

55. Zimny MH, Walters BL, Bahl A. Bedside ultrasound for hip dislocations. J Emerg Med 2012;43(6):1063–5.

56. Wu TS, Roque PJ, Green J, et al. Bedside ultrasound evaluation of tendon in-juries. Am J Emerg Med 2012;30(8):1617–21.

57. Berg K, Peck J, Boulger C, et al. Patellar tendon rupture: an ultrasound case report. BMJ Case Rep 2013;2013.

58. Phillips K, Costantino TG. Diagnosis of patellar tendon rupture by emergency ultrasound. J Emerg Med 2014;47(2):204–6.

59. Allemann Y, Sartori C, Lepori M, et al. Echocardiographic and invasive measure-ments of pulmonary artery pressure correlate closely at high altitude. Am J Physiol Heart Circ Physiol 2000;279(4):H2013–6.

60. Allemann Y, Hutter D, Lipp E, et al. Patent foramen ovale and high-altitude pul-monary edema. JAMA 2006;296(24):2954–8.

61. Hanaoka M, Kogashi K, Droma Y, et al. Myocardial performance index in sub-jects susceptible to high-altitude pulmonary edema. Intern Med 2011;50:2967–73.

62. Pagé M, Sauvé C, Serri K, et al. Echocardiographic assessment of cardiac per-formance in response to high altitude and development of subclinical pulmo-nary edema in healthy climbers. Can J Cardiol 2013;29(10):1277–84.

63. Fagenholz PJ, Gutman JA, Murray AF, et al. Chest ultrasonography for the diag-nosis and monitoring of high-altitude pulmonary edema. Chest 2007;131(4):1013–8.

64. Pratali L, Cavana M, Sicari R, et al. Frequent subclinical high-altitude pulmonary edema detected by chest sonography as ultrasound lung comets in recreational climbers. Crit Care Med 2010;38(9):1818–23.

65. Otto C, Hamilton DR, Levine BD, et al. Into thin air: extreme ultrasound on Mt Everest. Wilderness Environ Med 2009;20(3):283–9.

66. Frassi F, Gargani L, Tesorio P, et al. Prognostic value of extravascular lung water assessed with ultrasound lung comets by chest sonography in patients with dyspnea and/or chest pain. J Card Fail 2007;13(10):830–5.

67. Lichtenstein DA, Mezière GA. Relevance of lung ultrasound in the diagnosis of acute respiratory failure: the BLUE protocol. Chest 2008;134(1):117–25.

68. Volpicelli G, Elbarbary M, Blaivas M, et al. International evidence-based recommendations for point-of-care lung ultrasound. Intensive Care Med 2012;38(4): 577–91.

69. Fagenholz PJ, Gutman JA, Murray AF, et al. Optic nerve sheath diameter correlates with the presence and severity of acute mountain sickness: evidence for increased intracranial pressure. J Appl Physiol (1985) 2009;106(4):1207–11.

70. Sutherland AI, Morris DS, Owen CG, et al. Optic nerve sheath diameter, intracranial pressure and acute mountain sickness on Mount Everest: a longitudinal cohort study. Br J Sports Med 2008;42(3):183–8.

71. Ballantyne SA, O'Neill G, Hamilton R, et al. Observer variation in the sonographic measurement of optic nerve sheath diameter in normal adults. Eur J Ultrasound 2002;15(3):145–9.

72. Lochner P, Falla M, Brigo F, et al. Ultrasonography of the optic nerve sheath diameter for diagnosis and monitoring of acute mountain sickness: a systematic review. High Alt Med Biol 2015;16:195–203.

73. Kanaan NC, Lipman GS, Constance BB, et al. Optic nerve sheath diameter increase on ascent to high altitude: correlation with acute mountain sickness. J Ultrasound Med 2015;34(9):1677–82.

74. Lawley JS, Oliver SJ, Mullins P, et al. Optic nerve sheath diameter is not related to high altitude headache: a randomized controlled trial. High Alt Med Biol 2012; 13(3):193–9.

75. Rajajee V, Vanaman M, Fletcher JJ, et al. Optic nerve ultrasound for the detection of raised intracranial pressure. Neurocrit Care 2011;15(3):506–15.

76. Hylkema C. Optic nerve sheath diameter ultrasound and the diagnosis of increased intracranial pressure. Crit Care Nurs Clin North Am 2016;28(1):95–9.

77. Reissig A, Copetti R, Mathis G, et al. Lung ultrasound in the diagnosis and follow-up of community-acquired pneumonia: a prospective, multicenter, diagnostic accuracy study. Chest 2012;142(4):965–72.

78. Blaivas M. Lung ultrasound in evaluation of pneumonia. J Ultrasound Med 2012; 31(6):823–6.

79. Kurian J, Levin TL, Han BK, et al. Comparison of ultrasound and CT in the evaluation of pneumonia complicated by parapneumonic effusion in children. AJR Am J Roentgenol 2009;193(6):1648–54.

80. Rotte M, Fields JM, Torres S, et al. Use of ultrasound to diagnose and manage a five-liter empyema in a rural clinic in sierra Leone. Case Rep Emerg Med 2014; 2014:173810.

81. Chavez MA, Naithani N, Gilman RH, et al. Agreement between the World Health Organization algorithm and lung consolidation identified using point-of-care ultrasound for the diagnosis of childhood pneumonia by general practitioners. Lung 2015;193(4):531–8.

82. Heuvelings CC, Bélard S, Janssen S, et al. Chest ultrasonography in patients with HIV: a case series and review of the literature. Infection 2016;44(1):1–10.

83. Parlamento S, Copetti R, Di bartolomeo S. Evaluation of lung ultrasound for the diagnosis of pneumonia in the ED. Am J Emerg Med 2009;27(4):379–84.

84. Modi P, Glavis-bloom J, Nasrin S, et al. Accuracy of inferior vena cava ultrasound for predicting dehydration in children with acute diarrhea in resource-limited settings. PLoS One 2016;11(1):e0146859.

85. Levine AC, Shah SP, Umulisa I, et al. Ultrasound assessment of severe dehydration in children with diarrhea and vomiting. Acad Emerg Med 2010;17(10): 1035–41.

86. Pitman JT, Thapa GB, Harris NS. Field ultrasound evaluation of central volume status and acute mountain sickness. Wilderness Environ Med 2015;26(3): 319–26.

87. Guarracino F, Ferro B, Forfori F, et al. Jugular vein distensibility predicts fluid responsiveness in septic patients. Crit Care 2014;18(6):647.

88. Broilo F, Meregalli A, Friedman G. Right internal jugular vein distensibility appears to be a surrogate marker for inferior vena cava vein distensibility for evaluating fluid responsiveness. Rev Bras Ter Intensiva 2015;27(3):205–11.

89. Kent A, Patil P, Davila V, et al. Sonographic evaluation of intravascular volume status: can internal jugular or femoral vein collapsibility be used in the absence of IVC visualization? Ann Thorac Med 2015;10(1):44–9.

90. Çelebi yamanoğlu NG, Yamanoğlu A, Parlak İ, et al. The role of inferior vena cava diameter in volume status monitoring; the best sonographic measurement method? Am J Emerg Med 2015;33(3):433–8.

91. Feissel M, Michard F, Faller JP, et al. The respiratory variation in inferior vena cava diameter as a guide to fluid therapy. Intensive Care Med 2004;30(9): 1834–7.

92. Montalvo R, Wingard DL, Bracker M, et al. Morbidity and mortality in the wilderness. West J Med 1998;168(4):248–54.

93. Lippert SC, Nagdev A, Stone MD, et al. Pain control in disaster settings: a role for ultrasound-guided nerve blocks. Ann Emerg Med 2013;61(6):690–6.

94. Malchow RJ. Ultrasonography for advanced regional anesthesia and acute pain management in a combat environment. US Army Med Dep J 2009;64–6.

95. Sinatra R. Causes and consequences of inadequate management of acute pain. Pain Med 2009;10:957–8.

96. Di Gregorio G, Neal J, Rosenquist R, et al. Clinical presentation of local anesthetic systemic toxicity: a review of published cases, 1979 to 2009. Reg Anesth Pain Med 2010;35:181–7.

97. Costantino TG, Parikh AK, Satz WA, et al. Ultrasonography guided peripheral intravenous access versus traditional approaches in patients with difficult intravenous access. Ann Emerg Med 2005;46:456–61.

98. Sandhu NP, Sidhu DS. Mid-arm approach to basilic and cephalic vein cannulation using ultrasound guidance. Br J Anaesth 2004;93:292–4.

99. Blaivas M, Lyon M. The effect of ultrasound guidance on the perceived difficulty of emergency nurse-obtained peripheral IV access. J Emerg Med 2006;31: 407–10.

100. Panebianco NL, Fredette JM, Szyld D, et al. What you see (sonographically) is what you get: vein and patient characteristics associated with successful ultrasound-guided peripheral intravenous placement in patients with difficult access. Acad Emerg Med 2009;16(12):1298–303.

101. Stolz LA, Cappa AR, Minckler MR, et al. Prospective evaluation of the learning curve for ultrasound-guided peripheral intravenous catheter placement. J Vasc Access 2016;17(4):366–70.

102. Kagel EM, Rayan GM. Intravenous catheter complications in the hand and forearm. J Trauma 2004;56(1):123–7.

103. Shrestha D, Sharma UK, Mohammad R, et al. The role of ultrasonography in detection and localization of radiolucent foreign body in soft tissues of extremities. JNMA J Nepal Med Assoc 2009;48(173):5–9.

104. Graham DD Jr. Ultrasound in the emergency department: detection of wooden foreign bodies in the soft tissues. J Emerg Med 2002;22(1):75–9.

105. Horton LK, Jacobson JA, Powell A, et al. Sonography and radiography of soft-tissue foreign bodies. AJR Am J Roentgenol 2001;176(5):1155–9.

106. Soudack M, Nachtigal A, Gaitini D. Clinically unsuspected foreign bodies: the importance of sonography. J Ultrasound Med 2003;22(12):1381–5.

107. Paziana K, Fields JM, Rotte M, et al. Soft tissue foreign body removal technique using portable ultrasonography. Wilderness Environ Med 2012;23(4):343–8.

108. Blaivas M, Lyon M, Brannam L, et al. Water bath evaluation technique for emergency ultrasound of painful superficial structures. Am J Emerg Med 2004;22(7): 589–93.

109. Squire BT, Fox JC, Anderson C. ABSCESS: applied bedside sonography for convenient evaluation of superficial soft tissue infections. Acad Emerg Med 2005;12(7):601–6.

110. Adhikari S, Blaivas M. Sonography first for subcutaneous abscess and cellulitis evaluation. J Ultrasound Med 2012;31(10):1509–12.

111. Tayal VS, Hasan N, Norton HJ, et al. The effect of soft-tissue ultrasound on the management of cellulitis in the emergency department. Acad Emerg Med 2006; 13(4):384–8.

Is There a Doctor Onboard? Medical Emergencies at 40,000 Feet

Howard J. Donner, MD, CFI (Certified Flight Instructor)[a,b,*]

KEYWORDS

• Wilderness medicine • In-flight medical emergencies • Flight attendants • FAA

INTRODUCTION

It is estimated 2.75 billion people travel aboard commercial airlines every year and 44,000 in-flight medical emergencies occur worldwide each year.[1] Wilderness medicine requires a commonsense and improvisational approach to medical issues. A sudden call for assistance in the austere and unfamiliar surroundings of an airliner cabin may present the responding medical professional with a "wilderness medicine" experience. From resource management to equipment, this article sheds light on the unique conditions, challenges, and constraints of the flight environment.

THE FLIGHT ENVIRONMENT

Modern commercial aircraft fly at the interface between the troposphere and stratosphere, roughly equivalent to a cruising altitude of 32,000 to 45,000 feet. Above the troposphere, planes fly more smoothly and experience less turbulence and inclement weather. The height of the troposphere varies with altitude and season. Passengers are protected from high-altitude atmospheric conditions by a pressurized cabin environment that potentially creates its own medical ramifications.

CABIN ALTITUDE

The ambient atmospheric pressure at cruising altitude (30,000–40,000 feet) is about 200 to 300 hPa (roughly 0.2–0.3 atm). To allow passengers to survive and operate in this environment, the cabin must be pressurized. Despite pressurization, the internal cabin altitude is generally not maintained at sea level pressure because the aircraft structure required to maintain a sea level pressure would make the plane unacceptably heavy and expensive to build and operate. Thus, a compromise is made that is the most efficient for weight/strength/expense, while preventing passengers from

[a] National Wilderness Medicine Conferences, 3790 El Camino Real, Suite 2029, Palo Alto, CA 94306, USA; [b] Medical Operations, NASA Johnson Space Center, 2101 NASA Road 1 (SD3), Houston, TX 77058, USA
* 14375 Denton Avenue, Truckee, CA 96161, USA
E-mail address: hdonner24@gmail.com

Emerg Med Clin N Am 35 (2017) 443–463
http://dx.doi.org/10.1016/j.emc.2017.01.005
0733-8627/17/© 2017 Elsevier Inc. All rights reserved.

becoming hypoxic. The aircraft cabin is typically pressurized between 6000 and 8000 feet above sea level. Newer aircraft, such as the Airbus A380 and Boeing 787 Dreamliner, can pressurize the cabin to lower altitudes, equal to about 6000 feet, even in the upper flight levels. In the United States, Federal Aviation Administration (FAA) requirements allow a maximum cabin altitude of 8000 feet.

Many people with heart and lung disease travel by commercial aircraft, and are unaware of the risk that is incurred. The fractional oxygen content of the air in the cabin is the same as that at sea level, approximately 21%. What changes with increasing cabin altitude is the atmospheric pressure. At a typical cruising altitude, the atmospheric pressure in the cabin is decreased by about 25% to 30% and results in a similar decrease in the partial pressure of inspired oxygen. The lower partial pressure of oxygen in the aircraft cabin results in slight hypoxemia, with a corresponding decrease in oxygen saturation and a mild compensatory hyperventilation and tachycardia. Medical personnel responding to onboard medical events should not be surprised by decreases in arterial oxygen saturation in the range of 3% to 5%, even in healthy individuals.

PRESSURE AND DYSBARISM

Boyle's law states that in a perfect gas where mass and temperature are kept constant, the volume of the gas varies inversely with the absolute pressure.

$$(P \times V = P' \times V')$$

Reduction in aircraft cabin pressure can lead to volume expansion of closed gas-containing compartments in the human body.

Middle Ear

Expanding volumes of air in the paranasal and frontal sinuses may produce symptoms, but the most common manifestation of dysbarism associated with the flight environment is barotitis media resulting in ear pain. Barotitis media is commonly related to eustachian tube congestion secondary to upper respiratory infections, middle ear infections, chronic effusions, or allergies. Mild barotrauma may occur as either pressure increase caused by expansion of gases as the aircraft ascends, or by decreased pressure in the middle ear as the aircraft descends. Although mild discomfort is the typical presentation, in rare cases, the changes in pressure can produce rupture of the tympanic membrane.

The most simple and commonly used method to open the eustachian tube is to swallow. Chewing gum or sucking on hard candy may facilitate this process. Infants should be given a bottle or pacifier to suck on to facilitate swallowing, especially during descent.

Older children and adults may benefit from performing a Valsalva maneuver. This is achieved by pinching the nostrils and attempting exhalation through the nose. This maneuver is familiar to most scuba divers, because the same technique is used for equalizing ears during descent. Another useful technique is to have the patient swallow while pinching the nostrils closed. Other pressure equalization techniques[2] include the following:

- Voluntary tubal opening: Attempt to yawn or wiggle the jaw
- Valsalva maneuver: Pinch your nostrils, and gently blow through your nose
- Toynbee maneuver: Pinch your nostrils and swallow (good technique if equalization is needed during ascent)
- Frenzel maneuver: Pinch your nostrils while contracting your throat muscles, and make the sound of the letter "k"

- Lowry technique: Pinch your nostrils, and gently try to blow air out of your nose while swallowing
- Edmonds technique: Push your jaw forward, and use the Valsalva maneuver or the Frenzel maneuver

Dental

Cabin pressure changes may cause toothaches in patients with pre-existing dental disease, such as a dental abscess (barodontalgia).

Abdomen

Occasionally, intraluminal gas expansion caused by decreased cabin pressure may cause abdominal discomfort. The surgical literature contains references regarding complications during flight subsequent to recent abdominal surgery.[3,4] Travelers should be advised to check with their surgeon. The British Civil Aviation Authority publishes the following recommendations.[5]

- Travel should be avoided for 10 days following abdominal surgery.
- Following procedures, such as colonoscopy, where a large amount of gas has been introduced into the colon, it is advisable to avoid travel by air for 24 hours.
- It is advisable to avoid flying for approximately 24 hours after laparoscopic intervention, because of the residual CO_2 gas, which may be in the intra-abdominal cavity.
- Neurosurgical intervention may leave gas trapped within the skull, which may expand at altitude. It is therefore advisable to avoid air travel for approximately 7 days following this type of procedure.
- Ophthalmologic procedures for retinal detachment involve the introduction of gas by intraocular injections, which temporarily increase intraocular pressure. Depending on the gas, it may be necessary to delay travel for approximately 2 weeks if sulfur hexafluoride is used and 6 weeks pursuant to the use of perfluoropropane. For other intraocular procedures and penetrating eye injuries, 1 week should elapse before flying.

Gas Expansion and Medical Devices

Various medical devices that trap fixed quantities of expandable air must be considered when transporting patients aboard aircraft. Expanding trapped gas within these devices has been known to cause barotrauma during rapid ascent in unpressurized and pressurized aircraft. A partial list of these devices includes pneumatic splints (air splints), feeding tubes, urinary catheters, cuffed endotracheal tubes, and cuffed tracheostomy tubes.

If not contraindicated, the effects of gas expansion can be eliminated by installation of water rather than air during flight. These devices require careful monitoring; partial deflation should be considered if overexpansion is suspected. Feeding and infusion tubes should be capped off.

Pneumothorax

Travelers with pre-existing pulmonary disease are at risk for flight-related pneumothorax. A patient with a small, asymptomatic pneumothorax can develop a more significant pneumothorax as air expands within the pleural space during ascent. Risk of pneumothorax during air travel is increased in patients with cystic lung disease, recent pneumothorax, thoracic surgery, and chronic pneumothorax.[6]

FLYING AFTER SCUBA DIVING
Guidelines for Postdive Air Travel

The Divers Alert Network and the Undersea Hyperbaric Medical Society convened a workshop in 2002 to review the available data regarding postdive air travel. The published guidelines (**Table 1**) do not guarantee that one will avoid decompression sickness. Allowing even longer surface intervals than the recommended minimums further reduces the risk of decompression sickness.

There are additional considerations regarding the Divers Alert Network/Undersea Hyperbaric Medical Society flying after diving guidelines.[7] It is prudent to wait longer than the suggested minimum interval. Recent studies show that flying in a commercial aircraft, even after a 24-hour surface interval, can produce bubbles in a diver's blood; therefore, Divers Alert Network advises that one exercise caution by maintaining more conservative dive profiles during the final day of diving and plan for a 24-hour surface interval before flight. Any postdive ascent to a higher altitude—even using ground transportation—increases decompression stress, so one should follow the same guidelines if heading by car, bus, or foot from a dive site to the mountains.

CABIN AIR

Despite the pervasive antipathy expressed by airline passengers, there is little clinical evidence to suggest that cabin air quality on modern jets is potentially harmful. Many airline passengers have anecdotes about getting sick following a long duration flight. The risk of contracting an infection during a commercial flight arises from the close proximity to potentially germ-laden fellow passengers, and not from the quality of aircraft cabin air. A crowded airplane poses no greater risk than other enclosed spaces.

A portion of the cabin air (no more than 40%–50%) is recirculated and passes through high-efficiency particulate air filters. According to Boeing, between 94% and 99.9% of all airborne microbes are filtered during this process. The other source of cabin air is "bleed air" that is obtained when outside air is compressed by the aircraft's engines. The incoming bleed air is plumbed into air conditioning units for cooling. This mix of recirculated cabin air and outside bleed air makes it possible to efficiently regulate temperature and humidity.

Newer aircraft use high-efficiency particulate filters to remove gaseous contaminants, including some volatile organic compounds that may act as mild respiratory irritants.

Fume Events

In the event of an oil leak, bleed air may be exposed to gasses that could potentially expose passengers to neurotoxins. Such events are rare, but have reportedly

Table 1	
Divers Alert Network guidelines for flying after diving	
Dive Profile	**Minimum Preflight Surface Interval Suggestion**
Single no-decompression dive	12 h or more
Multiple dives in a day	18 h or more
Multiple days of diving	18 h or more
Dives requiring decompression stops	Substantially longer than 18 h

From Flying after scuba diving: how long should I wait? Divers Alert Network; 2016; and *Data from* DAN Medical Frequently Asked Questions. Available at: http://www.diversalertnetwork.org/medical/faq/Flying_After_Diving.

triggered neurologic symptoms, such as headaches and dizziness in crewmembers and passengers. Jet engine oils contain synthetic hydrocarbons and other additives, including the organophosphate tricresyl phosphate, which acts as a high-pressure lubricant. Most studies indicate that total tricresyl phosphate concentrations occurring during so-called fume events remain below threshold limits for causing neurologic symptomatology.[8] The concentration of organophosphates that aircraft crewmembers and passengers could be exposed to is insufficient to produce neurotoxicity.[9] A recent guide for health care providers concluded that "there are currently no tests of sufficient sensitivity and specificity to assess exposure/health effects outcomes."[10]

The newest Boeing airliner, the 787 Dreamliner, uses a no-bleed systems architecture that replaces the conventional pneumatic bleed air system with a high-power electrical compressor system that avoids any mixing of engine-based bleed air with internal cabin air.

Infectious Disease and Air Travel

Although modern airliners provide clean cabin air, air travelers are still subjected to long periods in enclosed spaces, which facilitates the spread of infectious disease. Multiple outbreaks of serious infectious diseases have been reported aboard commercial airlines including influenza, food poisoning, measles, tuberculosis, viral enteritis, severe acute respiratory syndrome, and smallpox.

The risk of cross-infection from airborne pathogens in aircraft cabins seems to be related to the duration of the flight (with 8 or more hours producing an increased risk), and proximity of the index passenger (seating within two rows associated with an increased risk).[11,12]

If a contagious disease is suspected, ask the ill passenger to use a facemask. A mask should be available in the medical kit and/or the first aid kit. Use of a facemask by the ill passenger is recommended by the World Health Organization.[13] Attempt to isolate the patient and relocate neighboring passengers. Discuss quarantining the passenger with the flight crew and any reporting requirements.

Low Humidity of Cabin Air

Airliner cabins are dry. Typical humidity levels in most airliners are about 2%. Airplane designers are happy to minimize moisture to help inhibit structural corrosion. Maintaining optimal cabin humidity (40%–70%) is prohibitive because of the increased cost and weight of equipment. The newer Boeing 787 does not use engine bleed air to pressurize the cabin. The 787 cabin contains 6% to 7% humidity, which according to studies done by Boeing improves the passenger experience. Low cabin humidity levels can lead to dehydration, so passengers are encouraged to increase water intake. Dry eyes can be especially problematic for travelers with pre-existing conditions and for soft contact lens wearers. Carrying "artificial tears" or contact rewetting drops is of benefit. Dry inflamed upper respiratory mucosa can produce cough and exacerbate reactive airway disease.

COSMIC-RADIATION EXPOSURE

Cosmic radiation originates from powerful events, such as star collisions, gamma ray bursts, black holes, and supernovae. Particles released by solar flares are another source. The earth's magnetic field and atmosphere shield the planet from 99.9% of cosmic radiation; however, for travelers outside the protection of Earth's magnetic field, space radiation becomes a more potential hazard. Exposure levels also rise when we travel by plane, especially at higher altitudes and latitudes.

In 1991, the International Commission on Radiological Protection declared cosmic radiation an occupational risk for flight crews. Since that time, exposure monitoring and maximum dose guidelines have been developed. Current recommendations are to limit annual crew exposure to 20 mSv/y averaged over 5 years (total of 100 mSv in 5 years).[14,15] Even frequent flyers and aircrews typically remain well below this limit.

Concerns increase when considering the developing fetus during pregnancy.[16] The National Council on Radiation Protection and Measurements recommends a monthly limit of 0.5 mSv, whereas the International Commission on Radiological Protection recommends a radiation limit of 1 mSv during the entire pregnancy. These recommendations would place limits on pregnant crewmembers and frequent air travelers, because flying roughly 15 long-haul round trips would expose a fetus to more than 1 mSv. To avoid risk to the fetus, the FAA recommends pregnant crewmembers take shorter, low-altitude, low-latitude flights.

The Centers for Disease Control and Prevention[17] recommends that if you are pregnant and aware of an ongoing solar particle event, that you reschedule your flight. A National Institute for Occupational Safety and Health (NIOSH) study found that flight attendants exposed to 0.36 mSv or more of cosmic radiation in the first trimester may have a higher risk of miscarriage. Although flying through a solar particle event is rare, a NIOSH and National Aeronautics and Space Administration study found that a pregnant flight attendant who flies through a solar particle event can receive more radiation than is recommended during pregnancy by national and international agencies.

How to Reduce Exposure

Ultimately the amount of cosmic radiation exposure received while flying depends on the amount of time in the air, altitude, latitude, and solar activity. Lowest dose rates at a given altitude are found close to the equator and intensify with increasing latitude. For any location at commercial flight altitudes, a higher altitude incurs a higher dose rate. Reducing aircraft altitude can significantly reduce radiation exposure during a solar radiation event in high-latitude areas.[18] With regard to solar particle events, the Centers for Disease Control and Prevention[17] states

- NIOSH has estimated that pilots fly through about six solar particle events in an average 28-year career.
- Avoiding exposure to solar particle events is difficult because they often happen with little warning. One can find out whether a solar particle event is currently active through these sources:
  - The National Aeronautics and Space Administration Nowcast of Atmospheric Ionizing Radiation System is being developed to report potentially harmful flight radiation levels to flight crews and passengers.
  - National Aeronautics and Space Administration Nowcast of Atmospheric Ionizing Radiation System: current radiation dose rate forecast.
  - A space weather app for the iPhone offers current information on solar activity (developed by Stellar North LLC).
  - The National Oceanic and Atmospheric Administration Space Weather Prediction Center's Aviation Community Dashboard includes a forecast for solar particle events.
  - A useful tool to estimate an individual's exposure to cosmic radiation from a specific flight is available from the FAA on its Web site (http://jag.cami.jccbi.gov/cariprofile.asp).

EMOTIONAL AND PHYSICAL STRESS DURING AIR TRAVEL

Travelers are often subject to conditions that increase anxiety and overall dysphoria during air travel, including the following:

- Time pressures of travel
- Airport congestion
- Rushing to make connecting flights
- Stress and anxiety associated with business travel
- Stress and anxiety associated with family-related events, such as reunions, weddings, and funerals
- Psychosocial disruptions in circadian rhythms (discussed next)
- Emotional effects of lack of sleep and dehydration
- Stress and anxiety associated with missed and canceled flights
- Unexpected layovers

JET LAG
Circadian Rhythm Sleep Disorder (Jet Lag)

Jet lag is a sleep disorder occurring in travelers who transit across three or more time zones. Jet lag occurs when the internal circadian rhythm "clock" adjusts slowly to the destination time. This disruption causes circadian rhythms to become out of synchronization with the destination time zone.

The pineal gland is highly involved with regulating the sleep-wake cycle by secreting melatonin. The synthesis and release of melatonin is stimulated by darkness and suppressed by light.[19]

Symptoms

Symptoms may include poor sleep, including sleep-onset insomnia, fractionated sleep, and early awakening; fatigue; mood changes; headache; irritability; poor concentration; depression; and mild anorexia.

Clinical Considerations

Although there is substantial individual variability in the severity of jet lag symptoms, the direction of travel and the number of time zones crossed are important factors to consider.[19,20] Specifically, westward travel generally causes less disruption than eastward travel.[21]

- Eastward travel is associated with difficulty falling asleep at the destination bedtime and difficulty arising in the morning.
- Westward travel is associated with early evening sleepiness and predawn awakening at the travel destination.
- Travelers flying within the same time zone typically experience the fewest problems, such as nonspecific travel fatigue.
- Crossing more time zones or traveling eastward generally increases the time required for adaptation.
- After eastward flights, jet lag lasts for the number of days roughly equal to two-thirds the number of time zones crossed; after westward flights, the number of days is roughly half the number of time zones.
- The intensity and duration of jet lag are related to the number of time zones crossed, the direction of travel, the ability to sleep while traveling, the availability and intensity of local circadian time cues at the destination, and individual differences in phase tolerance.

Prevention

Travelers can minimize jet lag by doing the following before travel[19]:

- Shift the timing of sleep to 1 to 2 hours later for a few days before traveling westward
- Shift the timing of sleep to 1 to 2 hours earlier for a few days before traveling eastward
- Shift mealtimes to hours that coincide with the previous changes
- Seek exposure to bright light in the evening if traveling westward, in the morning if traveling eastward
- Mobile apps, such as Jet Lag Rooster and Entrain, are available to help travelers calculate and adhere to a light/dark schedule
- Web sites, such as Jet Lag Advisor (http://www.britishairways.com/travel/drsleep/public/en_gb), offer similar services online; travelers answer a few simple questions regarding planned flights and advice is then calculated to minimize jet lag

Pharmacologic Treatment

The use of the nutritional supplement melatonin is controversial for preventing jet lag.[19] Some clinicians advocate the use of 0.5 to 5.0 mg of melatonin during the first few days of travel, and data suggest its efficacy.[22] The production of melatonin is not regulated by the Food and Drug Administration and commercially available products have demonstrated impurities. Additionally, current data also do not support the use of special diets to ameliorate jet lag. If used, timed treatment with melatonin in the early morning of the departure time zone (westward) or the very early evening of the departure time zone (eastward) preflight and postflight may improve initiation and maintenance of the desired phase shift.[23]

Newer melatonin receptor agonists, such as ramelteon, have recently been approved for the treatment of insomnia, but have not been well studied for use in jet lag.

The 2008 American Academy of Sleep Medicine[24] recommendations include the following:

- Promote sleep with hypnotic medication, although the effects of hypnotics on daytime symptoms of jet lag have not been well studied.
- Nonaddictive sedative hypnotics (nonbenzodiazepines), such as zolpidem, have been shown in some studies to promote longer periods of high-quality sleep. If a benzodiazepine is preferred, a short-acting one, such as temazepam, is recommended to minimize oversedation the following day. Because alcohol intake is often high during international travel, the risk of interaction with hypnotics should be emphasized with patients.
- If necessary, promote daytime alertness with a stimulant, such as caffeine in limited quantities. Avoid caffeine after midday.[25]
- Take short naps (20–30 minutes), shower, and spend time in the afternoon sun.

HEALTH ISSUES ASSOCIATED WITH COMMERCIAL AIR TRAVEL

Airlines are not required to report emergencies unless they require actual diversion of the flight. A recent article provides an extensive review of in-flight emergencies.[1] This article reviewed records of in-flight medical emergency calls from five domestic and international airlines to a physician-directed medical communication center from January 1, 2008, through October 31, 2010. During the study period there were approximately 744 million airline passengers who traveled on commercial airline flights. The communications center received 11,920 in-flight medical emergency calls (a rate of 16 medical emergencies per 1 million passengers). The incidence of in-flight medical emergencies was one in-flight medical emergency per 604 flights. The most common medical problems were syncope or presyncope (37.4%), respiratory symptoms (12.1%), and nausea or vomiting (9.5%).

Aircraft diversion occurred in 7.3% of cases, whereas 1.2% of patients resolved sufficiently before landing to negate the need for emergency medical service (EMS) services on landing. Only 37.3% of patients evaluated by EMS personnel after landing were transported to a hospital emergency department.

Medical problems that were associated with the highest rates of hospital admission were stroke-like symptoms (23.5%), obstetric or gynecologic symptoms (23.4%), and cardiac symptoms (21%). Although most of the medications that were used are available in the FAA emergency medical kit (EMK) (discussed later), some medications came from other passengers or the patient themselves. The most commonly used medications were oxygen (49.9%), intravenous (IV) normal saline (5.2%), and aspirin (5%).

Automated External Defibrillators

An automated external defibrillator (AED) was used on 137 patients (1.3%). An AED was applied in 24 cases of cardiac arrest but shock delivered in only five cases. The return of spontaneous circulation occurred in one patient receiving defibrillation. For eight other patients, an AED was used but no shock was indicated.

Death Rate

The death rate among all patients with in-flight medical emergencies was 0.3%. **Table 2** shows medical emergencies according to medical problem and outcome.

Ground-Based Consultation

For medical professionals responding to an in-flight emergency, their unfamiliarity with the flight environment can be anxiety provoking. Many physicians believe that they are inadequately trained or naive to operational aspects of the flight, such as indications for diversion, protocols, and equipment.

Health care providers should know that when they respond to an in-flight emergency, they are essentially never operating alone. There are multiple networks of ground-based consultants working closely with all domestic airlines in the United States and most foreign carriers.

The responsibility of deciding whether the plane needs to be rerouted is ultimately a decision made by the pilot. As a medical professional, your primary obligation is to offer your best medical opinion about the patient's condition and prognosis, including the degree of urgency.

In most cases, the pilot will probably have already contacted their own ground-based consultants before the flight attendant's call for assistance. You will be acting as the eyes and ears for the specialist on the ground that has familiarity with the environment and deals with these problems on a regular basis. The ground-based consultants can offer important information on resources, such as, medical kit contents, diagnostic capabilities, and airline operations.

Although the FAA does not officially require consultation with a ground-based consultant in the case of in-flight emergencies, all domestic airlines collaborate with specific agencies specializing in aeromedical emergency medical care. Most airline flight crews are advised to use these consultants for all in-flight medical emergencies. Additionally, most airlines require a consultation with the ground-based physician

Table 2
In-flight medical emergencies and outcome

Category	All Emergencies	Aircraft Diversion	Transport to a Hospital[a] n/N (%)	Hospital Admission[b]	Death, n
All categories	11,920/11,920 (100)	875/11,920 (7.3)	2804/10,877 (25.8)	901/10,482 (8.6)	36
Syncope or presyncope	4463/11,920 (37.4)	221/4463 (5.0)	938/4252 (22.1)	267/4123 (6.5)	4
Respiratory symptoms	1447/11,920 (12.1)	81/1447 (5.6)	311/1371 (22.7)	141/1336 (10.6)	1
Nausea or vomiting	1137/11,920 (9.5)	56/1137 (4.9)	243/1025 (23.7)	61/994 (6.1)	0
Cardiac symptoms	920/11,920 (7.7)	169/920 (18.4)	370/813 (45.5)	162/770 (21.0)	0
Seizures	689/11,920 (5.8)	83/689 (12.0)	224/626 (35.8)	75/602 (12.5)	0
Abdominal pain	488/11,920 (4.1)	50/488 (10.2)	164/412 (39.8)	41/391 (10.5)	0
Infectious disease	330/11,920 (2.8)	6/330 (1.8)	45/239 (18.8)	8/232 (3.4)	0
Agitation or psychiatric symptoms	287/11,920 (2.4)	16/287 (5.6)	38/249 (15.3)	17/244 (7.0)	0
Allergic reaction	265/11,920 (2.2)	12/265 (4.5)	40/233 (17.2)	8/229 (3.5)	0
Possible stroke	238/11,920 (2.0)	39/238 (16.4)	92/214 (43.0)	46/196 (23.5)	0
Trauma, not otherwise specified	216/11,920 (1.8)	14/216 (6.5)	34/185 (18.4)	5/180 (2.8)	0
Diabetic complication	193/11,920 (1.6)	15/193 (7.8)	45/181 (24.9)	13/172 (7.6)	0
Headache	123/11,920 (1.0)	10/123 (8.1)	23/108 (21.3)	4/107 (3.7)	0
Arm or leg pain or injury	114/11,920 (1.0)	6/114 (5.3)	27/100 (27.0)	4/98 (4.1)	0
Obstetric or gynecologic symptoms	61/11,920 (0.5)	11/61 (18.0)	29/53 (54.7)	11/47 (23.4)	0
Ear pain	49/11,920 (0.4)	1/49 (2.0)	2/43 (4.7)	1/43 (2.3)	0
Cardiac arrest	38/11,920 (0.3)	22/38 (57.9)	14/34 (41.2)	1/6 (16.7)	31
Laceration	33/11,920 (0.3)	1/33 (3.0)	3/26 (11.5)	0/25	0
Other	821/11,920 (6.9)	62/821 (7.6)	162/705 (23.0)	36/679 (5.3)	0
Unknown	8/11,920 (0.1)	0/8	0/8	0/8	0

[a] Postflight follow-up data on transport to a hospital by emergency medical service personnel were available for 10,877 of the 11,920 passengers with in-flight medical emergencies (91.2%).

[b] Postflight follow-up data on hospital admissions were available for 10,482 of the 11,920 passengers with in-flight medical emergencies (87.9%). Admitted patients were defined as those transported to the hospital who were admitted from the emergency department or who left the emergency department against medical advice, excluding patients who died.

From Peterson DC, Martin-Gill C, Guyette FX, et al. Outcomes of medical emergencies on commercial airline flights. N Engl J Med 2013;368(22):2077; with permission.

before the EMK is used. It should be noted that all communications with medical ground consultants are recorded.

Cockpit Coordination

Typically, the pilot in command or captain takes over the cockpit management of the medical emergency. This requires that the copilot or "First Officer" take over the responsibility of flying the aircraft. The pilot not flying would then notify air traffic controllers about the medical emergency. In the United States a pilot essentially always makes the decision to divert in consultation with a ground-based consultant.

Diversion

Diverting to a closer airport creates several logistical problems for the flight crew, including

- Medical capabilities and resources within close proximity to the landing airport
- Weather conditions
- Availability of instrument approaches in nonvisual flight conditions
- Runway size
- Availability of additional flight and cabin crew, if necessary, after landing to continue the flight
- Maintenance facilities and handling capabilities at the landing airport
- Availability of jet fuel
- Major inconvenience to the remaining passengers

When diversion is necessary during the early phase of a flight, the aircraft may still exceed maximum landing weight because of the additional fuel carried. Pilots can either land overweight, fly in circles or other holding patterns to burn off excess fuel, or dump fuel. Many modern aircraft have the capability to vent fuel overboard in the case of a grossly overweight landing situation.

According to Ruskin and colleagues[26] and Grendreau and DeJohn,[27] diversion should be recommended for the following:

- Unremitting chest pain
- Shortness of breath
- Severe abdominal pain
- Stroke
- Persistent unresponsiveness
- Refractory seizures
- Severe agitation

MEDICAL-LEGAL CONSIDERATIONS

In 1998 the US Congress enacted a federal statute to limit the liability of medically qualified individuals responding to medical emergencies aboard commercial airliners registered in the United States. The motivation of the Aviation Medical Assistance Act (AMAA) was to reduce concerns over the legal ramifications of assisting in an in-flight emergency should the outcome generate litigation. The AMAA, in its Section on Limitations on Liability, states[28]:

An individual shall not be held liable for damages in any action brought in a Federal or State court arising out of the acts or omissions of the individual in providing or attempting to provide assistance in the case of an in-flight medical emergency unless the individual, while rendering such assistance, is guilty of gross negligence or willful misconduct.

Gross negligence or willful misconduct constitute more than simple errors. This term indicates that a physician has departed substantially from minimally accepted medical care or has shown egregious behavior while providing care. An example of such flagrant disregard for the patient's health and safety is an intoxicated physician treating a patient.[29]

The immunities of the AMAA are not dependent on the care being provided without compensation; however, airlines recently have been sympathetic to the notion that compensation muddies the waters in regard to "Good Samaritan" law.

What if a health care provider is administering care on an international airline not registered in the United States? The inherent rule is that the laws of the country in which the carrier is based apply.[30] Other experts have argued that the laws of the country in (or over) which the incident occurs or where the parties are citizens could apply.[27] Some countries, such as Australia and countries in the European Union, impose a legal duty on the physician to respond. The United States, Canada, and the United Kingdom do not stipulate this requirement to act.[31]

The AMAA also extends immunity from liability to air carriers registered in the United States with regard to damages arising from assistance provided during an in-flight medical emergency. The AMAA, in its Section on Liability of Air Carriers, states[28]:

An air carrier shall not be liable for damages in any action brought in a Federal or State court arising out of the performance of the air carrier in obtaining or attempting to obtain the assistance of a passenger in an in-flight medical emergency, or out of the acts or omissions of the passenger rendering the assistance, if the carrier in good faith believes that the passenger is a medically qualified individual and not an employee or agent of the carrier.

Volunteers must be "medically qualified" and receive no monetary compensation to receive protection.[32] Airline employees meet the "in good faith" requirement by asking whether the person who volunteers to help is a health care provider (see the article on medical-legal issues in expedition and wilderness medicine elsewhere in this issue for more legal considerations).[30]

If a patient requires ongoing monitoring and therapy, the volunteer may need to stay by their side for the duration of the flight. Many airlines carry a "standard airline medical incident form." If this is available, use it for appropriate documentation. If there are no forms available, improvise using any means of documentation (**Table 3**).[33] When completed, request a copy, or photograph it with your smart phone for future

Table 3 Sample basic inflight report
Date
Airline
Flight #
History
Past medical history
Examination
Treatment
Disposition

reference. If the patient remains unstable, be prepared to continue offering assistance throughout the remainder of the flight. After landing, it is acceptable to hand over care to ground-based medical personnel for transfer to definitive care.

Emergency Medical Kits

FAA regulations regarding EMKs (**Fig. 1**) are as follows (see **Table 4** for the approved EMK[34] contents):

- The FAA has required EMKs and AEDs on all commercial airplanes with a maximum payload capacity of more than 7500 pounds and with at least one flight attendant since 1986.[34]
- The EMK is designed based on recommendations from the Aerospace Medical Association's Air Transport Medicine Committee.
- The medications that must be carried in all EMKs have an expiration date of approximately 1 year. The FAA advises that the best practice is to replace all of the medications annually.
- In 1994, examination gloves were added to the medical kits.
- In 2004, an updated kit, the enhanced EMK, was added to the requirement. The enhanced EMK added oral antihistamines, nonnarcotic analgesics, a bronchodilator, aspirin, injectable atropine, additional epinephrine, IV lidocaine, IV saline, and a bag valve mask. An AED was also required.
- FAA regulations state that a flight may not depart if it is missing the EMK or AED. By regulation, flight attendants may only use the equipment and medications under the direction of a licensed medical provider. For minor medical issues, flight attendants may use a simple "first aid" kit that is stowed separately without consulting a medical professional. The contents of an aircraft first-aid kit typically include[13]
  - Antiseptic swabs (10/packs)
  - Bandage adhesive strips
  - Bandage, gauze 7.5 cm × 4.5 cm

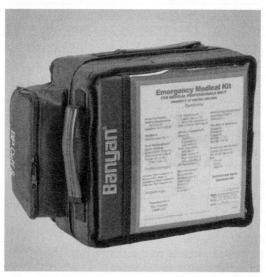

Fig. 1. United Airlines aviation emergency medical kit. (*Courtesy of* Healthfirst, Mountlake Terrace, WA and used with permission, Banyan Medical Systems, Inc.)

Table 4
Emergency medical kit required items

Contents	Quantity
Sphygmomanometer	1
Stethoscope	1
Airways, oropharyngeal (3 sizes): 1 pediatric, 1 small adult, 1 large adult or equivalent	3
Self-inflating manual resuscitation device with 3 masks (1 pediatric, 1 small adult, 1 large adult or equivalent)	1:3 masks
Cardiopulmonary resuscitation mask (3 sizes): 1 pediatric, 1 small adult, 1 large adult or equivalent	3
IV administration set: tubing with 2 Y-connectors	1
Alcohol sponges	2
Adhesive tape, 1-inch standard roll adhesive	1
Tape scissors	1 pair
Tourniquet	1
Saline solution, 500 mL	1
Protective nonpermeable gloves or equivalent	1 pair
Needles (2–18 gauge, 2–20 gauge, 2–22 gauge, or sizes necessary to administer required medications)	6
Syringes (1–5 mL, 2–10 mL, or sizes necessary to administer required medications)	4
Analgesic, nonnarcotic, 325-mg tablets	4
Antihistamine, 25-mg tablets	4
Antihistamine injectable, 50 mg (single-dose ampule or equivalent)	2
Atropine, 0.5 mg, 5 mL (single-dose ampule or equivalent)	2
Aspirin tablets, 325 mg	4
Bronchodilator, inhaled (metered dose inhaler or equivalent)	1
Dextrose, 50%/50 mL, injectable (single-dose ampule or equivalent)	1
Epinephrine 1:1000, 1 mL, injectable (single-dose ampule or equivalent)	2
Epinephrine 1:10,000, 2 mL, injectable (single-dose ampule or equivalent)	2
Lidocaine, 5 mL, 20 mg/mL, injectable (single-dose ampule or equivalent)	2
Nitroglycerine tablets, 0.4 mg	10
Basic instructions for use of the drugs in the kit	1

From FAA advisory circular. 2006. Available at: https://www.faa.gov/documentlibrary/media/advisory_circular/ac121-33b.pdf.

- o Bandage, triangular, 100-cm folded and safety pins
- o Dressing, burn 10 cm × 10 cm
- o Dressing, compress, sterile 7.5 cm × 12 cm approximately
- o Dressing, gauze, sterile 10.4 cm × 10.4 cm approximately
- o Adhesive tape, 2.5-cm standard roll
- o Skin closure strips
- o Hand cleanser or cleaning towelettes
- o Pad with shield or tape for eye
- o Scissors, 10 cm (if permitted by applicable regulations)
- o Adhesive tape, surgical 1.2 cm × 4.6 m
- o Tweezers, splinter
- o Disposable gloves (several pairs)

- ○ Thermometer (nonmercury)
- ○ Resuscitation mask with one-way valve
- ○ First-aid manual (an operator may decide to have one manual per aircraft in an easily accessible location)
- ○ Incident record form
- If the medical professional needs the kit, the flight attendant will procure it.
- The standard EMK may not be available on international flights with non-US carriers. The International Air Transport Association endorses the Aerospace Medical Association's recommendations, but does not regulate the contents of EMKs of international airlines.[35]

Automated External Defibrillators

- Before 1990, if there was a cardiac arrest on board, it was a standard airline practice to divert aircraft to the nearest major airport. If one considers the 20 to 30 minutes required for an emergency landing from cruising altitude, plus a 10-minute taxi time to the gate, it is clear that in the past, these patients rarely survived.
- The successful introduction of AEDs for use by personal outside of hospitals has resulted in vastly improved ventricular fibrillation survival rates.[36] These data have prompted many international airline organizations to introduce AEDs into their aircraft fleet.
- The FAA made it mandatory for all US-based commercial passenger aircraft with at least one flight attendant to carry on AEDs since 2001.[37]
- If an AED is on board, typically at least one cabin crew member will be trained in its use. Airline protocol requires a crewmember to manage the AED and assist or direct its use.
- If cardiopulmonary resuscitation (CPR) is indicated, begin CPR and ask the cabin crew to assist. One can expect that all cabin crew have been trained in basic CPR.
- Some on-board AEDs include an electrocardiographic display (monitor) that shows the cardiac rhythm. AEDs with monitoring capability are clinically useful because they allow better decision making when a passenger presents with chest pain, palpitations, dyspnea, or lightheadedness.[27,38]
- For monitoring only, a new device, the Tempus IC (Remote Diagnostic Technologies, Hampshire, United Kingdom), may be used by people with little or no medical training. It can monitor blood pressure, tympanic temperature, glucometry, oxygen saturation as measured by pulse oximetry, respiration and breath gas analysis, and electrocardiogram, and transmit these data to a remote physician for diagnosis.[39] It is being adopted by a few airlines at this time.
- A compact smart phone transducer, Kardia (AliveCor), is now available. The device allows monitoring of electrocardiogram when used in conjunction with a smart phone. Kardia's single lead electrocardiogram is comparable with Lead 1 of a standard electrocardiogram machines.[40]

Limitations of In-Flight Automated External Defibrillators

Limitations of in-flight AEDs include the following:

- Operator failure to deliver the shocks because of patient movements interfering with analysis[41]
- Operator turning off the AED prematurely
- Not following instructions to deliver shocks
- Not realizing that the AED leads are off
- Misreading the AED screen instruction to start CPR

- Vibrations of the aircraft while in flight; however, has not been borne out in real practice
- Some airlines only allow AED-trained cabin crew to operate on-board AEDs; volunteering health care professionals are often unfamiliar with the equipment and therefore less qualified than trained crew[42]

Approach to Patient Care During In-Flight Emergencies

- The isolated environment and unavailability of specialized equipment can make for a challenging experience. Maintaining a calm, competent, and professional demeanor can go a long way toward creating a less stressful environment for the patient, crew, and other airline passengers.
- Medical professionals should respond to a call only if they are a licensed, currently practicing medical provider.
- Be prepared to show a form of professional identification (eg, a medical license) that verifies your training.
- Do not respond if you have been drinking alcohol. If you have been drinking (eg, one drink) and no other provider responds, be sure to offer full disclosure to the flight crew and the patient.
- It is appropriate to ask the patient for consent before commencing in-flight care if they are not altered. This is generally best done with a crewmember as witness.[43]
- Ask for one flight attendant to continue assisting throughout the in-flight emergency. This helps to maintain continuity and ensures that you have access to needed equipment and cockpit communications.
- If the passenger seems to be severely ill, request ground-based consultation. On all US carriers and most international carriers you will have access to a ground-based consultant that greatly eases the pressure on any in-flight medical volunteer.
- You may legally speak to the flight crew about the medical issues.[29] The airline is not required to follow federal regulations regarding health care privacy, because airlines are not considered to be a covered entity as defined by HIPAA.
- History taking may be difficult because of language barriers. Family members or another available passenger may act as an interpreter. The flight crew may not offer this, and it may be up to you to request this via a simple cabin announcement.
- Obtain and record vital signs early in the event.
- Physical examination can be extremely limited because of limitations in space, vibration, and ambient cabin noise. Auscultation of the heart, lungs, or abdomen may be virtually impossible.
- Better conditions for the evaluation and care of a passenger may necessitate moving the patient to an open area, such as an aft galley. If a full resuscitation is indicated, such as bag mask ventilation or AED defibrillation, this can only be done with the patient moved to a larger area. Treating a patient in the aisle should be avoided when possible because it impedes normal flight crew operations.
- You may be able to find additional medical equipment from other passengers. For example, in the case of a suspected hypoglycemic or hyperglycemic emergency, ask the flight attendant to announce that you are in need of a glucometer, which a passenger with diabetes might have on board.
- Do not be afraid to request additional help. A common example might be a physician out of practice starting IV lines requesting an announcement for a nurse or emergency medical technician with IV skills. You should be ready to defer to

other providers who may have more experience delivering care in acute situations (ie, an office-based dermatologist deferring to an emergency physician).

- Do not to perform procedures that you are unfamiliar with.
- If the patient's presentation suggests a communicable disease, be sure to notify the cabin and/or flight crew.
- If you are presented with a "Do Not Resuscitate" order by an accompanying family member or friend, you need to make a decision on how to proceed. The cabin crew may decide to continue resuscitation if their company policy requires it, despite the Do Not Resuscitate order.[13]

DEATH ONBOARD

International Air Transport Association Guidelines for death on board (January 2016) state that cabin crew trained to perform CPR should continue CPR until one of the following occurs[44]:

1. Spontaneous breathing and circulation resume; or
2. It becomes unsafe to continue CPR (eg, heavy turbulence and/or forecasted difficult landing after liaising with the flight deck); or
3. All rescuers are too exhausted to continue; or
4. The aircraft has landed and care is transferred to EMS; or
5. The person is presumed dead. If CPR has been continued for 30 minutes or longer with no signs of life, and no shocks advised by an AED, the person may be presumed dead, and resuscitation ceased.

Airlines may choose to specify additional criteria, depending on the availability of ground to air medical support or an on board physician. According to some sources,[45] it may be prudent to avoid declaring death. This is because the legal implications of declaration of death vary from country to country. Therefore, limit involvement to advising the cabin crew regarding the presumption of death.

ON-BOARD MEDICAL OXYGEN (PORTABLE OXYGEN BOTTLES)

As stated in the Federal Aviation Regulations, 14 CFR 121.333 (E) (3)[46]:

For first-aid treatment of occupants who for physiological reasons might require undiluted oxygen following descent from cabin pressure altitudes above flight level 250, a supply of oxygen in accordance with the requirements of §25.1443(d) must be provided for two percent of the occupants for the entire flight after cabin depressurization at cabin pressure altitudes above 8000 feet, but in no case to less than one person. An appropriate number of acceptable dispensing units, but in no case less than two, must be provided, with a means for the cabin attendants to use this supply.

Many airlines carry a minimum of one portable oxygen bottle (POB) per flight attendant, which equals or exceeds the FAA minimum oxygen requirement discussed previously.

Flow Rates and Duration

If called to assist in an on-board emergency, keep in mind that POBs may have only two fixed settings: high (4 L/min) and low (2 L/min) constant flow. Selection is made via a knob mounted on top of the regulator. Do not confuse these settings with "low" and "high" flow used in most emergency departments and hospitals, where high flow implies 10 to 15 L per minute (or higher). The so-called "high flow" setting on aviation

POBs is therefore considerably lower than what is normally used in EMS settings. Alternatively, some airline POBs are adjustable between 2 and 8 L per minute.

Personal Portable Oxygen Bottles

The FAA prohibits the use of personal POBs during flight because they contain compressed gas or liquid oxygen that is considered hazardous material. Airlines are allowed to carry a passenger's filled oxygen cylinder in the aircraft cabin[47] but the passenger cannot use it. However, because written pilot notification and additional HAZMAT training and manual documentation are required, most US airlines do not offer this service. Passengers should check with the specific airline before planning on carrying their own oxygen cylinder to their destination.

Liquid oxygen is classified by the FAA as a hazardous material. Therefore, the use of liquid oxygen systems on commercial aircraft is prohibited. If necessary a portable liquid oxygen system can be checked as baggage if the oxygen reservoir has been emptied.

Passengers requiring a constant supply of compressed or liquid medical oxygen are either not be able to travel, or may request, from a licensed physician, verification that they can complete their flight without the use of medical oxygen.

Carrier-Supplied (Compressed) Oxygen (Portable Oxygen Bottles)

Some airlines provide, for a fee, compressed bottled oxygen during flight as a service to passengers who need oxygen therapy. Equipment specifics (eg, flow rates and available equipment, such as masks) vary among airlines. Airlines typically do not provide oxygen for passengers before or after a flight (eg, between connecting flights). Some oxygen suppliers can arrange to have a representative meet a passenger with portable oxygen at the airport when they arrive. Because of the red tape associated with carrying compressed oxygen on board, and the availability of portable oxygen concentrators (POCs), few airlines offer bottled oxygen.

Personal Portable Oxygen Concentrator

The FAA has recently issued guidelines permitting the onboard use of certain POCs. Most airlines allow POC devices to be brought onboard.[48] Check with the specific airline to see which POC models are approved for use during flight.[49] The FAA maintains up-to-date reference materials on approved portable oxygen concentrators.[50] Unlike carrier-supplied oxygen, POCs can be used by passengers during long layovers or delays. Travelers can also continue to use POCs at their final destination without the necessity for additional arrangements. Notes concerning use of POCs include the following[51]:

- If the system is not an FAA-approved POC, it is not permitted on the aircraft.
- Because POCs are considered assistive devices, they are not counted as carry-on luggage.
- The POC user is responsible for supplying sufficient spare batteries to power the device for the duration of the flight, including a contingency supply for any unanticipated delays.
- POC batteries may be recharged during layovers; however, airlines do not guarantee travelers access to electrical outlets during flight. Travelers with powered POCs should request a seat that offers them access to an electrical outlet (if available).

Continuous Positive Airway Pressure Devices

Note that patients with sleep apnea may require use of their continuous positive airway pressure devices during long-duration flights.[51] Portable continuous positive airway pressure devices are classified as "medical assist devices" and are permitted on most domestic and international flights.

FUTURE CHALLENGES

Challenges to be addressed in the future include the following:

- Lack of standardization of the onboard EMK contents. The FAA standard EMK offers an important foundation, but EMKs adopted by airlines may contain dissimilar items based on the individual airline's particular medical practice.
- Lack of mandatory and standardized reporting system for a better understanding of the overall incidence of in-flight emergencies.
- Lack of postflight follow-up to ascertain frequency of nonemergency medical issues (ie, venous thromboembolism).
- The FAA requires flight attendants to undergo training in AED and CPR every 24 months[52]; however, there is no standardized training in medical protocols for onboard emergencies.
- Most airlines do not have clear standardized medical protocols for flight attendants managing in-flight medical emergencies. This includes protocols for flight attendants on flights where no medical professionals are available to volunteer.[53]
- Modern telemedicine technologies remain out of reach for most airlines despite recent advances in this field.

SUMMARY

The author aspires to the notion that after reading this article and experiencing the dreaded "if there is a doctor on board please press your flight attendant button" (or some variation), the reader will raise their finger toward the daunting flight attendant button secure in the confidence that the mysteries of the flight environment, resources, and expectations have been transformed into something more tangible and familiar.

ACKNOWLEDGMENTS

The author thanks Brownie Schoene MD, Peter Lert CFI, Jim Bagian MD, Valerie Dobiesz, MD, Evan Donner, and Denise Lange.

REFERENCES

1. Peterson DC, Martin-Gill C, Guyette FX, et al. Outcomes of medical emergencies on commercial airline flights. N Engl J Med 2013;368:2075.
2. Ears & Diving Middle-Ear Equalization Divers Alert Network (DAN) Website. Available at: https://www.diversalertnetwork.org/health/ears/middle-ear-equalization. Accessed February 8, 2017.
3. Skjenna OW. Care in the air. CMAJ 1989;140:1126.
4. Kenfack R, Debaize S, Sztern B, et al. Perforation of a hiatal hernia after a high altitude flight. Rev Med Liege 2007;62:144–6.
5. Assessing fitness to fly; AviationHealthUnit, UKCivilAviationAuthority. 2012. Available at: http://www.caa.co.uk/Passengers/Before-you-fly/Am-I-fit-to-fly-/.
6. Hu X, Cowl CT, Baqir M, et al. Air travel and pneumothorax. Chest 2014;145(4): 688–94.

7. DAN Online Health Information Library, Health & Diving. Available at: http://www. diversalertnetwork.org/health/.

8. Nassauer S. New worries about cabin fume events - WSJ, Updated July 30, 2009. Available at: https://www.wsj.com/articles/SB100014240529702049009045743022930127 11628. Accessed February 8, 2017.

9. Bagshaw M. Cabin air quality: a review of current aviation medical understanding. London: King's College London and Cranfield University; 2013.

10. Harrison R, Murawski J, McNeely E, et al. Management of exposure to aircraft bleed-air contaminants among airline workers, a guide for health care providers, FAA; 2007. Available at: http://fdx.alpa.org/portals/26/docs/053116_ESC%20exposure.pdf. Accessed February 8, 2017.

11. Guidelines enable health authorities to assess risk of tuberculosis trans- mission aboard aircraft. Cabin Air Safety. Alexandria (VA): Flight Safety Foundation; 1998. Available at: http://www.flightsafety.org/ pubs/ccs_1998.html.

12. Select Committee on Science and Technology. Air travel and health: fifth report. London: United Kingdom House of Lords; 2000.

13. Aerospace Medical Association, Air Transport Medicine Committee. Medical emergencies: managing in-f light medical events. Alexandria (VA): Aerospace Medical Association; 2013.

14. Blettner M, Grosche B, Zeeb H. Occupational cancer risk in pilots and flight attendants: current epidemiological knowledge. Radiat Environ Biophys 1998;37:75–80.

15. The 2007 recommendations of the international commission on radiological protection. ICRP publication 103. Ann ICRP 2007;37:1–332.

16. Chen J, Lewis BJ, Bennett LG, et al. Estimated neutron dose to embryo and foetus during commercial flight. Radiat Prot Dosimetry 2005;114:475–80.

17. The National Institute for Occupational Safety and Health (NIOSH) AIRCREW SAFETY & HEALTH. Available at: http://www.cdc.gov/niosh/topics/aircrew/ cosmicionizingradiation.html.

18. Federal Aviation Administration. In-flight radiation exposure. Advisory Circular No. 120–61A. Washington, DC: FAA; 2006.

19. Ronnie Henry, Centers for Disease Control and Prevention Chapter 2Yellow Book The Pre-Travel Consultation.

20. Boulos Z, Campbell SS, Lewy AJ, et al. Light treatment for sleep disorders: consensus report. VII. Jet lag. J Biol Rhythms 1995;10(2):167–76.

21. Barion and Zee Page 10 Sleep Med. Author manuscript; available in PMC 2009 May 9. NIH-PA Author Manuscript NIH-PA Author Manuscript NIH-PA Author Manuscript.

22. Barion A, Zee PC. A clinical approach to circadian rhythm sleep disorders. Sleep Med 2007;8(6):566–77.

23. Arendt J. Managing jet lag: some of the problems and possible new solutions. Sleep Med Rev 2009;13:249–56.

24. Sack RL, Auckley D, Auger RR, et al. Circadian rhythm sleep disorders: part I, basic principles, shift work and jet lag disorders. An American Academy of Sleep Medicine review. Sleep 2007;30(11):1460–83.

25. Beaumont M, Batejat D, Pierard C, et al. Caffeine or melatonin effects on sleep and sleepiness after rapid eastward transmeridian travel. J Appl Physiol 2004; 96:50–8.

26. Ruskin KJ, Hernandez KA, Barash PA. Management of in-flight medical emergencies. Anesthesiology 2008;108:749–55.

27. Gendreau MA, DeJohn C. Responding to medical events during commercial airline flights. N Engl J Med 2002;346:1067–73.

28. Aviation Medical Assistance Act of 1998, pub. L. 105-170, Apr. 24, 1998, 112 Stat. 47, Sec. 5. Washington, DC: National Archives and Records Administration, 1998.
29. Nable JV, Tupe CL, Gehle BD. In-flight medical emergencies during commercial travel. N Engl J Med 2015;373(10):939–45.
30. Dachs RJ, Elias JM. What you need to know when called upon to be a good Samaritan. Fam Pract Manag 2008;15(4):37–40.
31. Sand M, Bechara FG, Sand D, et al. Surgical and medical emergencies on board European aircraft: a retrospective study of 10189 cases. Crit Care 2009;13(1):R3.
32. Public Law 105-170: Aviation Medical Assistance Act of 1998 (112 Stat. 47; April 24, 1998). Text from U.S. Government Printing Office. Available at: www.gpo.gov/fdsys/pkg/PLAW.../PLAW-105publ170.pdf.
33. Adapted from AirRx, Mobile reference guide for physicians and medical professionals during an in-flight emergency. IOS app, OSF Healthcare Systems.
34. Policy AC 121–33B — emergency medical equipment. Federal Aviation Administration, 2006. Available at: www.faa.gov/documentlibrary/media/advisory_circular/ac121-33b.pdf.
35. Available at: http://westjem.com/articles/in-flight-medical-emergencies.html.
36. Weaver WD, Hill D, Fahrenbruch CE, et al. Use of the automatic external de brillator in the management of out-of-hospital cardiac arrest. N Engl J Med 1988;319:661–6.
37. Federal Aviation Administration. Emergency Medical Equipment, Final Rule [online]. Available at: www.faa.gov/apa/pr/ pr.cfm?id=1262.
38. Page RL, Joglar JA, Kowal RC, et al. Use of automated external defibrillators by a U.S. airline. N Engl J Med 2000;343:1210–6.
39. Available at: http://www.rdtltd.com/commercial-aviation/l.
40. Available at: https://www.alivecor.com/.
41. Charles RA. Cardiac arrest in the skies. Singapore Med J 2011;52(8):582–5.
42. McKenas DK. Special report: cabin safety: bodily fluids a fact of life for inflight heart emergencies. Aviation Today 2000.
43. Silverman D, Gendreau M. Medical issues associated with commercial flights. Lancet 2009;373:2067–77.
44. International Air Transport Association Guidelines for Death On Board January 2016.
45. AirRx, Mobile reference guide for physicians and medical professionals during an in-flight emergency. IOS app, OSF Healthcare Systems.
46. ELECTRONIC CODE OF FEDERAL REGULATIONS §121.333. Supplemental oxygen for emergency descent and for first aid; turbine engine powered airplanes with pressurized cabins. Available at: http://www.ecfr.gov/cgi-bin/retrieveECFR?gp=&SID=018c23801b8359560674c41e18be7e04&r=SECTION&n=14y3.0.1.1.7.11.2.24.
47. FAA 49 CFR 175.501(e).
48. Special Federal Aviation Regulation (SFAR) No. 106, 14 CFR part 121.
49. FAA 14 CFR 135.91-Oxygen for medical use by passengers.
50. Available at: https://www.faa.gov/about/initiatives/cabin_safety/portable_oxygen.
51. "Traveling with portable oxygen" - Patient Education Guide American College of Chest Physicians.
52. US Federal Aviation Administration. Emergency medical equipment training: advisory circular 121–34B. Available at: http://www.faa.gov/regulations_policies/advisory_circulars/index.cfm/go/document.information/documentID/22519. Accessed February 6, 2017.
53. Mattison MD. Navigating the challenges of in-flight emergencies. JAMA 2011;305(19):2003–4.

Preparing for International Travel and Global Medical Care

Swaminatha V. Mahadevan, MD*, Matthew C. Strehlow, MD

KEYWORDS

- Travel • Immunization • Vaccination • Malaria prophylaxis • Preparation
- Travel medical kits

KEY POINTS

- Although more people are traveling, few seek pretravel consultation to mitigate avoidable health risks associated with traveling.
- A comprehensive pretravel medical consultation should include an individualized risk assessment, immunization review, and discussion of arthropod protective measures, malaria prophylaxis, traveler's diarrhea, and injury prevention.
- Travel with children and jet lag reduction require additional planning and prevention strategies.
- Travel and evacuation insurance is recommended when traveling to less resourced countries.
- Consideration should also be given to other high-risk travel scenarios, including the provision of health care overseas, adventure and extreme sports, water environments and diving, high altitude, and terrorism/unstable political situations.

INTRODUCTION

During the first 9 months of 2016, nearly 1 billion tourists had already traveled around the world, a 4% increase from the prior year.[1] The World Travel & Tourism Council projects that this number will increase to nearly 1.8 billion international travelers in 2025. Depending on their destination, approximately 22% to 64% of these travelers will experience some illness, most commonly diarrhea, respiratory infections, and skin conditions.[2] Some travelers may even develop life-threatening conditions (eg, malaria), which could have been avoided with proper pretravel preparation.

Disclosure: The authors have nothing to disclose.
Department of Emergency Medicine, Stanford University School of Medicine, 300 Pasteur Drive, Alway Building, M-121, Stanford, CA 94305, USA
* Corresponding author.
E-mail address: s.mahadevan@stanford.edu

Emerg Med Clin N Am 35 (2017) 465–484
http://dx.doi.org/10.1016/j.emc.2017.01.006
0733-8627/17/© 2017 Elsevier Inc. All rights reserved.

emed.theclinics.com

On a typical 2-week trip, travelers lose an average of 3 days because of illness, with nearly 20% remaining ill after their return home and 10% seeking medical care for their illnesses.[3]

For every 100,000 travelers visiting a developing country for 1 month[4]:

- 50,000 develop some health problem while abroad
- 8000 need to see a physician
- 5000 are confined to a bed
- 300 are admitted to a hospital
- 50 require air evacuation
- 1 dies

With prevention of these potential hazards in mind, this article explores the key elements of preparation for travel and global medical care.

PRETRAVEL CONSULTATION

Many travelers are unaware or unconcerned about the health and safety risks posed by travel, and few seek proper pretravel counseling.[5–9] Travelers visiting friends and relatives are at especially high risk for illness (specifically, malaria and food-borne illnesses); they tend to have a false sense of immunity, visit higher risk destinations, stay abroad longer, eat local food, and do not seek pretravel advice or use protective measures.[10–13] There is a known association between failing to seek pretravel consultation and the development of illnesses like malaria, which can have significant health and economic consequences.[13] The average health care payer cost to prevent malaria is $162, whereas the cost of treating an adult with malaria is $25,250 (with an additional 6–24 work days lost).[14]

A comprehensive pretravel medical consultation should include an individualized risk assessment; a review of immunizations; and a discussion of arthropod protective measures, malaria prophylaxis, traveler's diarrhea (TD), and other travel-related education and risk reduction practices. This approach is particularly important for travelers who are headed to developing countries; planning adventure travel; planning an extended trip; immune compromised or with chronic medical conditions; children; and pregnant or planning pregnancy.[2] Although consulting a specialist is advisable at any time before travel, a pretravel checkup should ideally occur at least six weeks in advance of the intended departure date to maximize the effect of immunizations and other preventive measures (eg, malaria chemoprophylaxis needs to be started in advance of travel).

INDIVIDUALIZED RISK ASSESSMENT

A traveler's individual risk of travel depends on several factors: medical history, itinerary (regions, season, dates), prior travel experience, activities (eg, adventure, mass gathering), accommodations, risk tolerance, and financial means. A traveler's medical history should also include current medications, disabilities, immune status, immunizations, surgeries, allergies, and pregnancy/breastfeeding status.

PRETRAVEL IMMUNIZATIONS

All travelers should be screened to determine their need for pretravel immunizations including a review of their current immunization history. In addition to routine or domestic vaccinations, additional destination-specific vaccinations may be required depending on the traveler's itinerary, anticipated activities, and duration of stay. Because of the associated health risks, pregnant women and immunocompromised patients should not receive live vaccines (eg, measles, mumps, rubella; polio [oral]; rotavirus; varicella-zoster; influenza [intranasal]; typhoid [oral]; yellow fever, and bacille Calmette-Guérin [for TB]).[15,16] Live vaccines should be administered on either the same day or four weeks apart to avoid vaccine failure.[15]

Routine Vaccinations

The risk of domestic vaccine-preventable diseases, such as influenza and hepatitis A, is higher in international travelers than that of more exotic vaccine-preventable illnesses, such as typhoid and Japanese encephalitis. Therefore, routine (domestic) immunizations should be reviewed to ensure that the traveler is up to date and booster doses should be provided as needed. A summary of recommendations for routine vaccinations is provided in **Table 1**.

Table 1
Routine vaccinations

	Indication	Route	Dosing Schedule
Haemophilus influenzae Type b	All infants; children/adults with asplenia or sickle cell disease, or following leukemia chemotherapy or BMT; ages 5–18 y with HIV	IM	3–4 doses: 2, 4, 6, 12–15 mo
Hepatitis A	All travelers >1 y old	IM	2 doses: day 0, 6–12 mo
Hepatitis B	All travelers	IM	3 doses: day 0, 1 mo, 6 mo
Herpes Zoster (Shingles)	Adults >60 y old	SC	Single dose
Human Papillomavirus	All children and young adults	IM	3 doses: day 0, 1–2 mo, 6 mo
Influenza	All travelers >6 mo old	IM, intranasal, or ID	Single dose
Measles, Mumps, Rubella	All travelers	SC	2 doses: day 0, 4 wk
Meningococcal Disease	Living in crowded conditions (eg, dormitory); routine at 11–12 y; booster at 16 y	IM	Single dose
Pneumococcal Disease	All infants and adults >65 y old	IM or SC	4 doses (infants): 2, 4, 6, 12–15 mo
Polio	All infants and children	SC	Single dose (if received primary childhood series)
Rotavirus	All infants	Oral	3 doses: 2, 4, 6 mo
Tetanus, Diphtheria, Pertussis	All travelers	IM	Single dose (if received primary childhood series)
Varicella (Chickenpox)	All travelers	SC	Two doses: (<13 y old) 12–15 mo, 4–6 y; (≥13 y old) 28 d apart

Abbreviations: BMT, bone marrow transplant; HIV, human immunodeficiency virus; ID, intradermal; IM, intramuscular; SC, subcutaneous.
Data from Ref.[2,15,16]

Travel-Specific Vaccinations

Some travel-specific vaccinations are indicated based on the traveler's anticipated itinerary, duration of travel, activities, and other risk factors. Some travelers may be required to show proof of vaccination (eg, yellow fever, meningococcal meningitis) to customs officials; therefore, it is advisable for travelers to carry their immunization records along with their passports. A summary of recommendations for travel-specific vaccinations is provided in **Table 2**.

ARTHROPOD PROTECTIVE MEASURES

Arthropods - mosquitoes, ticks, flies, and chiggers - can transmit infections such as malaria, dengue, and rickettsial diseases; some of these infections are only

Table 2 Travel-specific vaccinations				
	Indication	**Route**	**Dosing Schedule**	**Duration of Protection**
Cholera[a]	Adults 18–64 y at high risk	Oral	Single dose	3–6 mo
Japanese Encephalitis	Travelers to endemic areas	IM	2 doses: days 0 and 28	1–2 y after initial; >6 y if booster at 1–2 y
Meningococcal[b]	Travelers to meningitis belt of Africa or Saudi Arabia (pilgrimage)	IM	Single dose	3–5 y
Polio[b]	Travelers to country with ongoing transmission; >4 wk travel to Afghanistan or Pakistan	SC	Single dose (if received primary childhood series)	Lifelong (after primary series and booster as adult)
Rabies	Travelers to rabies enzootic areas (especially remote, rural, or extended stay)	IM	3 doses before exposure: 0, 7, and 21–28 d	2 additional doses (days 0 and 3) after exposure
Tick-borne Encephalitis[a]	Travelers to endemic areas (Europe, Soviet Union, Asia)	IM	3 doses: day 0, 1–3 mo, 5–12 mo	3 y
Tuberculosis (BCG)[a]	Consider in health workers traveling to areas with high TB resistance to both isoniazid and rifampin	ID	Single dose	10–15 y
Typhoid	All travelers to low-income nations	Oral or IM	4 doses (oral) Single dose (IM)	5 y (oral) 2–3 y (IM)
Yellow Fever	Travel to endemic areas (tropical Africa or South America); avoid in children <9 mo old	SC	Single dose	10 y

Abbreviation: BCG, bacille Calmette-Guérin.

[a] Not routinely given in the United States.

[b] Meningococcal and poliomyelitis are childhood vaccines that may require boosters in adult travelers with specific itineraries.

Data from Ref.[2,15,16]

preventable by anti-arthropod protective measures. Such vector-borne illnesses account for most systemic febrile illnesses in travelers presenting to travel and tropical medicine clinics.[17] Risk factors for vector-borne illnesses depend on the destination, setting (urban vs rural), length of stay, mode of transportation, season (dry vs rainy), and accommodation. Although some vectors, such as the female *Anopheles* mosquito, which transmits malaria, tend to bite from dusk to dawn, other vectors, such as mites and ticks, can bite day or night. Arthropod bites can be prevented through personal protective measures such as general avoidance techniques, insect repellents, and insecticide-treated materials (**Table 3**). Insecticide-treated clothing in association with topical insect repellents (eg, diethyltoluamide [DEET] or picaridin) provides very effective protection against arthropod bites.[18]

MALARIA CHEMOPROPHYLAXIS

The US Centers for Disease Control and Prevention (CDC) Web site (https://www.cdc.gov/malaria/) can help determine the risk of developing malaria based on travel destination. Because there currently is not a vaccine for malaria, all travelers to malaria-endemic areas should be given strong consideration for chemoprophylaxis.[19,20] Some patients

Table 3 Personal protective measures against arthropods	
Activity modification	Avoid areas with known outbreaks Avoid heavily vegetated areas (ticks, chiggers) Avoid outdoors from dusk to dawn (malaria-endemic regions)
Protected environment	Well-screened room, air conditioning, fan to reduce risk of malaria
Clothing: protective	Expose as little skin as possible (long sleeves, loose fitting, tucking shirt into pants, tucking pants into socks) Light colored (not blue) heavyweight clothing to reduce risk from mosquitoes, tsetse flies, and sand flies
Clothing/gear: insecticide treated	Apply permethrin to clothing, shoes, and camping gear, or purchase impregnated clothing May need reapplication after 5 washes
Insect repellent	Apply a repellent containing DEET (20%–50%) or picaridin (20%) to exposed skin Regularly reapply (DEET every 6–8 h, picaridin every 4 h) Apply daytime for *Aedes* mosquitoes, dusk/nighttime for *Anopheles* and *Culex* mosquitoes DEET is safe during second/third trimester of pregnancy and in children >2 mo old
Insecticide-treated bed nets	Sleeping under pyrethroid insecticide–impregnated bed nets (recommended for all travelers to malaria-endemic regions) Lasts months if not washed but needs retreatment to retain effectiveness
Spatial repellents	Impregnated plastic strips, coils, candles, fan emanators, heat-generating devices reduce nuisance biting Should not be used in lieu of other proven protective measures
Tick check	Full-body and clothing check after activity and at the end of the day, using a mirror or companion

Abbreviation: DEET, diethyltoluamide.
Data from Ref.[2,15,18]

are at higher risk for malaria than the general population, including those who are human immunodeficiency virus [HIV] positive, asplenic, or immunosuppressed.[21]

When taken properly, chemoprophylaxis is highly effective in preventing malaria.[21] Many chemoprophylactic agents need to be started before travel and continued for several weeks after returning (with duration depending on the agent) to be effective. Noncompliance is a significant risk factor for development of malaria; the most common reasons for nonadherence are forgetfulness, undesirable side effects, and not seeing mosquitoes.[22] Determining the appropriate chemoprophylactic agent depends on geographic considerations (especially chloroquine sensitivity vs resistance), duration of travel, dosing schedule, cost, and host factors (medical conditions, medications). The most commonly used agents are chloroquine, doxycycline, mefloquine, and atovaquone/proguanil (**Table 4**).

Some European authorities advocate the use of a standby self-treatment regimen in lieu of chemoprophylaxis,[23] especially for long-stay travelers. In such circumstances, a traveler self-treats if the symptoms are suggestive of malaria and there is no access to a qualified medical facility. A full course of atovaquone/proguanil or artemether-lumefantrine is recommended in these situations.[2]

TRAVELER'S DIARRHEA

TD is the most common travel-related ailment.[24] TD is defined as the passage of 3 or more unformed stools per day plus 1 additional enteric complaint (eg, vomiting, cramps, abdominal pain), either within 24 hours of travel or up to 7 days after returning. Between 10% and 40% of travelers develop TD, usually within the first 2 weeks of travel, with symptoms lasting a median of 3 days.[25,26] TD is predominantly transmitted by the fecal-oral route, with a bacterial cause in 80% to 90% of cases. Risk factors for TD include medications that reduce gastric acidity (antacids, proton pump inhibitors), pregnancy, young age, and immune compromise.[16,27]

For travelers to high-risk areas, several approaches can reduce but not eliminate the risk for TD. Because contaminated food and water cause most TD, the following are recommendations regarding food and water safety: (1) eating well-cooked, hot food while avoiding raw food, uncooked meat/fish/eggs, shellfish, and mayonnaise; (2) consuming peeled fruits and vegetables (and avoiding salads, salsas, and cold sauces); (3) consuming pasteurized dairy products; (4) consuming bottled or disinfected (boiled, filtered, treated) water and avoiding tap/well water and ice/juice made from the like; (5) avoiding foods from market stalls and street vendors; and (6) avoiding uncovered or unrefrigerated foods.[2,28] Hand washing before eating and after using the toilet can reduce risk by as much as 30%; if soap and water are not available, hand sanitizer (containing at least 60% alcohol) is advisable.[16,29]

Prophylactic antibiotics for TD are not routinely recommended (except in rare circumstances).[2] Bismuth subsalicylate (2 tablets 4 times a day for a maximum of 3 weeks) provides up to 65% protection.[30] Adverse effects of bismuth subsalicylate include black tongue, dark stools, and decreased absorption of doxycycline, and contraindications include aspirin/nonsteroidal antiinflammatory drug allergy, bleeding disorders, and breastfeeding. There is currently insufficient evidence to support the use of probiotics for TD prevention.[16,25]

The self-treatment of TD consists of oral rehydration, antimotility agents, and oral antibiotics. Adequate oral rehydration can prevent and treat dehydration. For mild dehydration, water or readily available liquids are sufficient, but avoid Gatorade, soft drinks, and juice because of their high sugar and low salt content.[25] For moderate to severe dehydration, use oral rehydration salts (ORS), either commercial or prepared

Table 4
Malaria chemoprophylactic agents

	Typical Adult Dosing	Typical Pediatric Dosing	Start (Pre-exposure)	Continue (Post-exposure)	Advantages	Disadvantages
Chloroquine	500 mg salt (300 mg base) oral once a week	8.3 mg salt (5 mg base)/kg/wk up to the adult dosage	2 wk	4 wk	• Safe and well tolerated • Can be used during pregnancy • Can be used in children (all ages)	• Global resistance outside of the Caribbean, Central America • May exacerbate psoriasis
Doxycycline	100 mg oral once a day	2 mg/kg/d up to adult dosage (for children ≥8 y) up to the adult dosage	2 d	4 wk	• Least expensive • Can prevent leptospirosis and rickettsia • Good last-minute choice • Widely available globally	• Esophageal irritation/ulceration • Skin photosensitivity • Vaginal yeast infections • Not for use in pregnancy and children <8 y old
Mefloquine	250 mg salt (228 mg base) oral once a week	≤9 kg: 5 mg/kg (4.6 mg/kg base) once per week >9–19 kg: one-fourth of 250-mg tablet weekly 20–30 kg: one-half of 250-mg tablet weekly 31–45 kg: three-fourths of 250-mg tablet weekly >45 kg: 250 mg once per week	2–3 wk	4 wk	• Weekly dosing • Good long-term regimen • Can be used during pregnancy • Can be used in children (all ages)	• Some areas of mefloquine resistance (southeast Asia) • Neuropsychiatric side effects • Avoid in patients with depression, psychosis, seizures, and atrioventricular conduction abnormalities
Atovaquone/proguanil	250 mg atovaquone/100 mg proguanil oral once a day	5–8 kg: one-half of a children's tablet (62.5 mg atovaquone/25 mg proguanil) daily 9–10 kg: three-fourths of a children's tablet daily 11–20 kg: 1 children's tablet daily 21–30 kg: 2 children's tablets daily 31–40 kg: 3 children's tablets daily >40 kg: 1 adult tablet daily	2 d	1 wk	• Well tolerated • Good for short trips • Good last-minute choice • Can be used in children (≥11 kg) and off label in children (≥5 kg)	• Expensive • Avoid with renal impairment • Not recommended for pregnant women, breastfeeding mothers, and children <5 kg

Data from Ref.[2,15,21]

at home. To make ORS at home, add half a teaspoon of salt and 6 level teaspoons of sugar to 1 L of safe water (bottled, sealed, or disinfected). Antimotility agents like loperamide are safe and effective for the treatment of nondysenteric TD, with or without concomitant antibiotics. Avoid antimotility agents in patients with blood in the stool or fever, or in children less than six years of age.[16] The early self-treatment of TD with antibiotics has been shown to reduce the duration of symptoms.[31,32] For severe diarrhea, consider a single dose of a quinolone (500 mg of ciprofloxacin or levofloxacin) or azithromycin (1 g) for more rapid cessation. Azithromycin is preferred in south and southeast Asia because of fluoroquinolone-resistant enteropathogens.[33]

INJURY PREVENTION

Travelers are 10 times more likely to die from an injury than an infection while overseas. Injuries, particularly road traffic accidents (57%) and drowning (25%), are the most common cause of death.[34,35] Travelers are three times more likely to drown abroad than at home,[36] and road traffic accidents are three times more common during rain, at night, or during national holidays.[37,38]

Despite the road safety hazards in low- and middle-income countries, travelers can reduce their risks by adhering to the following recommendations.[35] Bring child safety seats, select vehicles with functional seatbelts and wear them, and ride in the backseat (particularly when a vehicle lacks airbags). Avoid traveling when visibility is limited (eg, nighttime, fog, rain, snow) and riding in overcrowded or overweight vehicles (eg, minibuses, trucks). Avoid traveling on roads on 2-wheeled vehicles or bicycles, and, if you must, always wear a properly fitting helmet. Do not drive after drinking alcohol or ride with someone who has. In addition, take precautions when crossing roads as pedestrians often do not have the right of way and avoid walking on roads when visibility is limited (eg, nighttime).

Drowning is highly preventable and predominantly affects young children, but travelers can reduce their risks by taking the following precautions.[35] Bring personal flotation devices when planning water activities, especially for children and poor swimmers. Ensure that all children are supervised at all times by an adult who has not consumed alcohol. Do not operate or ride in watercraft or swim after consuming alcohol. Be familiar with the local water conditions and do not travel in overcrowded or undersized watercraft.

TRAVEL WITH CHILDREN

Children are the fastest growing population of travelers in the United States, with an estimated 2.2 million children and adolescents traveling to international destinations in 2010.[39] The causes of illness and injury are similar to those in adults but the risk is exacerbated in many circumstances, with 50% to 75% of children traveling to developing countries contracting some type of illness.[40,41] Further, pediatric patients account for a disproportionate number of travel-related hospitalizations.[41]

In general, child travelers should undertake additional planning and prevention strategies on top of those taken by adults. Illness prevention should focus on pretravel medical consultation to ensure that appropriate vaccinations and prophylaxis are administered; although TD prophylaxis is not recommended in children, malaria chemoprophylaxis is imperative for those traveling to endemic areas.[42] Preparation should also focus on exposure and bite prevention.

Acute diarrheal illnesses lasting less than 2 weeks are most common (28%), with bacterial causes accounting for approximately one-third of these infections.[43] Regular application of hand sanitizer and adhering to the mantra "Peel it, boil it, cook it, or forget it" can decrease the rate of children's TD.[42] ORS should be readily available for rehydration. Although strong evidence showing benefit is limited, antiemetics are recommended in children with vomiting to increase oral intake and combat dehydration. Antibiotic recommendations are similar to those for adults, with azithromycin preferred to fluoroquinolones for its lower resistance rate and its better safety profile in children.[26]

In malaria-endemic areas, bed netting is essential and netting, along with clothing, should be pretreated with permethrin. Skin should be covered with long, loose clothing, even in hot environments. DEET (25%–50%) or picaridin (KBR3023) (20%) should be applied to exposed areas of skin in children more than 2 months of age, with caution around hands and mucous membranes in the very young. A regimen of permethrin and insect repellants can be highly effective in preventing insect bites.[44] Malaria chemoprophylaxis is recommended in any location where recommended for adults; however, drug regimens can vary based on age (see **Table 4**).[42]

Many medications used for prophylaxis and treatment while traveling taste bitter and getting children to take medications can be challenging. Crushing pills and mixing with thin juices is generally ineffective. Crushing pills and mixing with peanut butter, yogurt, or other thicker, sweet foods that disguise the bitter flavor is more effective. Trialing different foods before travel to ensure compliance can avoid significant anxiety.

Modes of transport, whether by bicycle, car, boat, or airplane, are often poorly equipped to accommodate children's safety needs. Appropriately sized restraint and booster seats should be brought, because these are rarely available in developing nations. Confirm in advance with airlines which restraint seats may be used because they vary by airline and country. Many car seats have the added benefit of increasing child comfort and sleep during travel; sedating children during air travel is generally not recommended. Flotation devices for young children are often not available in developing countries and should be brought from home if needed. If bicycle or other 2-wheeled or 3-wheeled transportation is planned, correctly fitting helmets should be carried to the destination.

Air travel with children can be stressful and anxiety provoking. Toys, books, electronics, and games can reduce the stress and anxiety of travel. Although many international airlines have child meals that can be ordered in advance, bringing favorite foods can help. During ascent and descent, encouraging children to drink fluids or suck on fluids/food/pacifiers can prevent middle ear barotrauma and reduce pain.[45]

Motion sickness is common in children during travel. Symptoms often present differently in children less than 5 years of age, with ataxia being the predominant finding. Older children tend to experience more classic symptoms of nausea, vomiting, headaches, pallor, dizziness, and sweating.[46] There is little evidence to support the use of pharmacologic agents to combat motion sickness in children. Preventive measures such as a light meal at least three hours before travel; avoiding reading and excessive head movements; and focusing on distant, stable objects are recommended.[47]

JET LAG

Jet lag occurs when rapidly traversing times zones leads to the internal clock, circadian rhythm, being out of cycle with the external light-dark cycle. The result is disrupted sleep with wakefulness during dark hours and sleepiness during the day. The prevalence of jet lag is unknown but it is thought to increase with age.

The circadian rhythm is modifiable by several factors, the most powerful of which is exposure to light. Other factors include exercise, meals, and social contact. If appropriately timed, melatonin can be used in specific circumstances to increase the rate of adaptation to the new time zone. Caffeine can be used to combat daytime sleepiness;

however, caution must be used to avoid increasing sleep disruption. Other medications such as benzodiazepines and other benzodiazepine-receptor agonists are not recommended for routine use; however, short-term use may be appropriate on an individual basis.[48]

Recommendations for managing jet lag depend on the duration of the trip, number of time zones crossed, and direction of travel. For brief trips lasting less than 3 days, the recommendation is to remain on origin time, if feasible. Otherwise, general recommendations for managing jet lag when traveling across less than 8 time zones are listed here.[49]

Before travel
- Eastward travel: move bedtime and wake time to 30 minutes earlier per day for 3 days in advance of departure
- Westward travel: move bedtime and wake time to 30 minutes later per day for 3 days in advance of departure

During travel
- Avoid sedative-hypnotic medication in flight
- Set watch to destination time to follow below recommendations
- Sleep during destination nighttime
- Eastward travel: avoid early morning bright light and get late morning and early afternoon bright light
- Westward travel: get late afternoon and evening bright light and avoid light during nighttime

On Arrival
- Continue with the light pattern established during travel
- Short naps (<45 minutes)
- Caffeine as needed early in the daytime
- Take melatonin at bedtime for eastward travel; melatonin is not helpful for westward travel

When traveling eastward or crossing more than 8 times zones, avoid late afternoon and evening bright light and get morning light for the first few days after arrival. Mobile applications and Web-based programs may be helpful to time light exposure based on specific trip details.

TRAVEL AND TRIP INSURANCE

With up to 50% of travelers becoming ill or injured during their trips, travel insurance is imperative for travelers in the event of misadventure or illness.[4] Travel insurance provides coverage for travel, medical, and dental expenses incurred by travelers; expenses typically not covered by travelers' health or other insurance plans. Most importantly, travel insurance companies provide a 24-hour, 7-day-a-week contact in the event of emergencies, assisting with identifying qualified local practitioners and arranging for aeromedical evacuation when necessary. Coverage is available for individual trips and annual policies exist for frequent travelers.

Around 6 to 8 weeks before departure, travelers should review their current insurance policies, coverage through work, and potential coverage through their credit cards for trips purchased in this manner. In most instances, these are insufficient and further coverage is required. Travel insurance is readily available on the Internet and multiple sites allow comparison of costs and plan basics. Travel agencies, airlines, private health insurers, and doctors' offices can also provide application forms, and possibly plan recommendations. International coverage should include, at a minimum, the costs of medical care and aeromedical evacuation. Other coverage options are recommended, including dental care, personal liability, trip cancellation coverage, loss of personal effects, and carriage of body or ashes after death. Additional expenses, such as loss of income, transport of relatives, and daily allowance, are also available. Costs vary by plan attributes but experts recommend top-level plans, at least US$1.5 million in coverage for all expenses.[50,51] It is vital to ensure that insurance policies provide coverage for the specific locales and activities in the traveler's itinerary. Most standard plans do not cover activities such as travel to war zones, participation in adventure and extreme sports, certain infectious diseases, and pregnancy. In most situations, coverage can be obtained by contacting the insurance company directly, but surcharges apply. Travelers who are uninsurable because of advanced age or preexisting medical conditions should consider destinations where bilateral government health agreements exist and where airlines are prepared to transport travelers.

In advance of departure, travelers can contact insurance agencies for recommendations on specific facilities and recommended providers matching their itineraries. This information and other essential documents are critical to expediting care during emergencies. Travelers should carry a letter from their health care provider (HCP) detailing their medical history, medications, medication delivery devices (eg, syringes for administering insulin), and their travel insurance policy number and emergency contact information. Medications and key documents should always be in travelers' carry-on luggage to reduce the chance of loss because replacing essential medications abroad can be fraught with challenges. Emergency assistance companies often have their own network; however, medical assistance directories of professional organizations may also be referenced. Examples include the Clinic Directory of the International Society of Travel Medicine (http://www.istm.org/) and the Directory of the International Association of Medical Assistance to Travelers (https://www.iamat.org/).

SPECIFIC HIGH-RISK SCENARIOS
Health Care Providers

HCPs providing medical care or disaster relief face greater health risks than other international travelers. To remain healthy overseas, HCPs must protect themselves from travel-related illnesses and infectious diseases; they also need to be able to provide for their colleagues and the communities they are serving.

Clean potable water is essential for HCPs and their patients but may not be readily available in remote locations. Water may be disinfected with iodine tablets or chlorine, commercial water filters, or boiling to 70°C (160°F) for 30 minutes.[52] Solar radiation and ultraviolet filters may be used for clear water.[53]

HCPs have potential for exposure to patients and infectious materials, including body substances, contaminated medical supplies and equipment, contaminated environmental surfaces, and aerosols generated during certain procedures. To protect themselves, HCPs should bring personalized protective equipment (PPE), including gowns, gloves, masks or respirators, and boots, and use as appropriate for the clinical situation. Before putting on and after removal of PPE, proper hand hygiene (before and after contact) is essential to prevent transmission of infectious diseases.

HCPs providing direct patient care should try to avoid risky situations and should always be prepared for possible needle sticks. They should be vaccinated against hepatitis B, and have clean needles and syringes readily available as well as postexposure prophylaxis (PEP) for HIV. A commonly used HIV PEP regimen is 1 tablet of tenofovir 300 mg/emtricitabine 200 mg once a day and 1 tablet of raltegravir 400 mg twice a day, which should be started as soon as possible and continued for 4 weeks.[52]

Sports and Recreation

The risk of injury and illness during travel for adventure and extreme sports varies based on the activity and ranges from fairly benign to life threatening; the estimated risk for base jumping is 1 fatality for every 60 participants per year (1.7%).[54] More common adventure sports, such as snowboarding (6.1 incidents of injury/1000 visits) and alpine skiing (2.5 incidents of injury/1000 visits), carry lower but significant risks of serious injury.[55,56]

Accordingly, preparation and prevention of medical and traumatic emergencies depends on the activity undertaken. Education regarding common causes of injury and illness for a given environment and activity may decrease injury and allow earlier detection of illnesses related to high altitude, heat, and dehydration.[57] Before travel, confirming availability of proper safety equipment for the specific activity is imperative, including helmet use for skiers and snowboarders and wrist guards for snowboarders.[58] Proper training, pretravel medical evaluation, confirmation of access to seasoned medical professionals, and evacuation plans for austere environments are imperative to prevent serious morbidity and mortality. The use of licensed/certified guides can decrease risk, because studies have shown that the highest injury claim rates were observed for activities often undertaken independently, as opposed to commercially.[59]

Water Environments and Diving

Traveling for water recreation is exceedingly common. Water environments pose additional risks when traveling, with environmental, infectious, and traumatic injuries varying by location and activity. Cold water, sun exposure, seasickness, and hazardous marine life pose unique or intensified environmental hazards. Infection-causing organisms may be different from standard pathogens and require atypical therapy. Although traumatic injuries are less frequent (than with land-based sports), collisions with equipment and land may, along with submersion, pose serious risks.[60] Risks can be mitigated through proper equipment, training, and education (**Table 5**). Specific injury rates and injury types have been studied and depend on the activity undertaken.[60]

Among water activities, scuba diving is one of the most prevalent high-risk activities. There are more than 9 million recreational scuba divers in the United States alone, and the risk of death following diving has been estimated to be as high as 0.002%.[63] The most severe diving-related illnesses are caused by drowning and decompression sickness. The Diving Alert Network (www.diversalertnetwork.org) provides insurance and other safety information for divers, and well-recognized training organizations, such as Professional Association of Diving Instructors, Scuba Schools International, the World Underwater Federation, the National Association of Underwater Instructors, and the British Sub-Aqua Club, can help divers prepare and use appropriate safety precautions.

Air travel should be delayed from 12 to 48 hours after diving, depending on a variety of factors, including the number of dives along with the length and depth of dives, to avoid increasing the risk of decompression sickness.[64–66] However, evidence for time recommendations and individual risk prediction is limited; it is best to rely on established timetables for air travel after diving.[67] Mobile device applications are available making standardized timetables and recommendations easily referenced during travel.

Table 5
Common risks and preparation for water environment

Exposure: Risk	Preparation/Prevention	Notes
Environmental		
Sun exposure: burn	High-SPF, water-resistant sun screen	Apply sunscreen before application of DEET-containing insect repellant; use of DEET can decrease sunscreen's length of time effective
Cold water: hypothermia	Identify high-risk individuals (eg, children, elderly) Use of wetsuits or dry suits	Determine an appropriate exposure time before initiating activity
Boat travel: seasickness	Pretravel prescription and medication trial	Many medications are more effective if initiated before water travel
Marine life exposure: envenomation/ bite/sting	Pretravel education and training on local hazardous marine life Use of local, certified guide/ company Use of wetsuits and rash guards	Proper attire and behavior can prevent most exposures
Infectious		
Freshwater: schistosomiasis, leptospirosis	Avoid slow-moving and stagnant water Vigorous toweling and/or application of DEET after freshwater exposure Doxycycline prophylaxis (200 mg orally weekly) can be used for high-risk travelers (Sehgal SC,[61] Takafuji ET[62])	Exposure to wet plants and environments without immersion in water can lead to infection
Fresh, brackish, and salt water: AEEVM organisms	Avoid water with sewage contamination or algae Timely cleaning of wounds Early recognition of infection or a poor response to initial antibiotic regimen	
Injury		
Water submersion: drowning	Swim training Life preservers Avoid alcohol/drug use Check local conditions and recommendations Prescreen for high-risk conditions (eg, seizure disorder, cardiac disease)	Ensure that appropriately sized life preservers are available for all participants. Pediatric sizes and higher quality flotation devices are commonly not available on-site
Equipment/ environment: musculoskeletal and soft tissue injuries	Familiarize yourself with equipment Wear appropriate footwear when walking, wading, or swimming Carry basic wound care supplies First-aid training	Most injuries are caused by contact with the person's own equipment (eg, surfboard or sailboat boom)

Abbreviations: AEEVM, Aeromonas spp, Edwardsiella spp, Erysipelothrix rhusiopathiae, Vibrio vulnificus, Mycobacterium marinum; SPF, sun protection factor.

Acute Altitude Illness

Acute altitude illness, which includes acute mountain sickness (AMS), high-altitude cerebral edema (HACE), and high-altitude pulmonary edema (HAPE), is a consideration for travelers ascending to greater than 2000 m (6562 feet).[68] In general, acute altitude illness occurs at elevations greater than 2500 m (8202 feet), with 25% of travelers who ascend rapidly to this elevation developing symptoms of acute altitude illness. The greatest risk is in travelers ascending to more than 2800 m (9186 feet) but risk can be categorized into low, moderate, and high risk depending on factors identified by the Wilderness Medicine Society (**Table 6**); elevations are based on the height of sleeping as opposed to the maximum height achieved in a given day.[68]

In general, the key to altitude illness prevention is gradual ascent and, if at a moderate to high risk of AMS, prophylaxis with acetazolamide 125 mg twice daily (pediatric 2.5 mg/kg/dose) starting 24 hours before going greater than 2800 m and continuing for 2 days beyond highest altitude attained. Dexamethasone (2 mg every 6 hours or 4 mg every 12 hours started 24 hours before ascent and continued for a maximum of 10 days) is an alternative option for adult travelers with sulfa allergies or for those who cannot take acetazolamide for other reasons. These same agents can be carried to treat people with AMS and HACE, with the addition of nifedipine for climbers with HAPE. However, the definitive treatment of acute altitude illness remains pausing ascent for mild AMS and descending for moderate to severe AMS, HACE, and HAPE.[68]

Terrorism and Unstable Political Situations

Terrorism and politically unstable situations account for a very small percentage of deaths compared with illness and injury while traveling abroad. In 2015, the US Department of State reported that "terrorist action" accounted for only 17 of 912 (1.86%) US citizen deaths overseas and that almost half (8) of these deaths occurred in Kabul, Afghanistan.[69] However, concerns over terrorism remain, and travelers'

Table 6 Risk categories for acute mountain sickness	
Risk Category	**Description**
Low	Individuals with no prior history of altitude illness and ascending to ≤2800 m
	Individuals taking ≥2 d to arrive at 2500–3000 m with subsequent increases in sleeping elevation <500 m/d and an extra day for acclimatization every 1000 m
Moderate	Individuals with prior history of AMS and ascending to 2500–2800 m in 1 d
	No history of AMS and ascending to >2800 m in 1 d
	All individuals ascending >500 m/d (increase in sleeping elevation) at altitudes >3000 m but with an extra day for acclimatization every 1000 m
High	Individuals with a history of AMS and ascending to >2800 m in 1 d
	All individuals with a prior history of HACE
	All individuals ascending to >3500 m in 1 d
	All individuals ascending >500 m/d (increasing sleeping elevation) >3000 m without extra day for acclimatization
	Very rapid ascents (eg, <7 d ascents of Mt. Kilimanjaro)

Altitudes listed in the table refer to the altitude at which the person sleeps; ascent is assumed to start from elevations less than 1200 m; the risk categories described pertain to unacclimatized individuals.

From Luks AM, McIntosh SE, Grissom CK, et al. 2014 Wilderness Medical Society practice guidelines for the prevention and treatment of acute altitude illness: 2014 update. Wilderness Environ Med 2014;25(4 Suppl):S4–14; with permission.

Box 1
Travel medical kit considerations

Personal health documentation

- Allergy list
- Current medications
- Immunization record
- Medical/surgical history with list of diagnoses
- Emergency contact information
- Medical insurance information

Medications

Any prescription medicines

Allergy/antimotion
- Epinephrine autoinjector (0.3 mg)
- Short-acting antihistamine: diphenhydramine 25 mg, meclizine 25 mg
- Long-acting antihistamine: cetirizine 10 mg, loratadine 10 mg, fexofenadine 180 mg
- Scopolamine patch 1.5 mg

Altitude illness
- Acetazolamide 125 mg
- Dexamethasone 4 mg
- Nifedipine 30 mg

Antibiotics
- Amoxicillin 500 mg
- Ciprofloxacin 500 mg
- Azithromycin 250 mg
- Trimethoprim/sulfamethoxazole 160/800 mg
- Cephalexin 500 mg
- Amoxicillin/clavulanate potassium 875/125 mg
- Nitrofurantoin 100 mg

Antiemetic
- Ondansetron 4 to 8 mg oral dissolvable tablet
- Promethazine 25 mg rectal suppositories

Antifungal
- Fluconazole 150 mg
- Miconazole 2% cream
- Clotrimazole 1% cream
- Ketoconazole 2% cream

Antimalarial
- Chloroquine 500 mg salt (300 mg base)
- Mefloquine 250 mg salt (228 mg base)
- Atovaquone-proguanil 250/100 mg

Antiviral
- Oseltamivir 75 mg

Emergency contraception
- Levonorgestrel (Plan B One-Step) 1.5 mg
- Ulipristal (Ella) 30 mg

Eye care
- Saline drops
- Contact lens holder
- Spare glasses/contacts
- Polymyxin B sulfate/trimethoprim ophthalmic drops
- Erythromycin ophthalmic ointment

Gastrointestinal
- ORS
- Bismuth subsalicylate 262 mg
- Loperamide 2 mg
- Calcium carbonate 500 mg
- Ranitidine 150 mg
- Omeprazole 20 mg
- Calcium polycarbophil (FiberCon) 625 mg
- Docusate sodium 100 mg

Pain/antipyretic
- Acetaminophen 500 mg
- Ibuprofen 400 mg

Postexposure prophylaxis
- Tenofovir 300 mg/ emtricitabine 200 mg
- Raltegravir 400 mg

Respiratory
- Nasal saline drops
- Pseudoephedrine 60 mg
- Albuterol metered-dose inhaler

Skin
- Hydrocortisone 1%
- Triamcinolone 0.1%
- Mupirocin ointment
- Sunscreen
- Zanfel

Sleep aid
- *N*-acetyl-5-methoxy tryptamine (melatonin) 0.5-5 mg
- Zoldipem 5 to 10 mg

Arthropod avoidance
- DEET 20% to 50%
- Picaridin 20%
- Permethrin 0.5% solution

First-aid supplies

- Commercial first-aid kit
- Adhesive strips (SteriStrips)
- Adhesive tape
- Alcohol wipes
- Antiseptic cleanser
- Band-Aids
- Dental kit
- Disposable gloves
- Duct tape
- Elastic (Ace) bandages
- Gauze
- Hand sanitizer
- Hemostatic gauze
- Local anesthetic
- Moleskin/Molefoam

- Personal protective equipment
- Safety pins
- Scissors
- Splint
- Suture kit/sutures/stapler
- Syringe/needle
- Thermometer
- Tweezers
- Wound glue

Data from Terry AC, Haulman NJ. Travel Medical Kit. Med Clin North Am 2016;100(2):261–77.

concerns have a substantial impact on airline travel and tourism.[70,71] The US Department of State offers country-specific information on safety and security (https://travel.state.gov/content/passports/en/go.html) along with up-to-date travel advisories, a traveler checklist, vaccine and visa requirements, and embassy/consulate information. The associated Smart Traveler Enrollment Program allows travelers to quickly register their trips with the US Department of State, identify the closest location of a US embassy/consulate, and have the embassy/consulate notified of their upcoming travel to the country (https://step.state.gov/STEP/Index.aspx).

TRAVEL MEDICAL KIT

A properly stocked travel medical kit is an essential tool for treating travel-related illnesses and injuries. **Box 1** lists the items to consider in a creating a personalized travel medical kit.

REFERENCES

1. vol. 2016. Available at: http://media.unwto.org/press-release/2016-11-07/close-one-billion-international-tourists-first-nine-months-2016. Accessed December 28, 2016.
2. Freedman DO, Chen LH, Kozarsky PE. Medical considerations before international travel. N Engl J Med 2016;375(3):247–60.
3. Dick L. Travel medicine: helping patients prepare for trips abroad. Am Fam Physician 1998;58(2):383–98, 401–2.
4. Steffen R, Rickenbach M, Wilhelm U, et al. Health problems after travel to developing countries. J Infect Dis 1987;156(1):84–91.
5. Duval B, De Serre G, Shadmani R, et al. A population-based comparison between travelers who consulted travel clinics and those who did not. J Travel Med 2003;10(1):4–10.
6. Hamer DH, Connor BA. Travel health knowledge, attitudes and practices among United States travelers. J Travel Med 2004;11(1):23–6.
7. LaRocque RC, Rao SR, Tsibris A, et al. Pre-travel health advice-seeking behavior among US international travelers departing from Boston Logan International Airport. J Travel Med 2010;17(6):387–91.
8. Van Herck K, Van Damme P, Castelli F, et al. Knowledge, attitudes and practices in travel-related infectious diseases: the European Airport Survey. J Travel Med 2004;11(1):3–8.

9. Wilder-Smith A, Khairullah NS, Song JH, et al. Travel health knowledge, attitudes and practices among Australasian travelers. J Travel Med 2004;11(1):9–15.

10. 2016. Available at: https://wwwnc.cdc.gov/travel/page/vfr. Accessed December 28, 2016.

11. Bacaner N, Stauffer B, Boulware DR, et al. Travel medicine considerations for North American immigrants visiting friends and relatives. JAMA 2004;291(23): 2856–64.

12. LaRocque RC, Deshpande BR, Rao SR, et al. Pre-travel health care of immigrants returning home to visit friends and relatives. Am J Trop Med Hyg 2013;88(2): 376–80.

13. Leder K, Tong S, Weld L, et al. Illness in travelers visiting friends and relatives: a review of the GeoSentinel Surveillance Network. Clin Infect Dis 2006;43(9):1185–93.

14. 2016. Available at: http://www.cdcfoundation.org/businesspulse/travelers-health-infographic. Accessed December 28, 2016.

15. Sanford CA, Jong EC. Immunizations. Med Clin North Am 2016;100(2):247–59.

16. Sanford C, McConnell A, Osborn J. The pretravel consultation. Am Fam Physician 2016;94(8):620–7.

17. Freedman DO, Weld LH, Kozarsky PE, et al. Spectrum of disease and relation to place of exposure among ill returned travelers. N Engl J Med 2006;354(2): 119–30.

18. Alpern JD, Dunlop SJ, Dolan BJ, et al. personal protection measures against mosquitoes, ticks, and other arthropods. Med Clin North Am 2016;100(2):303–16.

19. Luthi B, Schlagenhauf P. Risk factors associated with malaria deaths in travellers: a literature review. Travel Med Infect Dis 2015;13(1):48–60.

20. Schlagenhauf P, Weld L, Goorhuis A, et al. Travel-associated infection presenting in Europe (2008-12): an analysis of EuroTravNet longitudinal, surveillance data, and evaluation of the effect of the pre-travel consultation. Lancet Infect Dis 2015;15(1):55–64.

21. Hahn WO, Pottinger PS. Malaria in the traveler: how to manage before departure and evaluate upon return. Med Clin North Am 2016;100(2):289–302.

22. Stoney RJ, Chen LH, Jentes ES, et al. Malaria prevention strategies: adherence among Boston area travelers visiting malaria-endemic countries. Am J Trop Med Hyg 2016;94(1):136–42.

23. Schlagenhauf P, Petersen E. Standby emergency treatment of malaria in travelers: experience to date and new developments. Expert Rev Anti Infect Ther 2012;10(5):537–46.

24. Harvey K, Esposito DH, Han P, et al. Surveillance for travel-related disease–Geo-Sentinel Surveillance System, United States, 1997-2011. MMWR Surveill Summ 2013;62:1–23.

25. Giddings SL, Stevens AM, Leung DT. Traveler's diarrhea. Med Clin North Am 2016;100(2):317–30.

26. Steffen R, Hill DR, DuPont HL. Traveler's diarrhea: a clinical review. JAMA 2015; 313(1):71–80.

27. Bavishi C, Dupont HL. Systematic review: the use of proton pump inhibitors and increased susceptibility to enteric infection. Aliment Pharmacol Ther 2011; 34(11–12):1269–81.

28. 2016. Available at: https://wwwnc.cdc.gov/travel/page/food-water-safety. Accessed December 28, 2016.

29. Henriey D, Delmont J, Gautret P. Does the use of alcohol-based hand gel sanitizer reduce travellers' diarrhea and gastrointestinal upset? A preliminary survey. Travel Med Infect Dis 2014;12(5):494–8.

30. Ericsson CD. Nonantimicrobial agents in the prevention and treatment of traveler's diarrhea. Clin Infect Dis 2005;41(Suppl 8):S557–63.
31. De Bruyn G, Hahn S, Borwick A. Antibiotic treatment for travellers' diarrhoea. Cochrane Database Syst Rev 2000;(3):CD002242.
32. Ericsson CD, Johnson PC, Dupont HL, et al. Ciprofloxacin or trimethoprim-sulfamethoxazole as initial therapy for travelers' diarrhea. A placebo-controlled, randomized trial. Ann Intern Med 1987;106(2):216–20.
33. Tribble DR, Sanders JW, Pang LW, et al. Traveler's diarrhea in Thailand: randomized, double-blind trial comparing single-dose and 3-day azithromycin-based regimens with a 3-day levofloxacin regimen. Clin Infect Dis 2007;44(3):338–46.
34. Hargarten SW, Baker TD, Guptill K. Overseas fatalities of United States citizen travelers: an analysis of deaths related to international travel. Ann Emerg Med 1991;20(6):622–6.
35. Stewart BT, Yankson IK, Afukaar F, et al. Road traffic and other unintentional injuries among travelers to developing countries. Med Clin North Am 2016; 100(2):331–43.
36. Tonellato DJ, Guse CE, Hargarten SW. Injury deaths of US citizens abroad: new data source, old travel problem. J Travel Med 2009;16(5):304–10.
37. Mogaka EO, Ng'ang'a Z, Oundo J, et al. Factors associated with severity of road traffic injuries, Thika, Kenya. Pan Afr Med J 2011;8:20.
38. Ngo AD, Rao C, Hoa NP, et al. Road traffic related mortality in Vietnam: evidence for policy from a national sample mortality surveillance system. BMC Public Health 2012;12:561.
39. Weinberg N, Weinberg M, Maloney S. CDC health information for international travel. New York: Oxford University Press; 2016.
40. Hendel-Paterson B, Swanson SJ. Pediatric travelers visiting friends and relatives (VFR) abroad: illnesses, barriers and pre-travel recommendations. Travel Med Infect Dis 2011;9(4):192–203.
41. Stauffer WM, Konop RJ, Kamat D. Traveling with infants and young children. Part I: anticipatory guidance: travel preparation and preventive health advice. J Travel Med 2001;8(5):254–9.
42. Stauffer W, Christenson JC, Fischer PR. Preparing children for international travel. Travel Med Infect Dis 2008;6(3):101–13.
43. Hagmann S, Neugebauer R, Schwartz E, et al. Illness in children after international travel: analysis from the GeoSentinel Surveillance Network. Pediatrics 2010;125(5):e1072–80.
44. Lillie TH, Schreck CE, Rahe AJ. Effectiveness of personal protection against mosquitoes in Alaska. J Med Entomol 1988;25(6):475–8.
45. Brown TP. Middle ear symptoms while flying. Ways to prevent a severe outcome. Postgrad Med 1994;96(2):135–7, 141–2.
46. Takahashi M, Ogata M, Miura M. The significance of motion sickness in the vestibular system. J Vestib Res 1997;7(2–3):179–87.
47. Polli JB, Polli I. Traveling with children: beyond car seat safety. J Pediatr (Rio J) 2015;91(6):515–22.
48. Suhner A, Schlagenhauf P, Höfer I, et al. Effectiveness and tolerability of melatonin and zolpidem for the alleviation of jet lag. Aviat Space Environ Med 2001; 72(7):638–46.
49. Goldstein CA. Jet lag. Waltham (MA): UpToDate; 2016.
50. Bewes PC. Trauma and accidents. Practical aspects of the prevention and management of trauma associated with travel. Br Med Bull 1993;49(2):454–64.

51. Leggat PA, Carne J, Kedjarune U. Travel insurance and health. J Travel Med 1999;6(4):243–8.
52. Kunin SB, Kanze DM. Care for the health care provider. Med Clin North Am 2016; 100(2):279–88.
53. 2016. Available at: https://wwwnc.cdc.gov/travel/page/water-disinfection. Accessed December 28, 2016.
54. Westman A, Rosén M, Berggren P, et al. Parachuting from fixed objects: descriptive study of 106 fatal events in BASE jumping 1981-2006. Br J Sports Med 2008; 42(6):431–6.
55. Gomez AT, Rao A. Adventure and extreme sports. Med Clin North Am 2016; 100(2):371–91.
56. Shealy JE, Ettlinger CF, Scher I, et al. 2010/2011 NSAA 10-year interval injury study, vol. 20. West Conshohocken (PA): ASTEM International; 2015.
57. Hume PA, Lorimer AV, Griffiths PC, et al. Recreational snow-sports injury risk factors and countermeasures: a meta-analysis review and Haddon matrix evaluation. Sports Med 2015;45(8):1175–90.
58. Hebert-Losier K, Holmberg HC. What are the exercise-based injury prevention recommendations for recreational alpine skiing and snowboarding? A systematic review. Sports Med 2013;43(5):355–66.
59. Bentley TA, Page SJ, Macky KA. Adventure tourism and adventure sports injury: the New Zealand experience. Appl Ergon 2007;38(6):791–6.
60. Nathanson AT, Young JM, Young C. Pre-participation medical evaluation for adventure and wilderness watersports. Wilderness Environ Med 2015;26(4 Suppl):S55–62.
61. Sehgal SC, Sugunan AP, Murhekar MV, et al. Randomized controlled trial of doxycycline prophylaxis against leptospirosis in an endemic area. Int J Antimicrob Agents 2000;13(4):249–55.
62. Takafuji ET, Kirkpatrick JW, Miller RN, et al. An efficacy trial of doxycycline chemoprophylaxis against leptospirosis. N Engl J Med 1984;310(8):497–500.
63. Ozdemir L, Duru-Aşiret G, Bayrak-Kahraman B, et al. Health-related adverse events and associated factors in recreational divers with different certification levels. J Travel Med 2013;20(5):289–95.
64. Cialoni D, Pieri M, Balestra C, et al. Flying after diving: in-flight echocardiography after a scuba diving week. Aviat Space Environ Med 2014;85(10):993–8.
65. Freiberger JJ, Denoble PJ, Pieper CF, et al. The relative risk of decompression sickness during and after air travel following diving. Aviat Space Environ Med 2002;73(10):980–4.
66. Sheffield PJ. Flying after diving guidelines: a review. Aviat Space Environ Med 1990;61(12):1130–8.
67. Naval Sea Systems Command, US Department of the Navy. U.S. Navy diving manual. Washington, DC: US Government Printing Office; 2008.
68. Luks AM, McIntosh SE, Grissom CK, et al. Wilderness Medical Society practice guidelines for the prevention and treatment of acute altitude illness: 2014 update. Wilderness Environ Med 2014;25(4 Suppl):S4–14.
69. US Department of State. Reports and statistics, vol. 2016. Washington, DC: US Department of State; 2016.
70. Chuang C, Khatri SH, Gill MS, et al. Medical and pharmacy student concerns about participating on international service-learning trips. BMC Med Educ 2015;15:232.
71. Rose A, Avetisyan M, Rosoff H, et al. The role of behavioral responses in the total economic consequences of terrorist attacks on U.S. air travel targets. Risk Anal 2016. [Epub ahead of print].

Medicolegal Issues in Expedition and Wilderness Medicine

Valerie A. Dobiesz, MD, MPH[a],*, William Sullivan, DO, JD[b,c,d]

KEYWORDS

- Medical malpractice • Professional liability • Medical clearance • Waiver of liability
- Good Samaritan laws • Duty to rescue

KEY POINTS

- There are unique liabilities inherent in wilderness trips that guides, organizers, and health care providers should understand to help mitigate risk and protect their clients and themselves.
- The elements of a medical malpractice claim in a wilderness medicine setting are the same as those in a hospital setting.
- There is variability in state statutes on licensing requirements and level of medical training mandated for guides and trip leaders.
- Good Samaritan laws immunize liability if there is no preexisting duty to treat, no established doctor–patient relationship, no compensation or expectation of compensation, and gross negligence did not occur.

INTRODUCTION

Wilderness activities are generally quite safe, especially when compared with other athletic activities, with the majority of injuries being minor musculoskeletal trauma and lacerations that can most often be addressed with basic first aid.[1–3] However, in recent years, there has been a significant increase in expeditions and wilderness trips to remote and austere environments. Wilderness enthusiasts and adventure seekers now encompass a wide range of ages, abilities, experience, and underlying medical conditions, which present many opportunities for tour organizations and outfitters, but also present several medicolegal challenges in the event of an accident, injury or medical emergency (**Box 1**).

Financial Disclosures: None.
[a] Department of Emergency Medicine, Harvard Humanitarian Initiative, Brigham & Women's Hospital, Harvard Medical School, Neville House, 75 Francis Street, Boston, MA 02115, USA; [b] Department of Emergency Medicine, University of Illinois, 1740 W Taylor St, Chicago, IL 60612, USA; [c] St. Margaret's Hospital, 600 E 1st St, Spring Valley, IL 61362, USA; [d] Law Office of William Sullivan, 21200 S La Grange Rd #365, Frankfort, IL 60423, USA
* Corresponding author.
E-mail address: vdobiesz@bwh.harvard.edu

Emerg Med Clin N Am 35 (2017) 485–494
http://dx.doi.org/10.1016/j.emc.2017.01.004
emed.theclinics.com

Box 1
Medicolegal scenarios to consider in wilderness and expedition medicine

A family practice physician is participating as a client in an organized rock climbing trip in a remote setting and comes upon an injured man who has an obvious limb-threatening injury associated with an open fracture.

  Is she legally obligated to help?

  Answer: It depends on where the accident occurs, but in general she is not legally obligated to help this victim in the United States or in many other common law countries. In some states, she would be required to at least call for assistance. Note that there may be a difference between legal actions and ethical actions.

The victim has full decisional capacity and refuses any and all care.

What should the physician do in that circumstance?

  Answer: She should respect the patient's personal autonomy. There has not been a physician–patient relationship established and those with decision-making capacity are entitled to refuse care.

The victim subsequently becomes disoriented and confused. The physician decides to render aid by splinting and suturing the gaping wound to the best of her ability. The wound later becomes infected and ultimately the victim loses his limb from gangrene. He sues for medical malpractice.

Is this physician protected by Good Samaritan laws?

  Answer: Yes, provided that there was an emergency situation, the physician had no preexisting duty to treat, there was no expectation of compensation, and the physician acted reasonably and prudently. It is important to understand the fundamental elements found in all Good Samaritan laws as well as the variations that occur by jurisdiction to be prepared when responding to a medical emergency in a wilderness setting.

Wilderness settings may pose increased risks of injury and illness to participants as compared with more urban settings for a variety of reasons, such as extremes in weather, adverse and rapidly changing environmental conditions, and delays and challenges in transport and evacuation, as well as limitations in readily available medical supplies and trained personnel.[4] These circumstances also increase the liability exposure to organizers and leaders of wilderness and adventure travel trips. Trip organizers, leaders, and medical personnel should be familiar with liability issues to mitigate risks and implement risk management strategies when planning trips.

Health care providers, guides, trip leaders, and organizers should have a fundamental understanding of basic medicolegal principles, such as the elements necessary for medical malpractice claims, professional liability, extent and geographic variability of immunity provided by Good Samaritan laws, waivers, and medical clearance, as well as duty to rescue and abandonment doctrines. It is important for trip health care providers and organizers to have a thorough understanding of the laws surrounding the duty to act and degree of medical training to which they must adhere to mitigate these increased liability risks, especially with clients who may have little to no wilderness experience or who may have unrealistic expectations of receiving the same standards of care and resources available in tertiary care settings.[5] Wilderness medicine malpractice claims are most often based on complaints of lack of proper health warnings, failure to provide medical services and facilities, and negligent delivery of medical care causing harm or injury.[4]

MEDICAL MALPRACTICE

Medical malpractice law in the United States is derived from English common law and has evolved over time subsequent to rulings in various state courts.[6] Tort law in common law jurisdictions, such as the United States, is a civil wrong or wrongful act causing an injury to another for which a remedy may be obtained, usually in the form of damages.[7] Tort laws include negligence cases and intentional wrongs that result in harm. Medical malpractice is a specific type of negligence occurring during the provision of medical care.[4,6] The injured party must show that the health care provider acted negligently in rendering care and that such negligence resulted in the injury incurring damages.

In the United States, as opposed to many other countries, medical malpractice law has traditionally been under the authority of individual states and not the federal government.[6] The elements of a medical malpractice claim in a wilderness medicine setting are the same as those in a hospital setting. To prevail, an injured party must prove duty, breach of duty, causation, and damages. Failure to prove even one of these elements is fatal to a plaintiff's malpractice case.

Duty can be created by actions or law. If no preexisting duty exists, there is generally no legal liability for failing to help another person, even if the help provided would create no risk to the rescuer. For example, there is generally no legal obligation to provide aid to a stranger drowning in a river. However, if one person places another into a dangerous situation (ie, pushes someone into the river), then the law creates a duty to rescue. A duty may also be created by one's profession. For example, by virtue of their job descriptions, public servants such as police and fire fighters have a duty to protect the public and would, therefore, be required to make reasonable attempts to rescue someone in danger. A physician hired by a cruise line to care for passengers on board the ship would have a similar duty. Finally, if one chooses to provide medical advice or medical care to another, then the law creates a duty to act reasonably. For example, advising someone on a hike that their chest pain is noncardiac or that a mushroom is safe to eat may result in liability if the person relies on that advice and later dies. Fear of liability has often caused medical personnel to avoid providing aid and was the impetus for development of Good Samaritan statutes, which are discussed elsewhere in this article.

Breach of duty is another way of saying "negligence." Once a duty to provide medical care is established, in most cases the provider must act reasonably. A typical definition of breach of duty would be "failing to exercise the skill, care and knowledge that a reasonably well-qualified practitioner in the same specialty would apply under the same or similar circumstances." There are several important points within that definition. First, any medical care provided must be "reasonable." The law does not require perfection, nor should any provider's actions be compared only with the best and brightest in the profession. Some states have also created statutes requiring that plaintiffs prove that a practitioner was "grossly negligent" before the practitioner can be held liable for medical malpractice. Breach of duty is also a situation-specific standard. The "standard of care" for treating an acute myocardial infarction is markedly different when comparing an emergency department at an urban center in the United States with an encampment at the summit of a mountain. In general, the most difficult thing to prove in malpractice claims involving wilderness activities is a breach of duty or violation of a standard.[5]

Medical malpractice not only requires that an injured party sustain actual damages; it also requires that another party's negligence caused those damages. For example, in a malpractice suit involving care rendered to a patient who fell from a cliff, the injured party would have to prove that the allegedly negligent medical care caused the injury rather than the fall from the cliff. The causation issue is sometimes clarified by the "but for test" where courts posit the question "but for the defendant's alleged negligence, would the plaintiff have suffered the injury?" Negligent acts will not support a malpractice lawsuit if they do not lead to a significant injury. For example, advising a hiker to rub poison sumac on a wound to prevent infection may inflame the tissues, delay healing, and could even precipitate a significant rash or infection. However, if the patient suffers no permanent damages, it is unlikely that a malpractice suit would come from the negligent advice.

Finally, compensable damages must occur for a lawsuit to be viable. De minimis damages such as a bruised leg, a sprained wrist, or time off of work, and solely "soft damages" such as emotional distress are generally insufficient to warrant the costs of filing and prosecuting a medical malpractice claim. Malpractice lawsuits are usually filed in a state trial court and usually adjudicated by jury trial. Because there may be significant state-to-state variability in malpractice case law, each health care provider, guide, or trip organizer should have some familiarity with laws in their own states and in the state or country where the trip will take place.

PROFESSIONAL LIABILITY

Outfitters and wilderness organizations should ideally review and follow industry norms for health care services provided by similar companies in similar locations. Industry norms often follow state and/or federal laws governing wilderness activities.[5] One study reviewing state laws found that only 22 states required a license for individuals taking clients into the wilderness for compensation and only 10 (45%) of those states also required some form of first aid training as a condition of acquiring and maintaining such licensure.[1] State statutes may also dictate necessary first aid training for guides and outfitters. For example, Colorado has a statute dictating the first aid requirements for white water outfitters and guides, C.R.S. §§ 33 to 32 to 105.5, which requires a standard first aid card to work on a river.[5] Many state statutes require a regulatory agency such as the Department of Fish and Game to specify the type and level of first aid training required of guides.[5] Similarly, organizations such as the Boy Scouts of America have national standards for high adventure programs requiring leaders to have first aid and cardiopulmonary resuscitation training with a minimum of an 8-hour course through a community agency (standard No. 20–120).[1]

In general, companies have a duty to staff trips to remote areas with personnel who have "significant training to provide adequate first aid and medical care until evacuation can be arranged."[4] These providers are most often emergency medicine technicians or laypersons with basic first aid training and are held to the standard of a "reasonably prudent layperson." If a company elects to voluntarily staff a physician on a trip, and publicizes this fact in promotional materials, it may create an implied or express contract for the availability of medical services and the company may be held to a higher standard because a physician would have more training and capability, and potentially more resources to evaluate and manage emergencies that might otherwise occur on these type of trips. Litigation over first aid care provided by outfitters and guides is rare, but litigation against search and rescue groups and volunteers is increasing and generally associated with other claims.[5]

MEDICAL CLEARANCE OF TRIP PARTICIPANTS

In general, wilderness trip operators have no duty to screen trip participants medically.[4] It is up to the individual travelers to exercise due caution in their own safety as well as to understand the personal health risks of a wilderness trip. Despite having no obligation to medically screen participants, the participants' medical screening information may be beneficial to trip organizers. This information may serve to inform clients about the health hazards involved in the planned trip and alert trip organizers to better anticipate and prepare for any special needs or necessary accommodations.

It is important to provide physicians performing a medical screening examination or preparticipation evaluation (PPE) with adequate information regarding trip environmental conditions, health hazards, level and amount of activity required, and the level of access to medical care that will be available.[8] Medical screening forms should emphasize the functional requirements of the trip.[4] Organizers of wilderness activities may restrict participation if the decision is individualized, reasonable, and based on sound medical evidence.[8,9]

When medical screening is requested of participants, physicians preforming a PPE for wilderness activities should follow the same general principles as those for sports with a few caveats.[8] In addition to documenting a complete examination, it is important to consider and document the additional environmental and personal health issues relative to the wilderness activity being proposed and refer the participants to a specialist for further screening as deemed necessary. Travel medicine principles including vaccinations, prophylactic medications, recommendations for travel, and adventure insurance should be considered.[8] The clinician performing the PPE has a responsibility to clear or restrict the participant for the planned activity and should understand that, because of the remote settings, wilderness activities may pose greater risks and involve different group dynamics than more controlled sports environments.[8] When faced with the risk of not being allowed to participate in a wilderness activity owing to a medical issue, some participants may falsify medical information, putting them at an increased risk of injury or illness. This type of behavior has been well-documented by the Dive Alert Network, which recorded many cases of dive accidents that were potentially preventable had participants not falsified medical forms.[10] It is recommended that a PPE occur a minimum of 6 weeks before the trip so that the patient has time to address and correct any potential concerns before the trip.[8]

WAIVER OF LIABILITY
Duty to Warn and Educate Trip Participants

In general, there is no duty to warn trip participants of obvious dangers.[4] For example, if a trip includes an airplane flight, then the risks associated with air travel do not need to be disclosed to the participants because such risks are considered common knowledge. There is, however, a duty for travel agents or trip organizers to warn travelers of known unreasonable risks or dangers.[4] For example, such circumstances might include political instability or high crime rates that are foreseeable and/or likely to occur near a trip location. There is no duty to warn about speculative or undetermined risks. Even in the absence of a duty, it may be in the best interest for trip organizers to provide additional information on unique weather and environmental conditions, the activity level needed, necessary safety equipment, recommended immunizations, water and food safety concerns, and any known risks to keep participants healthy, well-informed, and injury free. Injured participants often cite a lack of proper health warnings when filing claims.[4]

GOOD SAMARITAN LAWS IN WILDERNESS MEDICINE

All travel expenses were waived for you in exchange for providing emergency medical care as a physician on a mountain climbing trip. During the trip you treat a client suffering high altitude cerebral edema. There is a bad outcome. Can you successfully invoke protection from the Good Samaritan law in this situation?

Answer: Probably not, because, by agreeing to provide emergency medical care before the trip, you had a preexisting duty to care for clients on the trip.

A physician is on a rafting trip with her family and friends. During the trip she diagnoses a friend with a wound infection and prescribes antibiotics. The patient suffers an anaphylactic reaction to the medication and develops long-term complications. The physician is sued.

Is the physician protected by the Good Samaritan law?

Answer: Probably. A wound infection would likely be considered an "emergency" and the physician acted reasonably by prescribing antibiotics. If there was no previous knowledge about anaphylaxis to the prescribed antibiotics, the Good Samaritan statute would likely shield the physician from liability.

The term "Good Samaritan" is synonymous with a compassionate person who helps strangers. The meaning was derived from the Bible parable in the Book of Luke 10:33 in which a man is beaten, robbed, and left for dead on the side of the road. A priest and a Levite both passed by the man, but a Samaritan stopped to render first aid, transported the injured man to an inn, and offered to pay for the cost of his care.[11–13] Good Samaritan laws were enacted to encourage medical providers to render aid during medical emergencies by protecting them from liability. The Utah Supreme Court explained that good Samaritan laws attempt to prevent a situation where "the Good Samaritan who tries to help may find himself [mired] in damages, while the priest and the Levite who pass by on the other side go on their cheerful way rejoicing."[14]

California was the first state in the United States to enact a Good Samaritan statute in 1959.[12] Before these statutes, physicians who chose to provide emergency care to a stranger in an emergency could be held liable for damages caused by any negligence. Good Samaritan laws were intended to encourage anyone to provide care at the scene of an emergency by precluding civil suits for ordinary negligence.[12,15,16] Now every state in the United States provides some type of statutory Good Samaritan protection. In addition, federal statutes also afford protections to medical personnel to provide emergency medical care under certain circumstances. For example, the Aviation Medical Assistance Act of 1998 provides that any individual providing assistance during an in-flight medical emergency shall not be liable for damages in federal or state court unless the person is guilty of gross negligence or willful misconduct.[17]

The US legal system is based on common law originating from England, which stipulates that a stranger is generally under no legal duty to provide aid to someone in peril. In the United States and in other common law countries, physicians do not generally have a legal obligation to render emergency aid to strangers. One California Supreme Court decision noted that, "No one is obliged by law to assist a stranger, even though he can do so by a mere word, and without the slightest danger to himself."[18] However, ethical and moral imperatives sometimes conflict with legal dicta. For example, Section (D) (3) (d) of the American College of Emergency Physicians Code of Ethics for Emergency Physicians states that "Because of their unique expertise, emergency physicians have an ethical duty to respond to emergencies in the community and offer assistance."[19] Because ethical imperatives to provide emergency medical care sometimes conflict with legal ramifications in the event of a bad outcome resulting from this care, it is important that physicians, health care providers, and trip guides and leaders who render medical treatment have an understanding of both the existence and the variability of laws protecting them from liability.

There are few data on the frequency and location of Good Samaritan events encountered by health care providers outside of the hospital, especially with regard to assistance provided in wilderness settings. One study surveying a convenience sample of emergency physicians in Colorado reported a median frequency of 2 Good Samaritan acts per 5 years of practice, with the most common locations being sports and entertainment events (25%), road traffic accidents (21%), and wilderness settings (19%).[20] The study also aimed to determine which emergency kit supplies and medications were most commonly used by physicians responding to these emergencies as Good Samaritans. The most useful supplies needed were reported to be gloves (54%), dressings (34%), and a stethoscope (20%), and the most useful medications were oxygen (19%), intravenous fluids (17%), and epinephrine (14%).[20] This study demonstrated that most physicians can expect to respond many times during a career as Good Samaritans. It also alluded to the potential benefits of carrying an emergency kit and the supplies that may be most helpful when planning emergency kits for responding to these situations.[20]

Another survey done on a convenience sample of 253 licensed physicians residing in North Carolina reported that 4 out of 5 physicians (79.4%) reported previous opportunities to act as Good Samaritans and that 93% of respondents intervened as a Good Samaritan during their last opportunity.[15] The most common location of assistance was an airplane. There was no difference between sexes, practice setting, specialty type, or experience level in response rates. Most notably, those physicians with a greater perceived knowledge of Good Samaritan law were more likely to have intervened.[15] The most commonly cited reasons for not intervening was that another person was in control (42.2%), lack of emergency training (20.4%), and concern for legal liability (13.3%).[15]

In general, Good Samaritan laws immunize liability for rendering emergency medical care if there is no preexisting duty to treat, if no established doctor–patient relationship exists, if there was no compensation or expectation of compensation, and if no gross negligence has occurred.[14] Physicians and health care providers should also always respect patient autonomy and informed consent should be obtained even in emergency situations if the victim has decision-making capacity.[19] Patients have the right to refuse emergency care if they have decisional capacity. If victims are unresponsive, an implied consent will be assumed.[12]

Each state has unique Good Samaritan statutory language. Despite this variability, there are several themes common to most Good Samaritan statutes. First, the care provided must be necessary to treat an emergency condition. Routine medical care or offhand medical advice while casually sitting around a camp site would likely not invoke Good Samaritan statute protections in the event of a bad outcome. Note that the definition of an "emergency" for purposes of the Good Samaritan statues is intended to be fairly liberal. For example, an Oklahoma Supreme Court decision stated that "[k]eeping in mind that the [Good Samaritan] Act's purpose is to invite medical providers to intervene, the term 'emergency' must be given the broadest sense possible."[21]

To be covered under the Good Samaritan statute, the care provided must also be gratuitous. In other words, there cannot be compensation or the expectation of compensation in return for the provision of medical care. Billing a patient for care or a prior agreement to serve in an official capacity as a medical provider during any activity would likely negate a Good Samaritan defense. Similarly, waiving one's compensation as a camp physician after a bad outcome has occurred would still negate a Good Samaritan defense because there was a preexisting expectation of compensation. Small tokens of gratitude received for providing gratuitous care would likely not be considered "compensation" under the law, but as the value of a gift increases, the more likely it is that courts may consider the gift "compensation" for purposes of Good Samaritan statutes.

Finally, Good Samaritan statutes immunize care that is negligent, but do not protect against care that is deemed "grossly negligent." Although the definition of gross negligence varies between states, it is a high bar to overcome. Definitions used by some courts include actions that were taken with a reckless disregard for another's safety, that were "less than careless," and that were willful, wanton, or malicious.[22] As a general rule, basic first aid, basic life support, automatic external defibrillator use, and advanced cardiac life support (performed by those who have been trained in advanced cardiac life support) would almost certainly be covered by the Good Samaritan umbrella. The further one strays from these protocols, the less likely that the care will be covered under Good Samaritan statutes. Using sticks and twine to splint a broken arm would likely invoke Good Samaritan protections. Using the same sticks to attempt an appendectomy at a camp site likely would not.

A 2013 survey of Good Samaritan statutes across the United States noted that all states have Good Samaritan laws protecting physicians licensed in their own jurisdictions and that only Kentucky failed to extend this immunity to physicians licensed in other states.[12] However, Kentucky does extend immunity to a person certified by the American Heart Association or the American Red Cross to perform cardiopulmonary resuscitation.[12] This same survey also noted some additional nuances with certain state Good Samaritan statutes. For example, several states provide varying forms of conditional immunity to physicians who render voluntary care at an athletic event (AZ, AR, CA, CO, KS, MI, MO, NC, OR, TN, VA, WI).[12] Colorado and Maine specifically provide immunity to physicians volunteering for ski patrol.[12]

Although there is a general rule abrogating a duty to provide aid to a stranger in an emergency, there are also exceptions to that rule. Rhode Island (Rhode Island General Laws 11–56–1),[23] Minnesota (Minnesota Stat. Ann. § 604A.01),[24] and Vermont (Vermont Stat. Ann. tit. 12, § 519)[25] statutes contain language requiring that any person provide reasonable assistance to another person who is "exposed to or has suffered grave physical harm," provided that the assistance does not cause peril to the rescuer or others. Failure to do so may subject the violator to various penalties including fines of $100 to $500, petty misdemeanors, or, in Rhode Island, up to 6 months' imprisonment. It is important to note that these statutory duties to rescue are not absolute. They do not apply to those who are not in "grave danger" and also do not apply if providing assistance may put the rescuer or others in peril. For example, the statutes (and moral decency) would require that a bystander throw a drowning victim a life preserver. However, the statutes would likely not require that the bystander jump into water to help the drowning victim, because doing so may place the bystander in peril.

SUMMARY

Wilderness trips and expeditions are increasingly popular to remote settings, predisposing participants to accidents and medical illness unique to these settings. Although these activities are generally safe, there is increased liability exposure to trip guides, organizers, and health care providers that should be accounted for in planning these trips. When care is provided in wilderness settings, it is important to understand that medical malpractice has the same fundamental elements in the wilderness as in any practice setting. Each wilderness trip guide, leader, and organization should follow state and federal statutes on licensing requirements and level of medical training needed for the activity being planned. There is generally no requirement for medical clearance for wilderness trips, but the information can be useful to participants and trip organizers. PPEs, when performed, are similar to those done for sports but should also take into consideration the unique setting, level of activity, group dynamics, and travel involved when making recommendations.

Good Samaritan laws exists in every state in the United States and in general immunize those that render aid in emergencies when there is no preexisting duty, no physician–patient relationship, no compensation or expectation of compensation, and no gross negligence. There is state-to-state and country variability in Good Samaritan laws that should be understood before embarking on any wilderness expedition to understand the nuances of coverage and whether a duty to act may exist. In emergency situations there are moral and ethical considerations for health care providers that may not align with the law but in general, acting within your scope of practice in a manner consistent with what a reasonable person would do in a similar situation is a judicious and commendable approach.

REFERENCES

1. Welch TR, Clement K, Berman D. Wilderness first aid: is there an "industry standard"? Wilderness Environ Med 2009;20:113–7.
2. McIntosh SE, Leemon D, Visitacion J, et al. Medical incidents and evacuations on wilderness expeditions. Wilderness Environ Med 2007;18:298–304.
3. Flores AH, Haileyesus T, Greenspan AI. National estimates of outdoor recreational injuries treated in emergency departments, United States, 2004–2005. Wilderness Environ Med 2008;19:91–8.
4. Langer C, Baine J. Medical liability and wilderness emergencies. Wilderness medicine Auerbach PS. 6th edition. Philadelphia: Elsevier; 2012.
5. Moss JH. Response to "Wilderness first aid: is there an 'industry standard?'". Wilderness Environ Med 2010;21:79–81.
6. Bal BS. An introduction to medical malpractice in the United States. Clin Orthop Relat Res 2009;467(2):339–47.
7. Garner BA. Black's law dictionary. 10th edition. St. Paul (MN): Thomson West; 2014.
8. Young CC, Campbell AD, Lemery J, et al. Ethical, legal, and administrative considerations for preparticipation evaluations for wilderness sports and adventures. Wilderness Environ Med 2015;26:S10–4.
9. Bernhardt DT, Roberts WO. PPE preparticipation physical evaluation. 4th edition. Elk Grove Village (IL): American Academy of Pediatrics; 2010.
10. Nord D. To lie or not to lie? Alert Diver; 2010. Available at: http://www.alertdiver.com/To_Lie_or_Not_to_Lie. Accessed August 31, 2016.
11. DeGuerre C. Good Samaritan statues: are medical volunteers protected? Virtual Mentor 2004;6(4).
12. Stewart PH, Agin WS, Douglas SO. What does the law say to Good Samaritans? A review of Good Samaritan statutes in 50 states and on US airlines. Chest 2013; 143(6):1774–83.
13. The parable of the Good Samaritan. The Holy Bible. New Revised Standard editionLuke 10. Nashville (TN): Thomas Nelson Publishers; 1990. p. 30–6.
14. Court Listener Hirpa v. IHC Hospitals, Inc. 948 P.2d 785 (Utah 1997). Available at: https://www.courtlistener.com/opinion/1125437/hirpa-v-ihc-hospitals-inc/. Accessed September 4, 2016.
15. Sullivan W. The Good Samaritans. Emergency Physicians Monthly 2010;17.
16. Garneau WM, Harris DM, Viera AJ. Cross-sectional survey of Good Samaritan behavior by physicians in North Carolina. BMJ Open 2016;6:e010720.
17. H.R. 2843 (105th): Aviation Medical Assistance Act of 1998. Available at: https://www.govtrack.us/congress/bills/105/hr2843/text. Accessed September 6, 2016.

18. Stanford Law School Supreme Court of California Resources Malloy v. Fong, 37 Cal.2d 356(1951). Available at: http://scocal.stanford.edu/opinion/malloy-v-fong-29492. Accessed September 4, 2016.
19. American College of Emergency Physicians Clinical & Practice Management. Code of ethics for emergency physicians. Available at: https://www.acep.org/Clinical--Practice-Management/Code-of-Ethics-for-Emergency-Physicians/. Accessed September 6, 2016.
20. Burkholder TW, King RA. Emergency physicians as Good Samaritans: survey of frequency, locations, supplies and medications. West J Emerg Med 2016;17(1): 15–7.
21. Weaver, JC. AHC Media Good Samaritan laws: are you protected when you render aid in a crisis. Jackson v. Mercy Health Center, Inc., 864 P.2d 839 (Okla.1993). Available at: https://www.ahcmedia.com/articles/117923-good-samaritan-laws-are-you-protected-when-you-render-aid-in-a-crisis. Accessed September 4, 2016.
22. Dachs R, Elias J. Family practice management. What you need to know when called upon to be a Good Samaritan. 2008. Available at: www.aafp.org/fpm. Accessed August 31, 2016.
23. Justia US Law. Rhode Island General Laws 11-56-1. Available at: http://law.justia.com/codes/rhode-island/2012/title-11/chapter-11-56/chapter-11-56-1. Accessed September 4, 2016.
24. The Office of the Revisor of Statutes Minnesota Stat. Ann. § 604A.01. Available at: https://www.revisor.mn.gov/statutes/?id=604a.01. Accessed September 5, 2016.
25. Vermont General Assembly Vermont Stat. Ann. tit. 12, § 519. Available at: http://legislature.vermont.gov/statutes/section/12/023/00519. Accessed September 4, 2016.

Index

Note: Page numbers of article titles are in **boldface** type.

Emerg Med Clin N Am 35 (2017) 495–502
http://dx.doi.org/10.1016/S0733-8627(17)30032-9
0733-8627/17

Moving?

Make sure your subscription moves with you!

To notify us of your new address, find your **Clinics Account Number** (located on your mailing label above your name), and contact customer service at:

Email: journalscustomerservice-usa@elsevier.com

800-654-2452 (subscribers in the U.S. & Canada)
314-447-8871 (subscribers outside of the U.S. & Canada)

Fax number: 314-447-8029

**Elsevier Health Sciences Division
Subscription Customer Service
3251 Riverport Lane
Maryland Heights, MO 63043**

*To ensure uninterrupted delivery of your subscription, please notify us at least 4 weeks in advance of move.

Printed and bound by CPI Group (UK) Ltd, Croydon, CR0 4YY

08/05/2025

01864699-0005